Oncology Imaging and Intervention in the Abdomen

Editors

ROBERT J. LEWANDOWSKI
MATTHEW S. DAVENPORT

RADIOLOGIC CLINICS OF NORTH AMERICA

www.radiologic.theclinics.com

Consulting Editor
FRANK H. MILLER

September 2015 • Volume 53 • Number 5

ELSEVIER

1600 John F. Kennedy Boulevard • Suite 1800 • Philadelphia, Pennsylvania, 19103-2899

http://www.theclinics.com

RADIOLOGIC CLINICS OF NORTH AMERICA Volume 53, Number 5
September 2015 ISSN 0033-8389, ISBN 13: 978-0-323-39583-0

Editor: John Vassallo (j.vassallo@elsevier.com)
Developmental Editor: Donald Mumford

Radiologic Clinics of North America (ISSN 0033-8389) is published bimonthly by Elsevier Inc., 360 Park Avenue South, New York, NY 10010-1710. Months of issue are January, March, May, July, September, and November. Periodicals postage paid at New York, NY and additional mailing offices. Subscription prices are USD 460 per year for US individuals, USD 709 per year for US institutions, USD 220 per year for US students and residents, USD 535 per year for Canadian individuals, USD 905 per year for Canadian institutions, USD 660 per year for international individuals, USD 905 per year for international institutions, and USD 315 per year for Canadian and foreign students/residents. To receive student and resident rate, orders must be accompanied by name of affiliated institution, date of term and the signature of program/residency coordinator on institution letterhead. Orders will be billed at individual rate until proof of status is received. Foreign air speed delivery is included in all *Clinics* subscription prices. All prices are subject to change without notice. **POSTMASTER:** Send address changes to *Radiologic Clinics of North America*, Elsevier Health Sciences Division, Subscription Customer Service, 3251 Riverport Lane, Maryland Heights, MO 63043. **Customer Service: Telephone: 1-800-654-2452** (U.S. and Canada); **1-314-447-8871** (outside U.S. and Canada). **Fax: 1-314-447-8029. E-mail: journalscustomerservice-usa@ elsevier.com (for print support); journalsonlinesupport-usa@elsevier.com (for online support).**

Reprints. For copies of 100 or more of articles in this publication, please contact the Commercial Reprints Department, Elsevier Inc., 360 Park Avenue South, New York, New York 10010-1710. Tel.: +1-212-633-3874; Fax: +1-212-633-3820; E-mail: reprints@elsevier.com.

Radiologic Clinics of North America also published in Greek Paschalidis Medical Publications, Athens, Greece.

Radiologic Clinics of North America is covered in *MEDLINE/PubMed (Index Medicus), EMBASE/Excerpta Medica, Current Contents/Life Sciences, Current Contents/Clinical Medicine, RSNA Index to Imaging Literature, BIOSIS, Science Citation Index,* and *ISI/BIOMED.*

Printed in the United States of America.

Contributors

CONSULTING EDITOR

FRANK H. MILLER, MD
Chief, Body Imaging Section and Fellowship
Program; Medical Director of MRI; Professor,
Department of Radiology, Northwestern
University Feinberg School of Medicine,
Chicago, Illinois

EDITORS

ROBERT J. LEWANDOWSKI, MD, FSIR
Associate Professor of Radiology, Director of
Interventional Oncology, Department of
Radiology, Northwestern University
Feinberg School of Medicine, Chicago,
Illinois

**MATTHEW S. DAVENPORT, MD, FSAR,
FSCBTMR**
Assistant Professor of Radiology and Urology,
Michigan Radiology Quality Collaborative,
Department of Radiology, University of
Michigan Health System, Ann Arbor, Michigan

AUTHORS

SHARON Z. ADAM, MD
Department of Radiology, Northwestern
Memorial Hospital, Northwestern University
Feinberg School of Medicine, Chicago,
Illinois

MAHMOUD M. AL-HAWARY, MD
Division of Abdominal Imaging, Department of
Radiology, University of Michigan Hospitals,
Ann Arbor, Michigan

BRIAN C. ALLEN, MD
Abdominal Imaging, Department of Radiology,
Duke University Medical Center, Durham,
North Carolina

MICHELLE A. ANDERSON, MD, MSc
Division of Gastroenterology, Department of
Internal Medicine, University of Michigan
Hospitals, Ann Arbor, Michigan

THOMAS D. ATWELL, MD
Associate Professor of Radiology, Department
of Radiology, Mayo Clinic College of Medicine,
Rochester, Minnesota

MUSTAFA R. BASHIR, MD
Director of MRI; Associate Professor of
Radiology, Division of Abdominal Imaging,
Department of Radiology, Center for
Advanced Magnetic Resonance Development,
Duke University Medical Center, Durham,
North Carolina

CHRISTOPHER L. BRACE, PhD
Associate Professor, Departments of
Radiology and Biomedical Engineering,
University of Wisconsin, Madison, Wisconsin

DANIEL B. BROWN, MD
Department of Radiology and Radiological
Sciences, Vanderbilt University Medical
Center, Nashville, Tennessee

RICHARD H. COHAN, MD
Professor, Department of Radiology, University of Michigan Hospital, University of Michigan Health System, Ann Arbor, Michigan

JAMES H. ELLIS, MD
Professor, Department of Radiology, University of Michigan Hospital, University of Michigan Health System, Ann Arbor, Michigan

ISAAC R. FRANCIS, MD, MBBS
Melvyn Korobkin Collegiate Professor of Radiology, Division of Abdominal Imaging, Department of Radiology, University of Michigan Hospitals, Ann Arbor, Michigan

GREGORY T. FREY, MD
Instructor in Radiology, Department of Radiology, Mayo Clinic College of Medicine, Jacksonville, Florida

J. LOUIS HINSHAW, MD
Associate Professor, Department of Radiology, University of Wisconsin, Madison, Wisconsin

HERO K. HUSSAIN, MD
University of Michigan Health System, Ann Arbor, Michigan

FRED T. LEE Jr, MD
Professor, Departments of Radiology and Biomedical Engineering, University of Wisconsin, Madison, Wisconsin

ROBERT J. LEWANDOWSKI, MD, FSIR
Section of Interventional Radiology, Department of Radiology, Division of Interventional Oncology, Department of Radiology, Robert H. Lurie Comprehensive Cancer Center, Robert H. Lurie Comprehensive Cancer Center, Northwestern University Feinberg School of Medicine, Chicago, Illinois

ANDREW J. LIPNIK, MD
Department of Radiology and Radiological Sciences, Vanderbilt University Medical Center, Nashville, Tennessee

PETER S. LIU, MD
Assistant Professor of Radiology and Vascular Surgery, Division of Abdominal Imaging, University of Michigan Medical Center, Ann Arbor, Michigan

MEGHAN G. LUBNER, MD
Associate Professor, Department of Radiology, University of Wisconsin, Madison, Wisconsin

FRANK H. MILLER, MD
Chief, Body Imaging Section and Fellowship Program; Medical Director of MRI; Professor, Department of Radiology, Northwestern University Feinberg School of Medicine, Chicago, Illinois

JEET MINOCHA, MD
Division of Interventional Radiology, Department of Radiology, University of California San Diego, San Diego, California

CHRISTOPHER MOLVAR, MD
Section of Vascular and Interventional Radiology, Department of Radiology, Loyola University Medical Center, Maywood, Illinois

DAVID M. SELLA, MD
Assistant Professor of Radiology, Department of Radiology, Mayo Clinic College of Medicine, Jacksonville, Florida

SHANE A. WELLS, MD
Assistant Professor, Department of Radiology, University of Wisconsin, Madison, Wisconsin

TIMOTHY J. ZIEMLEWICZ, MD
Assistant Professor, Department of Radiology, University of Wisconsin, Madison, Wisconsin

Contents

> Liver MR imaging is the test of choice for lesion characterization in patients without a history of chronic liver disease. Multiple pulse sequences are used in combination to reach a diagnosis. The individual/incremental value of sequences encountered in modern clinical MR imaging with respect to several commonly encountered lesions in the noncirrhotic liver is reviewed.

> There have been major changes in the management and reporting of hepatocellular carcinoma (HCC) in the last decade. Cross-sectional imaging is now pivotal in the management of cirrhotic patients, in particular in the diagnosis and staging of HCC. Although diagnostic systems have become relatively well developed, approximately one-third of HCC nodules may have an atypical appearance, necessitating ancillary testing, close follow-up, or biopsy. The introduction of standardized diagnostic and reporting systems has improved communication between radiologists and clinicians, but there remains substantial disagreement between radiologists in feature assignment and nodule characterization.

> Tumor ablation in the liver has evolved to become a well-accepted tool in the management of increasingly complex oncologic patients. At present, percutaneous ablation is considered first-line therapy for very early and early hepatocellular carcinoma and second-line therapy for colorectal carcinoma liver metastasis. Because thermal ablation is a treatment option for other primary and secondary liver tumors, an understanding of the underlying tumor biology is important when weighing the potential benefits of ablation. This article reviews ablation modalities, indications, patient selection, and imaging surveillance, and emphasizes technique-specific considerations for the performance of percutaneous ablation.

> The liver is a common site of metastatic and primary disease, as well as a site of benign masses. Given the import of liver containing tumor, its treatment draws from a variety of cancer specialists. Potentially curative options exist for primary and metastatic liver disease; however, advanced disease presentation often prevents cure. The current level of evidence for embolotherapy targeting hepatocellular carcinoma and liver metastatic colorectal cancer is examined, along with

intra-arterial treatment options for focal nodular hyperplasia and hepatic adenoma. More specifically, chemoembolization, both conventional and drug-eluting bead, and ^{90}Y radioembolization are reviewed.

This article illustrates the imaging characteristics of cystic and solid renal masses, along with a summary of identified imaging criteria that may be of use to differentiate masses that are more likely to be benign from those that are more likely to be malignant. In addition, important features of known or suspected renal cancers that should be identified before treatment are summarized, including staging of renal cancer and RENAL nephrometry. Finally, the imaging appearance of patients following treatment of renal cancer, including after partial or total nephrectomy, thermal ablation, or chemotherapy for metastatic disease, is reviewed.

The role of interventional radiology in the management of renal malignancy has expanded in the last 2 decades, largely because of the efficacy of image-guided ablation in treating renal cell carcinoma (RCC). Clinical guidelines now incorporate ablation into standardized RCC management algorithms. Importantly, both radiofrequency ablation and cryoablation have shown long-term durability in the definitive treatment of RCC, and early outcomes following microwave ablation are equally promising. While selective renal artery embolization has a role in the palliation in select patients with RCC, it can also be used to minimize complications in the ablation of larger renal masses.

The adrenal glands are a common site for primary benign and malignant tumors and metastatic disease. Computed tomography (CT), MR imaging, and fluorine-18 fluorodeoxyglucose PET combined with CT are the most common imaging modalities used to assess the adrenal glands. There are established morphologic criteria for both CT and MR imaging that can be used to assess whether an adrenal mass is benign or malignant, and whether follow-up, biopsy, or resection should be performed. In the setting of a known primary malignancy, CT, MR imaging, and PET can help differentiate most benign masses from metastasis.

High-resolution imaging modalities, such as multi-detector computed tomography, MR imaging, and endoscopic ultrasound, are frequently used alone or in combination to characterize focal solid and cystic pancreatic neoplasms. Imaging in solid pancreatic neoplasms, typically adenocarcinoma and neuroendocrine tumors, is primarily used to detect and stage the extent of the tumor and to determine if complete surgical resection for cure is feasible. In cystic pancreatic masses, imaging aims to differentiate benign nonmucinous cystic lesions from potentially or frankly malignant mucin-producing cysts. Several noninvasive and invasive treatment options can be performed if surgical resection is not possible or contraindicated.

Image-guided percutaneous biopsy of abdominal masses is a safe, minimally invasive procedure with a high diagnostic yield for a variety of pathologic processes. This article describes the basic technique of percutaneous biopsy, including the different modalities available for imaging guidance. Patient selection and preparation for safe performance of the procedure is emphasized, and the periprocedural management of coagulation status as well as basic indications and contraindications of the procedure are briefly discussed. In particular, the role of biopsy in the diagnosis of liver and renal masses is highlighted.

Locoregional therapies for hepatic neoplasms have distinctive imaging features after treatment, different from those observed after systemic therapy. As these therapies are becoming more common, it is important that radiologists be aware of the imaging appearance of tumors after locoregional therapies to correctly diagnose treatment response or failure and potential complications. This article reviews the imaging recommendations and findings after intra-arterial therapies (chemoembolization and radioembolization) and ablative therapies.

Locoregional therapies (LRTs) have proved valuable in the treatment of patients with cancer, most commonly in the liver. Accurate assessment of response to these therapies is crucial because objective response can be a surrogate of improved survival. Imaging plays an essential role in the objective evaluation of tumor response to most cancer therapies, including LRTs. Assessing imaging response to LRTs, however, can be challenging and is evolving. This article reviews the different criteria used to assess radiologic response to LRTs, with special attention to imaging assessment following treatment of hepatocellular carcinoma.

PROGRAM OBJECTIVE

The objective of the *Radiologic Clinics of North America* is to keep practicing radiologists and radiology residents up to date with current clinical practice in radiology by providing timely articles reviewing the state of the art in patient care.

TARGET AUDIENCE

Practicing radiologists, radiology residents, and other health care professionals who provide patient care utilizing radiologic findings.

LEARNING OBJECTIVES

Upon completion of this activity, participants will be able to:
1. Review methods of evaluation and intervention in renal masses.
2. Discuss the role of imaging in diagnosis and evaluation of disorders of the kidneys, liver, and pancreas.
3. Recognize the uses of ablation and intra-arterial therapies in the treatment of liver masses.

ACCREDITATION

The Elsevier Office of Continuing Medical Education (EOCME) is accredited by the Accreditation Council for Continuing Medical Education (ACCME) to provide continuing medical education for physicians.

The EOCME designates this enduring material for a maximum of 15 *AMA PRA Category 1 Credit*(s)™. Physicians should claim only the credit commensurate with the extent of their participation in the activity.

All other health care professionals requesting continuing education credit for this enduring material will be issued a certificate of participation.

DISCLOSURE OF CONFLICTS OF INTEREST

The EOCME assesses conflict of interest with its instructors, faculty, planners, and other individuals who are in a position to control the content of CME activities. All relevant conflicts of interest that are identified are thoroughly vetted by EOCME for fair balance, scientific objectivity, and patient care recommendations. EOCME is committed to providing its learners with CME activities that promote improvements or quality in healthcare and not a specific proprietary business or a commercial interest.

The planning committee, staff, authors and editors listed below have identified no financial relationships or relationships to products or devices they or their spouse/life partner have with commercial interest related to the content of this CME activity:

Sharon Z. Adam, MD; Mahmoud M. Al-Hawary, MD; Brian C. Allen, MD; Michelle A. Anderson, MD, MSc; Thomas D. Atwell, MD; Richard H. Cohan, MD; James H. Ellis, MD; Anjali Fortna; Isaac R. Francis, MD; Gregory T. Frey, MD, MPH; Hero K. Hussain, MD; Robert J. Lewandowski, MD, FSIR; Andrew J. Lipnik, MD; Peter S. Liu, MD; Meghan G. Lubner, MD; Frank H. Miller, MD; Jeet Minocha, MD; Christopher Molvar, MD; Erin Scheckenbach; David M. Sella, MD; Karthikeyan Subramaniam; John Vassallo; Shane A. Wells, MD; Timothy J. Ziemlewicz, MD.

The planning committee, staff, authors and editors listed below have identified financial relationships or relationships to products or devices they or their spouse/life partner have with commercial interest related to the content of this CME activity:

Mustafa R. Bashir, MD is a consultant/advisor for Bristol-Meyers Squibb Company, receives research support from Siemans Corporation; GE Healthcare, a unit of General Electric Company; Bayer HealthCare AG; and Guerbet Group.

Christopher L. Brace, PhD is a consultant/advisor for, with stock ownership in, NeuWave Medical, Inc.

Daniel B. Brown, MD is a consultant/advisor for Cook Medical, a division of Cook Group Incorporated; and Medtronic plc.

Matthew S. Davenport, MD, FSAR, FSCBTMR receives royalties/patents from Wolters Kluwer.

J. Louis Hinshaw, MD is a consultant/advisor for, with stock ownership in, NeuWave Medical, Inc.

Fred T. Lee Jr, MD receives royalties/patents from Covidien plc, and has stock ownership in and is a member of the board of directors for NeuWave Medical, Inc.

UNAPPROVED/OFF-LABEL USE DISCLOSURE

The EOCME requires CME faculty to disclose to the participants:
1. When products or procedures being discussed are off-label, unlabelled, experimental, and/or investigational (not US Food and Drug Administration [FDA] approved); and
2. Any limitations on the information presented, such as data that are preliminary or that represent ongoing research, interim analyses, and/or unsupported opinions. Faculty may discuss information about pharmaceutical agents that is outside of FDA-approved labelling. This information is intended solely for CME and is not intended to promote off-label use of these medications. If you have any questions, contact the medical affairs department of the manufacturer for the most recent prescribing information.

TO ENROLL

To enroll in the *Radiologic Clinics of North America* Continuing Medical Education program, call customer service at 1-800-654-2452 or sign up online at http://www.theclinics.com/home/cme. The CME program is available to subscribers for an additional annual fee of USD 315.

METHOD OF PARTICIPATION

In order to claim credit, participants must complete the following:

1. Complete enrolment as indicated above.
2. Read the activity.
3. Complete the CME Test and Evaluation. Participants must achieve a score of 70% on the test. All CME Tests and Evaluations must be completed online.

CME INQUIRIES/SPECIAL NEEDS

For all CME inquiries or special needs, please contact elsevierCME@elsevier.com.

RADIOLOGIC CLINICS OF NORTH AMERICA

FORTHCOMING ISSUES

November 2015
The Acute Abdomen
Richard M. Gore, *Editor*

January 2016
CT Angiography
Peter S. Liu and Joel F. Platt, *Editors*

March 2016
Topics in Transplantation Imaging
Puneet Bhargava and Matthew T. Heller, *Editors*

RECENT ISSUES

July 2015
Emergency and Trauma Radiology
Savvas Nicolaou, *Editor*

May 2015
Advanced MR Imaging in Clinical Practice
Hersh Chandarana, *Editor*

March 2015
Coronary Artery Disease and the Myocardial Ischemic Cascade
U. Joseph Schoepf and James C. Carr, *Editors*

ISSUE OF RELATED INTEREST

Surgical Oncology Clinics of North America, October 2014 (Vol. 23, No. 4)
Imaging in Oncology
Vijay P. Khatri, *Editor*

THE CLINICS ARE AVAILABLE ONLINE!
Access your subscription at:
www.theclinics.com

Preface

Imaging and Image-guided Intervention Are Irrevocably Linked

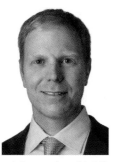

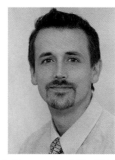

Robert J. Lewandowski, MD, FSIR   Matthew S. Davenport, MD, FSAR, FSCBTMR

Editors

We humbly submit this text on abdominal imaging and related image-guided interventions to the readership. The authors who constructed these articles are experts in their fields and have worked tirelessly to present to you cutting-edge information in an easily digestible and relevant format. The intended audience is health care practitioners dedicated to providing maximally informative imaging results and/or minimally invasive interventional techniques to patients with abdominopelvic disease states.

In the pages that follow, you will learn the skills needed to diagnose liver masses in the noncirrhotic and cirrhotic liver, current best practices on liver ablative techniques and intra-arterial hepatic therapies, how to differentiate and triage a variety of benign and malignant renal masses, interventional approaches to the diagnosis and management of renal and adrenal masses, imaging and interventional algorithms in the management of patients with pancreatic disease, advanced image-guided biopsy technique, and how best to interpret imaging findings following interventional therapies.

As medicine continues to accelerate into the twenty-first century, we have observed an increasing reliance on advanced imaging to guide patient management, and an increasing dependence on minimally invasive image-guided techniques to diagnose and cure disease. We fully anticipate this trend to continue and believe that a superior understanding of imaging translates directly into superior technical performance with image-guided interventions. In the articles that follow, we hope to demonstrate to you that these fields (imaging-based diagnostics, imaging-based therapeutics) are irrevocably linked, and to bring you, the reader, up to speed on the latest in these disciplines so that you are best positioned to provide superior care to your patients.

Sincerely,

Robert J. Lewandowski, MD, FSIR
Department of Radiology
Northwestern University Feinberg School of
Medicine
676 North St. Clair Street, Suite 800
Chicago, IL 60611, USA

Matthew S. Davenport, MD, FSAR, FSCBTMR
Department of Radiology
University of Michigan Health System
1500 East Medical Center Drive B2-A209P
Ann Arbor, MI 48109, USA

E-mail addresses:
r-lewandowski@northwestern.edu (R.J. Lewandowski)
matdaven@med.umich.edu (M.S. Davenport)

Radiol Clin N Am 53 (2015) xi
http://dx.doi.org/10.1016/j.rcl.2015.06.001
0033-8389/15/$ – see front matter © 2015 Published by Elsevier Inc.

Liver Mass Evaluation in Patients Without Cirrhosis: A Technique-Based Method

Peter S. Liu, MD

KEYWORDS

- Liver • MR imaging • T2-weighted • Opposed-phase • Dynamic postcontrast
- Diffusion-weighted imaging

KEY POINTS

- MR imaging is the test of choice for liver lesion detection and characterization. Multiphase computed tomography (CT) can also be used in patients who cannot undergo MR imaging.
- No single MR imaging sequence in a panacea for lesion characterization; rather, incremental specificity is gained by using the various sequences in concert with one another.
- T2-weighted imaging can be performed with moderate, heavy, and very heavy/extreme degrees of T2 weighting. Intralesional signal changes between the degrees of T2 weighting offers some characterization benefit.
- Dual echo in-phase and opposed-phase T1-weighted gradient echo imaging can delineate the presence of intralesional lipid, which can greatly focus the differential diagnosis of a liver mass.
- Dynamic postcontrast T1-weighted imaging is the most commonly used tool for liver lesion characterization, with distinct patterns seen for several common liver masses. Extracellular gadolinium contrast agents (MR imaging) and iodinated contrast agents (CT) show similar patterns of enhancement.
- Diffusion-weighted imaging aids in the detection and characterization of hepatic metastases.
- Hepatocyte-specific contrast agents aid in lesion characterization primarily when there is some intralesional accumulation on hepatobiliary phase imaging. This finding is most frequently seen in focal nodular hyperplasia.

INTRODUCTION

The characterization of a known or suspected liver mass is a common indication for cross-sectional imaging, such as computed tomography (CT) or MR imaging. Although many patients with chronic liver disease require advanced imaging to better characterize lesions found on surveillance imaging, these examinations are increasingly being required for patients who lack a history of chronic liver disease or cirrhosis. In part, this change may be related to the increased use of cross-sectional imaging for the workup of abdominal-related symptoms, leading to incidentally discovered liver lesions. Incidental small liver lesions are found in approximately 12% to 17% of CT examinations, and these figures may be underestimated given technical advances that have resulted in increased imaging resolution.[1,2] Most of these lesions are benign, even in patients with a known history of extrahepatic malignancy. Nonetheless, a small percentage of these incidentally discovered lesions do represent an unexpected malignancy or disease progression of a known malignancy.

Expert recommendations have been developed to aid clinicians in the management of incidentally

Division of Abdominal Imaging, University of Michigan Medical Center, 1500 East Medical Center Drive, Ann Arbor, MI 48109-0030, USA
E-mail address: peterliu@med.umich.edu

Radiol Clin N Am 53 (2015) 903–918
http://dx.doi.org/10.1016/j.rcl.2015.05.008
0033-8389/15/$ – see front matter © 2015 Elsevier Inc. All rights reserved.

radiologic.theclinics.com

discovered liver lesions.[3] Although the clinical data of background liver disease or known extrahepatic malignancy can influence the pretest probability of malignancy, it does not greatly alter the technical recommendation; generally, contrast-enhanced MR imaging is considered the test of choice for focal liver lesion characterization. In situations in which MR imaging cannot be performed, multiphase contrast-enhanced CT can be considered as an alternative option. In this article, the imaging technique used in modern liver imaging is reviewed, with a particular focus on MR imaging and the incremental benefit of various sequences for liver lesion characterization in the noncirrhotic liver. In particular, the added characterization benefit for some of the most common liver lesions (including hepatic cysts, hemangioma, focal nodular hyperplasia [FNH], hepatic adenoma, and metastasis) are highlighted in line with the sequence discussion. Although some lesion behavior may overlap with entities seen in the cirrhotic liver, the reader is directed to an article by Bashir and Hussain elsewhere in this issue for a more detailed discussion about cirrhosis and hepatocellular carcinoma (HCC).

IMAGING OVERVIEW
Ultrasonography

The liver may be imaged using a variety of cross-sectional techniques, including ultrasonography, CT, and MR imaging. For initial imaging/screening of the liver, ultrasonography is an excellent modality; it is fast, readily available, relatively inexpensive, and uses no ionizing radiation.[4] Ultrasonography can be operator dependent and is often limited in patients with large body habitus. Moreover, ultrasonography performed without ultrasound-based contrast agents has low sensitivity and specificity for focal hepatic masses, particularly small lesions less than 10 mm.[5,6] Beyond liver lesion detection, ultrasonography without ultrasound-based contrast agents also has limited value for lesion characterization, because there is substantial overlap in the appearance of benign and malignant solid hepatic masses. Ultrasonography is good at differentiating solid from cystic lesions and is implemented in this role for patients who cannot tolerate CT or MR imaging.[3] Ultrasonography is also an excellent modality for real-time imaging to guide percutaneous biopsy.

Computed Tomography

Liver CT offers better diagnostic sensitivity than ultrasonography for the detection of focal hepatic masses, with a reported sensitivity of 75% to 96%.[7] In addition, liver CT offers diagnostic advantage over ultrasonography without ultrasound-based contrast agents in regards to liver lesion characterization. Similar to ultrasonography, CT is able to differentiate solid and cystic lesions (when large enough, eg, >15 mm), primarily based on the observed or measured attenuation of a lesion in Hounsfield units. However, CT also allows discrimination between various solid hepatic masses. This characterization is often performed using a multiphase contrast-enhanced CT technique after administration of an iodinated contrast material, which diffuses from the intravascular space to the extracellular space. The dynamic behavior of a liver lesion during the various phases of imaging can show characteristic patterns of enhancement that may permit accurate characterization. This multiphase postcontrast CT technique is akin to dynamic postcontrast MR imaging performed with extracellular gadolinium-based contrast agents (GBCA) and offers similar dynamic information for lesion characterization. Unenhanced CT images are generally not required but may be useful in specific situations, such as assessing intralesional calcification or acute hemorrhage.

Liver CT is an excellent choice for patients who cannot undergo contrast-enhanced MR imaging because of implanted device compatibility, a metallic foreign body in a dangerous location, a severe allergiclike reaction to GBCA, or chronic dialysis. CT is an ionizing imaging technique that delivers radiation to the patient, estimated to average 10 to 30 mSv for adult patients using typical multiphase liver CT protocols.[3] Newer dose reduction techniques, such as iterative reconstruction, can significantly reduce the radiation dose to the patient, particularly in multiphase protocols.[8] The standard liver CT protocol at our institution is listed in **Table 1**.

Table 1 Multiphase hepatic CT parameters	
Slice thickness: 2.5 mm	Slice interval: 1.25 mm
Pitch: 1.371:1	Speed: 55
Noise Index: 21.6–24.84	ASIR: 30%
kVp: 120	mA: Auto (minimum 100/maximum 575)
Field of View: optimized — to body habitus	

Contrast material: 125 mL of iodinated contrast material (370 mg iodine/mL), followed by a 50-mL flush of normal saline (0.9 NS).
Scan timing (all times from injection start): arterial phase, 35 s; venous phase, 65 s; delayed phase, 180 s.
Abbreviation: ASIR, adaptive statistical iterative reconstruction.

MR Imaging

Contrast-enhanced liver MR imaging is considered the test of choice for the detection and characterization of a liver lesion relative to other imaging techniques. Liver MR imaging is often performed using a variety of sequences and planes, which can vary between institutions. Generally, a combination of T1-weighted, T2-weighted, and postcontrast imaging is used to provide accurate lesion characterization.[9] Postcontrast imaging is often accomplished using a dynamic imaging technique, similar to the multiphase technique used in CT. However, because MR imaging does not deliver ionizing radiation to the patient, numerous imaging phases can be acquired without harm to the patient; generally, these phases provide added value by imaging the liver at multiple time points after contrast material administration. GBCA are used commonly in MR imaging. Typically, GBCA are extracellular agents, which, once administered, reside in the intravascular space and interstitial space. Complementary techniques such as diffusion-weighted imaging (DWI) may offer additional value and are frequently encountered in clinical practice. Alternative contrast agents that show specific uptake by hepatocyte cell transport proteins can also be used, which may offer additional lesion characterization benefit.[10] The high diagnostic accuracy of MR imaging for liver lesion characterization results from the various tissue properties that are highlighted using the individual MR imaging sequences. The standard liver MR imaging protocol used at our institution is listed in **Table 2**.

TECHNIQUE-BASED METHODS FOR LESION CHARACTERIZATION

The final diagnosis of a lesion in the noncirrhotic liver is often based on the radiologist's assimilation of several features into a single best diagnosis. Using MR imaging, multiple characteristics of a lesion can be shown using different pulse sequences. Therefore, understanding the incremental value of each sequence is critical for lesion characterization and is explored in a stepwise fashion. Because CT can be used in patients who cannot receive MR imaging, understanding the characterization principles of dynamic postcontrast imaging is doubly important, because this is the primary characterization technique for CT. The kinetic enhancement pattern of lesions is similar between CT performed with iodinated contrast material and MR imaging performed with extracellular GBCA. Therefore, the dynamic contrast-enhancement patterns described in the following sections can be applied to both multiphase CT and MR imaging.

MR IMAGING
T2-Weighted Images

T2-weighted imaging is routinely included in most liver MR imaging protocols and typically highlights entities that have a fluid or cystic component. T2-weighted images often have high tissue contrast given that background liver has relatively short T2 relaxation times relative to various liver masses, including liver cysts, hemangiomas, and metastases.[11,12] Although conventional spin-echo imaging can be used for T2-weighted images elsewhere in the body, an accelerated multiecho technique is often required for T2 weighting in abdominal imaging given the long acquisition times required by spin-echo techniques for even modest T2 weighting.[13] Techniques such as rapid acquisition with relaxation enhancement (also called turbo spin-echo and fast spin-echo) or half-Fourier acquisition single-shot turbo spin-echo (also called single-shot fast spin-echo) are often used for liver imaging. Sometimes, these techniques are paired with respiratory tracking or triggering systems to synchronize image acquisition to phase of respiration, thereby increasing the overall image signal that can be used to improve tissue contrast or spatial resolution.[12,13]

Lesions can be assessed on T2-weighted images by looking at the signal intensity relative to other structures. Most commonly, this comparison is made between hepatic cysts and markers of simple fluid in the abdomen, such as cerebral spinal fluid or simple bile in the gallbladder lumen. However, there is an additional characterization value of T2-weighted images that relies on the relative difference in signal intensity within a lesion as the degree of T2 weighting is increased through images with higher echo times (TEs). Many modern MR imaging protocols use T2-weighted images that have at least 2 different TEs, as described in **Table 2**. Moderate T2-weighted images should have an TE of approximately 60 to 120 milliseconds and heavily T2-weighted images should have an TE greater than 160 milliseconds (ideally in the 180–200 millisecond range).[9,14] A third weighting can also be considered: a very heavy/extreme T2 weighting with TEs greater than 500 to 600 milliseconds, which clinically is applicable for magnetic resonance cholangiopancreatography (MRCP) sequences.

At 1.5 T, the mean T2 relaxation times of liver, solid malignancies, hemangiomas, and cysts have been reported as 51 to 54 milliseconds, 80 to 85 milliseconds, 155 to 178 milliseconds, and 517 to 583 milliseconds, respectively.[15,16] Thus, as the degree of T2 weighting is increased, the relative loss of signal within a lesion is a visual

Table 2
Liver MR imaging protocol

Sequence name	Coronal and axial T2W	Axial heavy T2W	Coronal T2W MRCP/ very heavy T2W	In-phase/opposed-phase T1W	Dynamic Postcontrast T1W	DWI
Sequence type	SSFSE	FSE	FRFSE	SPGR	SPGR	2D echo planar imaging
Repetition time (TR) (ms)	Minimum	4000	Minimum	150	Minimum	6000
Echo time (TE/TE effective) (ms)	180	90	650	2.3 Opposed-phase/ 4.6 In-phase	Minimum	Minimum
Field of view (cm)	To fit, often 36–40	To fit	36	To fit	To fit, often 28–40	To fit
Slice thickness (mm)	8	6	1.4	6	4	6
Matrix	128 x 256	192 x 320	256 x 256	160 x 256	160 x 320	128 x 128
Number of excitations (NEX)	0.5	1	2	1	0.5	8
Fat suppression?	—	Yes	—	—	Yes	—
Additional comments	—	+ Respiratory triggering	—	Flip angle 70°	Flip angle 12°	—

Contrast material: 0.2 mL/kg body weight gadobenate dimeglumine or 0.1 mL/kg body weight gadoxetic acid.
Scan timing determined by bolus-tracking software: arterial phase; venous and delayed to follow.
Abbreviations: 2D, two-dimensional; FSE, fast spin-echo; MRCP, magnetic resonance cholangiopancreatography; SPGR, spoiled gradient recalled echo; SSFSE, single-shot fast spin-echo; T1W, T1-weighted; T2W, T2-weighted.

representation of the T2 relaxation times. When there is a dramatic change in relative signal, this can offer some insight as to the underlying diagnosis for lesion characterization. For example, solid hepatic malignant lesions often have some high signal intensity relative to background liver on moderate (TE = 60–120 milliseconds) T2-weighted images but show only minimal increased signal versus background liver on heavily (TE = 180–200 milliseconds) T2-weighted images (**Fig. 1**).[14,16] The behavior of malignant solid hepatic masses between moderately (TE = 60–120 milliseconds) and heavily (TE = 180–200 milliseconds) T2-weighted images is similar to that of normal splenic tissue, which has been attributed to the similar T2 relaxation time of splenic parenchyma.[11,17] As a result, the spleen can serve as an internal imaging control for identifying potentially malignant solid hepatic masses such as metastases. Because there is little relative signal left in malignant solid lesions on heavily (TE = 180–200 milliseconds) T2-weighted images, the amount of signal expected in very heavily/extremely (TE >500–600 milliseconds) T2-weighted images is low, often rendering solid hepatic metastases inconspicuous on such pulse sequences.

In contrast to malignant solid hepatic lesions, hemangiomas and cysts have higher T2 relaxation times and therefore tend to show relatively little observed signal loss between moderately and heavily T2-weighted images. To differentiate these 2 entities on T2-weighted imaging, one must look for signal changes as the degree of T2 weighting increases from heavy (TE = 180–200 milliseconds) to very heavy/extreme (TE >500–600 milliseconds). Typically, hemangiomas show a substantial reduction in relative signal intensity between heavily (TE = 180–200 milliseconds) and very

heavily/extremely (TE >500–600 milliseconds) T2-weighted sequences, becoming nearly inconspicuous (**Fig. 2**).[18] This decrease in relative signal intensity is similar to the reduction encountered in malignant solid hepatic masses between moderately (TE = 60–120 milliseconds) and heavily (TE = 180–200 milliseconds) T2-weighted images.

On the other hand, hepatic cysts remain high signal intensity relative to background liver on extremely (TE >500–600 milliseconds) T2-weighted sequences, because of the inherent long T2 relaxation time of hepatic cysts (**Fig. 3**). Compared with moderately (TE = 60–120 milliseconds) and heavily (TE = 180–200 milliseconds) T2-weighted images, the relative signal intensity of hepatic cysts on very heavy/extremely (TE >500–600 milliseconds) T2-weighted images is only minimally diminished. Therefore, a lesion characterization benefit can be found by examining the loss of relative signal intensity within a lesion between moderately (TE = 60–120 milliseconds), heavily (TE = 180–200 milliseconds), and very heavily/extremely (TE >500–600 milliseconds) T2-weighted sequences; in particular, one should look for a stepwise significant decrease in signal intensity within a lesion between sequences that have stepwise increases in T2 weighting.

In-Phase and Opposed-Phase T1-Weighted Images

Clinical applications of MR imaging use signal generated from protons, which may be associated with either fat-based or water-based molecules.[19] Slight differences in the electron structure between fat-based and water-based protons result in a subtle variance in the precessional frequency between these species. This precessional frequency difference is approximately 3.5 ppm, or

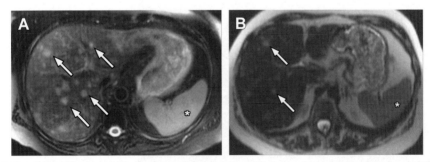

Fig. 1. Axial T2-weighted images with moderate T2 weighting (TE approximately 90 milliseconds [*A*]) and heavy T2 weighting (TE approximately 180 milliseconds [*B*]). There are numerous lesions (*arrows*) throughout the liver that show high signal intensity on moderate T2-weighted images but become less conspicuous in overall degree and number on heavily T2-weighted images. This pattern of signal loss between moderate and heavily T2-weighted images is frequently seen in malignant lesions such as metastases. Note the similar relative loss of signal intensity in the spleen (*asterisk*).

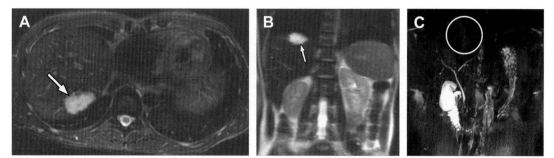

Fig. 2. Axial T2-weighted image with moderate T2 weighting (TE approximately 90 milliseconds [A]), coronal T2-weighted image with heavy T2 weighting (TE approximately 180 milliseconds [B]), and maximum intensity projection image from coronal three-dimensional T2-weighted MRCP sequence with very heavy/extreme T2 weighting (TE approximately 675 milliseconds [C]). There is a lobulated mass in the right hepatic dome with high signal on both moderate and heavily T2-weighted images (*arrow*), but there is little appreciable signal in this area on very heavy/extreme T2-weighted images (*circle* denotes expected location of lesion). This pattern of signal loss is commonly seen in hepatic hemangiomas.

approximately 210 to 225 Hz at a field strength of 1.5 T and 420 to 450 Hz at a field strength of 3.0 T.[9,10,19] Because of this slight offset in the precessional frequency, specific imaging phenomena may occur as artifacts of this frequency difference. Chemical shift artifact of the first kind or chemical shift misregistration artifact is a spatial artifact that occurs in the frequency encode direction as a result of the difference in precessional frequency.[12] Because the observed precessional frequency of fat-based protons differs slightly from the expected resonance frequency for the magnet field strength, the data are spatially misregistered, resulting in dark and bright bands at fat–water interfaces.[9] However, determination of macroscopic fat–water interfaces can also be performed using fat-suppression imaging, yielding more obvious depiction of the interface through differences in tissue contrast. The use of fat suppression also nullifies this chemical shift artifact of the first kind and renders its value somewhat moot.

On the other hand, chemical shift artifact of the second kind, also called chemical shift phase cancellation, is an expected artifact that occurs when specific imaging times/TEs are used with a gradient echo sequence. In this setting, the net transverse magnetization of fat-based and water-based protons may be summative (in-phase) or cancelling (opposed-phase) depending on the selected TE. For a 1.5-T magnet, opposed-phase imaging can occur at approximately 2.1 to 2.3 milliseconds and in-phase imaging can occur at approximately 4.2 to 4.6 milliseconds.[12] These times are halved for a 3.0-T magnet (eg, approximately 1.1 milliseconds for the first opposed-phase and approximately 2.2 milliseconds for the

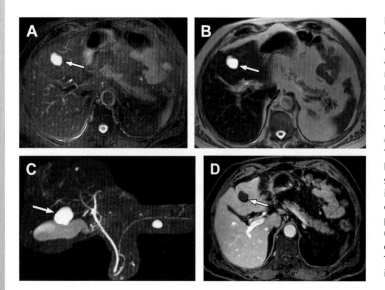

Fig. 3. Axial T2-weighted images with moderate T2 weighting (TE approximately 90 milliseconds [A]) and heavy T2 weighting (TE approximately 180 milliseconds, [B]), and maximum intensity projection image from coronal three-dimensional T2-weighted MRCP sequence with very heavy/extreme T2 weighting (TE approximately 740 milliseconds). There is a well-defined lesion in left hepatic lobe with high signal intensity seen on all T2 weightings (*arrow* in A–C), which is highly suggestive of simple fluid in a hepatic cyst. Axial postcontrast T1-weighted image (venous phase [D]) shows no internal enhancement in this lesion (*arrow*). These imaging features are compatible with a hepatic cyst.

first in-phase). The imaging manifestation of this chemical shift phase cancellation is 2-fold. First, at macroscopic fat–water interfaces, there is a dark signal border that forms on opposed-phase images, sometimes referred to as India ink artifact or etching artifact. This dark border is the result of cancelling magnitude vectors from fat-based and water-based protons within the same voxel, such as at the edge/interface of the renal parenchyma with the retroperitoneal fat. This dark border is present in both phase and frequency encoding directions, as opposed to chemical shift artifact of the first kind.[9] Second, this artifact may also be encountered in lesions or tissue with cells that contain a mixture of fat-based and water-based protons (ie, at a microscopic level). This phenomenon generally manifests as patchy or uniform loss of signal within a lesion on opposed-phase imaging versus in-phase imaging, in contrast to loss of signal only at the edge as encountered in macroscopic fat–water interfaces. Thus, the presence of microscopic lipid can be identified within lesions, which may substantially aid in lesion characterization.

For the liver, the most common usefulness of chemical shift phase cancellation artifact is the identification of hepatic steatosis. Many different patterns of steatosis have been described, including diffuse, geographic, and nodular; other unique patterns have also been seen in select patients, such as those undergoing peritoneal dialysis.[20,21] From a lesion detection perspective, the presence of background hepatic steatosis in the liver may aid in the detection of hepatic masses, because the diffuse steatosis on opposed-phase images often highlights the lesion as a result of intralesional or perilesional sparing.[12] More importantly, the presence of intralesional lipid can be a helpful finding that greatly restricts the differential diagnosis for a hepatic mass. The primary hepatic lesions that contain microscopic lipid include focal steatosis, regenerative nodules with steatosis (steatotic nodules), HCC, hepatic adenomas, and FNH in the setting of existing hepatic steatosis.[22,23] There are other reportable instances of lesions that contain microscopic lipid; however, these do not merit consideration for a pragmatic differential diagnosis given the rarity of the lipid-containing variants of these entities.[23] Often, the primary differential entities may be split in 2 based on the presence of arterial hyperenhancement, which is typically present in HCC, hepatic adenoma, and FNH, but lacking in focal steatosis and regenerative nodules.

Approximately 35% to 77% of adenomas show loss of signal on opposed-phase T1-weighted imaging (Fig. 4).[23,24] More recent work on hepatocellular adenomas has shown 3 subtypes based on pathologic analysis: hepatocyte nuclear factor (HNF) 1α inactivation, β-catenin inactivation, and lesions with acute inflammatory features, including inflammatory infiltrates and dilated sinusoids.[25] Although definite characterization can be made only by pathologic specimen analysis, the HNF-1α subtype is most often associated with intralesional steatosis (encountered in >90% of

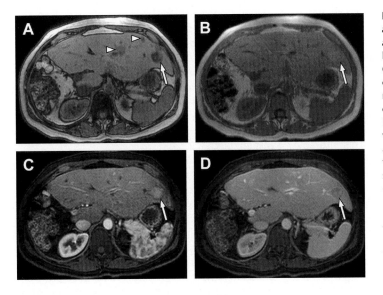

Fig. 4. Axial opposed-phase (A) and in-phase (B) T1-weighted images show a rounded mass in the lateral segment left hepatic lobe (arrow) with internal loss of signal on the opposed-phase image relative to the in-phase image, compatible with intralesional lipid. Other lesions are denoted with arrowheads in (A). On arterial phase postcontrast T1-weighted imaging (C), the lesion shows hypervascularity with avid enhancement (arrow). On venous phase postcontrast T1-weighted imaging (D), the lesion is isointense to slightly hypointense (arrow) versus the background liver. These imaging features are often seen in hepatic adenomas, particularly if there is no history of chronic liver disease. Note that HCC can overlap with these imaging features, although HCC is more frequently encountered in the cirrhotic population.

such lesions in 1 study).[26] On the other hand, intralesional lipid is seen less frequently in HCC. One histopathologic analysis showed that approximately 20% of all HCCs were found to have intralesional lipid, and this rate increased to 36% in larger lesions.[27] Some investigators[23] have commented that the distribution of lipid may be more patchy or heterogeneous in HCC versus adenomas, although this is not necessarily reliable. Therefore, although intralesional lipid is a feature that can tremendously limit the differential diagnosis of a hepatic mass lesion, the presence of intralesional lipid alone cannot reliably distinguish between benign (eg, adenoma) and malignant (eg, HCC) entities.

COMPUTED TOMOGRAPHY AND MR IMAGING: DYNAMIC POSTCONTRAST IMAGING

Multiphase dynamic postcontrast imaging is the primary method for lesion characterization in hepatic CT and plays a major role in lesion characterization in liver MR imaging. Hepatic CT may be used in patients who have a contraindication to MR imaging or lack access to high-quality liver MR imaging. Hepatic CT relies on iodinated contrast material to show the enhancement kinetics of a lesion but suffers from lower tissue contrast than gadolinium-enhanced MR imaging. Moreover, because hepatic CT is an imaging technique that uses ionizing radiation, protocol selection is particularly important to limit patient dose. Most frequently, a 3-phase protocol is used, with timing similar to liver MR imaging (see later discussion). Occasionally, a noncontrast series may be obtained for identification of hyperdense elements such as calcification or hemorrhage.

In MR imaging, dynamic postcontrast imaging is typically performed using a T1-weighted three-dimensional (3D) spoiled gradient echo sequence, which is an accelerated 3D gradient echo sequence that destroys residual transverse magnetization at the end of each repetition time, preventing any buildup of magnetization that could later influence signal on subsequent excitations.[13] This strategy allows the sequence to be performed as fast as possible, with minimum repetition time and minimum TE. As a result, the sequence is often performed during a single breath hold. Fat suppression is often used to maximize tissue contrast and improve the visibility of enhancing structures. Often, the multiphase technique begins with a precontrast data set that is used for lesion characterization (ie, identification of intrinsic T1 hyperintensity) and to permit subtraction imaging. Entities that can be hyperintense to background liver on precontrast T1-weighted imaging include blood products from previous treatment (eg, thermal ablation), intralesional hemorrhage (eg, hepatic adenoma, HCC, hemorrhagic metastasis), other paramagnetic substances such as melanin (eg, melanoma metastasis), fat (usually suppressed with fat suppression), and proteinaceous material (eg, mucinous cystadenoma, proteinaceous cysts). Most abdominal MR imaging studies are performed with traditional extracellular GBCA, which diffuse from the intravascular space to the interstitial space after injection and are excreted via the kidneys, similar to iodinated contrast agents used in CT.

Dynamic postcontrast imaging for both CT and MR imaging often uses 3 phases, including an arterial-dominant phase, a venous phase, and an equilibrium phase. The arterial-dominant phase is also referred to as the late hepatic arterial phase and occurs slightly later than a traditional arterial angiographic phase; proper timing is confirmed by observing uniform enhancement in the hepatic artery, some enhancement in the portal vein, and no enhancement in the hepatic veins.[9] The rationale for using a late hepatic arterial phase is that this phase maximizes conspicuity of hypervascular liver lesions relative to background liver.[12,28] A variety of timing methods may be chosen for obtaining a well-timed, reproducible arterial phase, including fixed delay, timing bolus, and bolus-tracking techniques. At our institution, the bolus-tracking technique is preferred for liver MR imaging and produces relatively consistent results; with this method, the delivery of contrast material to the abdominal aorta is actively monitored and triggers the initiation of the late hepatic arterial phase after a 7- to 8-second fixed delay. Bolus tracking accounts for intrinsic patient factors (ie, cardiovascular output, circulation time) and technician fluctuations that would otherwise be estimated or ignored. On the other hand, the fixed delay technique is used at our institution for hepatic CT, because the larger volume of administered iodinated contrast material for CT aids in overcoming the patient and technical factors that can frequently affect dynamic timing with liver MR imaging.

Hepatic cysts show no internal enhancement on dynamic postcontrast imaging, because they are filled with fluid and lack a substantial solid component (see **Fig. 3**).[29] Occasionally, cysts may show high signal intensity on precontrast T1-weighted MR imaging or increased attenuation on noncontrast CT images as a result of intralesional hemorrhage or protein content. This factor can simulate enhancement but is easily differentiated from true enhancement with subtraction imaging on MR imaging and measurement of attenuation change on CT.

Hepatic hemangiomas have been classified into 3 subtypes differentiated by their dynamic post-contrast imaging features.[30] The type 1 pattern of enhancement is characterized by uniform, intense arterial phase hyperenhancement with similar to slightly higher signal intensity versus background liver on later phases of dynamic post-contrast imaging (**Fig. 5**). This pattern of enhancement may be encountered in tiny hemangiomas. In such cases of type 1 enhancement, corroborative features of hemangioma should be sought, such as high signal intensity on moderately and heavily T2-weighted images. A type 2 pattern of enhancement is associated with most conventional hemangiomas and is characterized by peripheral, nodular, discontinuous enhancement that progresses centripetally across the dynamic phases of imaging, with complete fill-in on delayed imaging (**Fig. 6**). A type 3 pattern of enhancement is similar to type 2, but shows incomplete fill-in on delayed phase imaging and is generally seen in giant hemangiomas that exceed 5 cm.[31]

The dynamic postcontrast behavior of FNH is well described and often used as a primary diagnostic feature, but many FNH cannot be definitively distinguished from other entities (eg, adenoma) by the dynamic postcontrast enhancement pattern alone. FNH is histologically composed of abnormally arranged hepatocytes, typically around a central scar/nidus, which is theorized to arise as a response to a congenital vascular malformation.[29,30] Although FNH can be nearly occult on precontrast images (T1-weighted images and T2-weighted images in MR imaging, noncontrast images in CT), FNH shows rapid, intense arterial phase hyperenhancement, which subsequently becomes nearly isointense/isoattenuating to background hepatic parenchyma on later phases of dynamic postcontrast imaging (**Fig. 7**). When the central scar is present (~50% of cases), it may manifest as conspicuous central delayed enhancement on postcontrast imaging or mild hyperintensity on T2-weighted imaging.[30]

Hepatic metastases have a variety of appearances based on the histology of the primary tumor. Most are classified as hypovascular relative to liver, show abnormal continuous rim enhancement in the arterial-dominant phase, and show low-level/incomplete central internal enhancement on delayed phase imaging with perilesional enhancement (**Fig. 8**).[32] This pattern of enhancement is commonly seen in metastases from primary sites such as colon, breast, and lung. On the other hand, small hypervascular metastases (eg, neuroendocrine malignancies) are often well seen only on the late hepatic arterial phase and occult on other postcontrast phases. Cystic metastases are often difficult to characterize by CT but may show faint peripheral rim enhancement on dynamic postcontrast MR imaging. This differing appearance by modality relates to the superior contrast resolution of MR imaging compared with CT.

Hepatic adenomas have traditionally been recognized as heterogeneous, hypervascular masses that show strong hyperenhancement in the arterial-dominant phase and relative isointensity on later phases of dynamic postcontrast imaging (see **Fig. 4**).[29] With the recognition of pathologic subtypes of hepatic adenomas, increased scrutiny has been paid to their dynamic postcontrast features. Adenomas of the

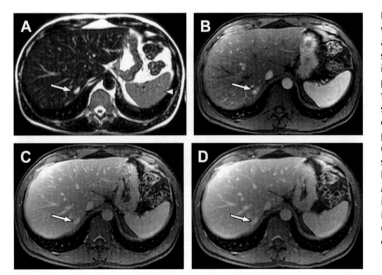

Fig. 5. Axial T2-weighted image with heavy T2 weighting (TE approximately 235 milliseconds [A]) shows a rounded small mass (*arrow*) in the posterior segment right hepatic lobe with very high signal intensity, greater than that of the spleen (*arrowhead*), suggesting a cyst or hemangioma. Axial dynamic postcontrast T1-weighted images (arterial, *B*; venous, *C*; delayed, *D*) show relatively uniform hypervascularity on arterial phase images (*arrow* in *B*) with similar high signal intensity on later phases of dynamic imaging as background blood pool (*arrow* in *C, D*). These features are compatible with a flash-filling/type 1 hepatic hemangioma.

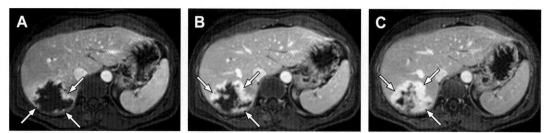

Fig. 6. Axial dynamic postcontrast T1-weighted images (arterial, *A*; venous, *B*; delayed, *C*) show a large mass in the posterior segment right hepatic lobe with peripheral, nodular, discontinuous enhancement (*arrows* in *A*) with progressive centripetal enhancement on later phases of dynamic postcontrast imaging (*arrows* in *B, C*). This behavior is characteristic of a hepatic hemangioma and can be seen in either type 2 or type 3 lesions.

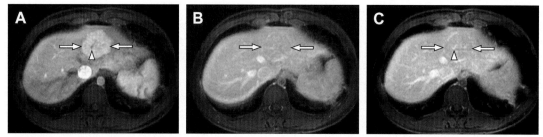

Fig. 7. Axial dynamic postcontrast T1-weighted images (arterial, *A*; venous, *B*; delayed, *C*) show a large mass in left hepatic dome (*arrows*) that enhances avidly in the arterial phase but becomes relatively isointense to background hepatic parenchyma on venous and delayed phase imaging. Note presence of a central scar, which is hypointense on arterial phase imaging (*arrowhead* in *A*) but shows delayed enhancement (*arrowhead* in *C*). This dynamic imaging appearance is characteristic of FNH.

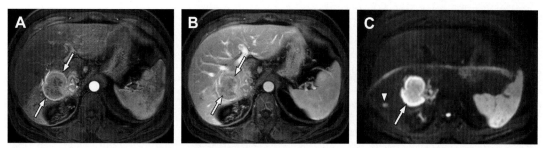

Fig. 8. Axial dynamic postcontrast T1-weighted images (arterial, *A*; venous, *B*) show a rounded mass in right hepatic lobe near the inferior vena cava, with rim enhancement on arterial phase imaging (*arrows* in *A*) and some solid internal enhancement on later phases of dynamic imaging that is less than that of background liver (*arrows* in *B*). Axial DWI (*C*) shows very high signal in the lesion (*arrow*) as well as conspicuous additional lesion in the right hepatic lobe (*arrowhead*), which that is more easily seen on DWI than on the dynamic postcontrast images. This imaging pattern is often seen with metastases, as was the case in this patient with renal cell carcinoma.

inflammatory subtype often show marked, intense hyperenhancement in the arterial-dominant phase, with some persistent enhancement on the later phases of dynamic postcontrast imaging.[26] The degree of enhancement is usually more modest in the HNF-1α subtype lesions, with little persistent enhancement in the later phases of dynamic postcontrast imaging.[33] These 2 subtypes (inflammatory and HNF-1α) account for approximately 70% to 85% of all adenomas, whereas the β-catenin subtype and a variety of unclassified subtypes comprise the remainder.

The β-catenin adenoma subtype is important, because it shares a similar dynamic postcontrast behavior to HCC, with avid arterial-dominant phase hyperenhancement and delayed phase hypoenhancement (ie, washout).[26] The risk for malignant transformation to HCC seems to be highest for the β-catenin subtype.[33] This similarity serves to reinforce the concept that hepatic adenomas can be HCC mimics. Biopsy or resection are sometimes performed in such cases.

MR IMAGING
Diffusion-Weighted Imaging

DWI is an MR imaging technique that is predicated on differences in the microscopic free motion of water molecules. In vivo water molecules may be constrained by interactions with cell membranes, macromolecules, and dense cell packing, which varies based on tissue type and location, resulting in an in vivo apparent diffusion rather than a single theoretic diffusion.[10] The use of diffusion MR imaging was pioneered in 1965 and became a viable clinically relevant tool for stroke imaging more than 20 years ago. The use of DWI in the liver has lagged behind applications in the brain, because of difficulty in applying the technique in the moving abdomen, but has recently gained increasing interest as a result of improved ultrafast techniques, including single-shot spin-echo echo planar imaging. The detailed physics of DWI is beyond the scope of this review, but a summary is provided.

DWI was originally performed by adding a symmetric pair of diffusion-sensitizing gradients around the 180° refocusing pulse of a T2-weighted sequence.[34] Because of the gradient symmetry, water molecules in highly constrained environments (ie, impeded diffusion) would not be allowed to change phase appreciably between the 2 gradients, and therefore would create little rephasing difference. As a result, little difference to the underlying T2 signal would be generated, resulting in high signal intensity on DWI.[9,10,34] On the other hand, water molecules with free diffusion would be expected to have substantial phase change between the 2 diffusion gradients, leading to a resultant net phase difference that reduces the underlying T2 signal and manifests as low signal on DWI. The sensitivity to water diffusion can be varied by changing the b factor or b value, which is proportional to the diffusion gradient applied, including the gradient amplitude, duration, and timing relationship of the paired pulses.[10,34] Although the b value can be selected arbitrarily, most liver applications use only b values less than 1000 s/mm^2 because of the relatively low signal intensity in the background liver (caused by the short T2 relaxation time of hepatic parenchyma) and reasonable imaging times relative to signal achieved. Several b values are often used in clinical practice, including a b value of 0 s/mm^2, a low b value series (b = 20–150 s/mm^2), and a high b value series (b = 500–800 s/mm^2). A b value of 0 s/mm^2 means that no diffusion-sensitizing gradient is applied, resulting in a T2-weighted image. A low b value series (typically b = 20–150 s/mm^2) can be used to nullify the perfusional effects on DWI signal created by moving protons in the blood stream.[9,34] A high b value series (typically b = 500–800 s/mm^2) more selectively isolates impeded diffusion such as that seen in lymphatic tissue and cellular tumors.[9,10] When 2 or more b values are used, an apparent diffusion coefficient (ADC) can be calculated to quantify the observed in vivo diffusion and to aid in differentiating intrinsic residual high T2 signal (ie, T2 shine-through) from true impeded diffusion.

In clinical liver applications, the use of DWI is often limited to qualitative metastasis detection, although some lesion characterization benefits have been described. DWI has been shown to be vastly superior to routine T2-weighted sequences for the detection of metastatic liver lesions (particularly small liver lesions), with detection rates of 78% to 100% depending on the published series.[35] Moreover, DWI has been shown to have similar sensitivity to dynamic postcontrast MR imaging for the detection of hepatic metastases and is of particular use in identifying small lesions and hypervascular metastases (eg, neuroendocrine tumors).

From a lesion characterization perspective, the qualitative assessment of lesions can be performed by examining the various b value DWI series and the computed ADC map. Benign lesions, including cysts and hemangiomas, show a pattern of high signal on the low b value series (ie, predominantly T2 weighted), with diminished signal on the high b value series (ie, predominantly diffusion weighted). This situation results in high signal/high values on the ADC map (**Fig. 9**).[33] In contrast, malignant lesions often show more pronounced/higher signal

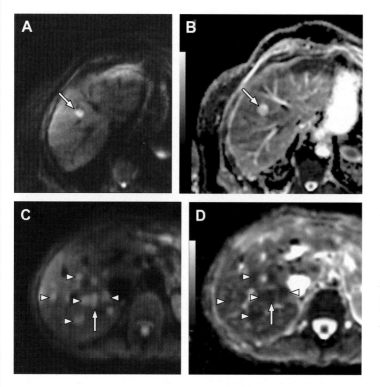

Fig. 9. Axial DWI and ADC map corresponding to a hepatic cyst (*A*, *B*, respectively) and axial DWI and ADC map corresponding to hepatic metastasis (*C*, *D*, respectively). Note the pattern of high signal on both DWI and ADC map in hepatic cysts, indicating T2 shine-through (*arrows* in *A*, *B*). This finding contrasts the true restricted diffusion pattern of a hepatic metastasis with high signal on DWI and low signal on ADC map (*arrows* in *C*, *D*). The quantitative ADC value for this cyst was 3.0 (x 10^{-3} mm^2/s), which is higher than the postulated threshold of 1.60 to 1.63 (x 10^{-3} mm^2/s) that can be used to discriminate a benign entity from a potential malignant lesion. The quantitative ADC value for this metastasis was 0.9 (x 10^{-3} mm^2/s). Note multiple other hepatic metastases (*arrowheads* in *C* and *D*) with similar imaging characteristics.

on the high b value series (ie, predominantly diffusion weighted) with low signal/low values on the ADC map (ie, corresponding to impeded diffusion). Small studies have validated the qualitative use of DWI for lesion characterization, including a reported 93% accuracy for differentiating lesions 1 cm or smaller as benign or malignant.[36] DWI has been described as a quantitative technique for lesion characterization, noting that threshold ADC values of 1.60 to 1.63 (x 10^{-3} mm^2/s) have yielded reported accuracies of 75% to 88% for discrimination of malignant lesions (low ADC value) from benign lesions (high ADC value).[10] The ADC values have been shown to vary between MR imaging scanner systems and acquisition parameters/technique, and there is a reported 14% coefficient of variation within an individual lesion/patient. This variation and the overlap that exists between some benign and malignant lesions limit the practical application of quantitative DWI for specific lesion characterization.[37,38]

Hepatocyte-Specific Contrast Agents

In addition to extracellular GBCA, several other contrast agents exist in MR imaging that have targeted uses or additional characterization benefit. For liver imaging, this category most recently includes agents that are tailored to have active uptake into hepatocytes via the OATP1 transport protein and excretion into the biliary system via the MRP2 protein.[10] These compounds are often referred to as hepatocyte-specific contrast agents (HSCA) and include gadobenate dimeglumine (Gd-BOPTA, Multihance, Bracco Diagnostics, Princeton, NJ) and gadoxetic acid (Gd-EOB-DTPA, Eovist/Primovist, Bayer Healthcare Pharmaceuticals, Wayne, NJ). These GBCA have a dual pharmacokinetic behavior. Soon after intravenous injection, these compounds behave similarly to traditional extracellular compounds as they diffuse from the intravascular space into the interstitial space. However, the active accumulation and excretion of contrast material by the hepatobiliary system results in different delayed imaging characteristics from traditional extracellular GBCA. Specifically, a hepatobiliary imaging phase may be added using a T1-weighted spoiled gradient echo sequence, similar to that used for the earlier time points and sometimes with a higher flip angle (eg, 20°–30°). The hepatobiliary phase provides superior contrast resolution, which can be used to discriminate structures with and without functioning hepatocytes.[9] Because the hepatic extraction of contrast agent differs between the 2 compounds (approximately 5% for Gd-

BOPTA and 50% for Gd-EOB-DTPA), the timing of the hepatobiliary phase also differs: 45 to 120 minutes for Gd-BOPTA versus 20 minutes for Gd-EOB-DTPA.[10]

The primary benefit for hepatobiliary phase imaging for lesion characterization is the identification of intralesional uptake of contrast material in the hepatobiliary phase; this indicates that the lesion in question contains functional hepatocytes with specific transport proteins. The degree of uptake can be variable, ranging from mild (ie, isointense or even minimally hypointense to background liver) to marked (ie, hyperintense to background liver). The pattern of uptake may also be heterogeneous, including uniform uptake, inhomogeneous internal hyperintensity, and peripheral rimlike uptake with central hypointensity.[39] However, the interpretation of functional information is more binary, either present (regardless of degree of uptake) or absent.[10] Most focal liver lesions lack functioning transport proteins and appear very dark versus background liver because of absent uptake. Although the lack of uptake is often used to corroborate a metastatic focus, this appearance overlaps with most other liver lesions, including benign (eg, hemangioma, cyst, most adenomas) and malignant (eg, cholangiocarcinoma, HCC) entities.

Therefore, identification of positive uptake within a lesion on hepatobiliary phase images is more helpful, because it can greatly narrow the differential diagnosis. This situation is most commonly seen in FNH, with 90% to 96% of FNH showing some degree of uptake (**Fig. 10**).[39,40] However, FNH occasionally shows little uptake on hepatobiliary phase images.[39] Although contrast material uptake in the hepatobiliary phase restricts the differential diagnosis to that of masses containing functioning hepatocytes, both benign and malignant entities can have this pattern. Approximately 2.5% to 8.5% of HCCs may show uptake on hepatobiliary phase imaging, which may be related to variable expression of transport proteins.[10] One recent study indicated that 9% of hepatocellular adenomas may also show uptake on hepatobiliary phase imaging, although the individual adenoma subtypes were not specifically analyzed for cohort differences.[41] The lack of specificity of hepatobiliary phase uptake (or lack thereof) has limited the generalizability of hepatobiliary phase imaging for lesion characterization. Paradoxically, the primary benefit of hepatobiliary phase imaging seems to be lesion detection (eg, identifying the number and location of potentially resectable colon cancer metastases).

SUMMARY

The emergence of modern cross-sectional imaging techniques permits both identification and detailed analysis of liver lesions, particularly through MR imaging. Numerous benign and malignant lesions have been described in the noncirrhotic liver. No specific sequence or postcontrast imaging phase in MR imaging or CT is a single panacea for lesion characterization. Rather, the characterization of liver lesions is best accomplished by tabulating the relative imaging features of a lesion across several imaging sequences and understanding the individual value of certain sequences for specific diagnoses (**Tables 3–7**). By combining traditional imaging sequences (including various T2-weighted sequences, in-phase/opposed-phase T1-weighted imaging, and dynamic postcontrast imaging) with adjunct applications such as DWI and HSCA, a confident diagnosis can often be made in many cases in the noncirrhotic liver.

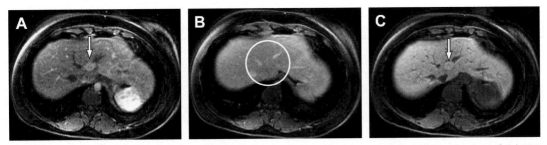

Fig. 10. Axial dynamic postcontrast T1-weighted images (arterial, *A*; venous, *B*) after administration of Gd-EOB-DTPA show a hypervascular mass in the left hepatic dome between the middle and left hepatic veins (*arrow* in *A*). This lesion is relatively isointense to background liver on venous phase images (*circle* denotes expected location of lesion). Axial hepatobiliary phase images obtained 20 minutes after Gd-EOB-DTPA administration (*C*) show uptake within the lesion, similar or slightly more than the background liver. This finding confirms the presence of functioning transport proteins within this lesion. The imaging features are compatible with FNH.

Table 3
Characterization value of T2-weighted sequences

Cyst	High signal intensity across all degrees of T2 weighting, including moderate, heavy, and very heavy/extreme T2 weighting
Hemangioma	High signal intensity on moderate and heavy T2-weighted sequences, greater than spleen and liver. Substantial loss of signal occurs at transition from heavy to very heavy/extreme T2 weighting
Metastasis	High signal intensity on moderate T2-weighted images, substantial loss of signal occurs at transition from moderate to heavy T2 weighting. Follows relative signal intensity of spleen on most T2-weighted sequences

Table 4
Characterization value of in-phase/opposed-phase T1-weighted sequence

Adenoma	Lesion most often associated with signal loss on opposed-phase imaging, particularly HNF-1α subtype. Few HCC can show loss of signal, often more patchy/heterogeneous
Metastasis	Rarely may show uptake if primary tumor contains intralesional lipid, such as clear-cell subtype of renal cell carcinoma

Table 5
Characterization value of dynamic postcontrast imaging

Cyst	No internal enhancement
Hemangioma	Depends on subtype. Type 1 shows uniform arterial enhancement and delayed phase hyperintensity that is similar to background blood pool. Types 2 and 3 show peripheral, nodular, discontinuous enhancement with centripetal fill
FNH	Intense arterial-dominant phase enhancement, nearly isointense to background liver on later phases of dynamic imaging. Central scar in 50%, shows delayed enhancement with extracellular GBCM
Metastasis	Depends on primary tumor type, most are hypovascular relative to liver with continuous rim enhancement on arterial-dominant phase and low-level internal enhancement on later dynamic imaging. Hypervascular metastases may be seen only in arterial phase
Adenoma	Arterial-dominant phase enhancement in almost all, although degree of enhancement can vary with subtype (highest in inflammatory subtype). Generally isointense or slightly hyperintense on delayed phase imaging. Some may show intralesional washout, simulating HCC, particularly β-catenin subtype

Table 6
Characterization value of DWI

Metastasis	Qualitatively depicted true impeded diffusion with high signal on DWI, low signal on ADC map. Quantitatively low on ADC but number varies with system/protocol
Cyst	Qualitatively depicted as T2 shine-through with high signal on DWI and matching high signal on ADC map
Hemangioma	Qualitatively depicted as T2 shine-through with high signal on DWI and matching high signal on ADC map

Table 7
Characterization value of HSCA

FNH	Most (≥90%) show some degree of uptake, although pattern of uptake does vary, including homogeneous, heterogeneous/patchy, and peripheral rimlike uptake
Adenoma	Few (9%) show some degree of uptake. Small percentage of HCC can also show uptake
Metastasis	Uniform very low signal intensity because of lack of uptake

REFERENCES

1. Jones EC, Chezmar JL, Nelson RC, et al. The frequency and significance of small (less than or equal to 15 mm) hepatic lesions detected by CT. AJR Am J Roentgenol 1992;158(3):535–9.

2. Schwartz LH, Gandras EJ, Colangelo SM, et al. Prevalence and importance of small hepatic lesions found at CT in patients with cancer. Radiology 1999;210(1):71–4.

3. Saini S, Ralls PW, Balfe DM, et al. Liver lesion characterization. American College of Radiology. ACR Appropriateness Criteria. Radiology 2000;215(Suppl):193–9.

4. Liu PS, Francis IR. Hepatic imaging for metastatic disease. Cancer J 2010;16(2):93–102.

5. Böhm B, Voth M, Geoghegan J, et al. Impact of positron emission tomography on strategy in liver resection for primary and secondary liver tumors. J Cancer Res Clin Oncol 2004;130(5):266–72.

6. Wernecke K, Rummeny E, Bongartz G, et al. Detection of hepatic masses in patients with carcinoma: comparative sensitivities of sonography, CT, and MR imaging. AJR Am J Roentgenol 1991;157(4):731–9.

7. Mainenti PP, Mancini M, Mainolfi C, et al. Detection of colo-rectal liver metastases: prospective comparison of contrast enhanced US, multidetector CT, PET/CT, and 1.5 Tesla MR with extracellular and reticulo-endothelial cell specific contrast agents. Abdom Imaging 2010;35(5):511–21.

8. Shuman WP, Chan KT, Busey JM, et al. Standard and reduced radiation dose liver CT images: adaptive statistical iterative reconstruction versus model-based iterative reconstruction-comparison of findings and image quality. Radiology 2014;273(3):793–800.

9. Guglielmo FF, Mitchell DG, Roth CG, et al. Hepatic MR imaging techniques, optimization, and artifacts. Magn Reson Imaging Clin N Am 2014;22(3):263–82.

10. Liu PS, Hussain HK. Contemporary and emerging technologies in abdominal magnetic resonance imaging. Semin Roentgenol 2013;48(3):203–13.

11. Siegelman ES, Chauhan A. MR characterization of focal liver lesions: pearls and pitfalls. Magn Reson Imaging Clin N Am 2014;22(3):295–313.

12. Wile GE, Leyendecker JR. Magnetic resonance imaging of the liver: sequence optimization and artifacts. Magn Reson Imaging Clin N Am 2010;18(3):525–47.

13. Boyle GE, Ahern M, Cooke J, et al. An interactive taxonomy of MR imaging sequences. Radiographics 2006;26(6):e24.

14. Ito K, Mitchell DG, Outwater EK, et al. Hepatic lesions: discrimination of nonsolid, benign lesions from solid, malignant lesions with heavily T2-weighted fast spin-echo MR imaging. Radiology 1997;204(3):729–37.

15. Goldberg MA, Hahn PF, Saini S, et al. Value of T1 and T2 relaxation times from echoplanar MR imaging in the characterization of focal hepatic lesions. AJR Am J Roentgenol 1993;160(5):1011–7.

16. Cieszanowski A, Szeszkowski W, Golebiowski M, et al. Discrimination of benign from malignant hepatic lesions based on their T2-relaxation times calculated from moderately T2-weighted turbo SE sequence. Eur Radiol 2002;12(9):2273–9.

17. Thomsen C, Josephsen P, Karle H, et al. Determination of T1- and T2-relaxation times in the spleen of patients with splenomegaly. Magn Reson Imaging 1990;8(1):39–42.

18. Kiryu S, Okada Y, Ohtomo K. Differentiation between hemangiomas and cysts of the liver with single-shot fast-spin echo image using short and long TE. J Comput Assist Tomogr 2002;26(5):687–90.

19. Bley TA, Wieben O, François CJ, et al. Fat and water magnetic resonance imaging. J Magn Reson Imaging 2010;31(1):4–18.

20. Wells SA. Quantification of hepatic fat and iron with magnetic resonance imaging. Magn Reson Imaging Clin N Am 2014;22(3):397–416.

21. H'ng MW, Kwek JW. Imaging appearance of severe subcapsular hepatic steatosis: mimicking hepatic embolic infarcts. Br J Radiol 2010;83(989):e98–100.

22. Morii K, Nakamura S, Yamamoto T, et al. Steatotic regenerative nodules mimicking hepatocellular carcinoma. Liver Int 2014;34(3):477.

23. Prasad SR, Wang H, Rosas H, et al. Fat-containing lesions of the liver: radiologic-pathologic correlation. Radiographics 2005;25(2):321–31.

24. Chung KY, Mayo-Smith WW, Saini S, et al. Hepatocellular adenoma: MR imaging features with

pathologic correlation. AJR Am J Roentgenol 1995; 165(2):303–8.

25. Rebouissou S, Bioulac-Sage P, Zucman-Rossi J. Molecular pathogenesis of focal nodular hyperplasia and hepatocellular adenoma. J Hepatol 2008;48(1): 163–70.

26. Laumonier H, Bioulac-Sage P, Laurent C, et al. Hepatocellular adenomas: magnetic resonance imaging features as a function of molecular pathological classification. Hepatology 2008;48(3):808–18.

27. Kutami R, Nakashima Y, Nakashima O, et al. Pathomorphologic study on the mechanism of fatty change in small hepatocellular carcinoma of humans. J Hepatol 2000;33(2):282–9.

28. Van Beers BE, Materne R, Lacrosse M, et al. MR imaging of hypervascular liver tumors: timing optimization during the arterial phase. J Magn Reson Imaging 1999;9(4):562–7.

29. Horton KM, Bluemke DA, Hruban RH, et al. CT and MR imaging of benign hepatic and biliary tumors. Radiographics 1999;19(2):431–51.

30. Ba-Ssalamah A, Baroud S, Bastati N, et al. MR imaging of benign focal liver lesions. Magn Reson Imaging Clin N Am 2010;18(3):403–19.

31. Danet IM, Semelka RC, Braga L, et al. Giant hemangioma of the liver: MR imaging characteristics in 24 patients. Magn Reson Imaging 2003;21(2):95–101.

32. Danet IM, Semelka RC, Leonardou P, et al. Spectrum of MRI appearances of untreated metastases of the liver. AJR Am J Roentgenol 2003;181(3): 809–17.

33. Lewis S, Dyvorne H, Cui Y, et al. Diffusion-weighted imaging of the liver: techniques and applications. Magn Reson Imaging Clin N Am 2014;22(3):373–95.

34. Katabathina VS, Menias CO, Shanbhogue AK, et al. Genetics and imaging of hepatocellular adenomas: 2011 update. Radiographics 2011;31(6): 1529–43.

35. Taouli B, Koh DM. Diffusion-weighted MR imaging of the liver. Radiology 2010;254(1):47–66.

36. Holzapfel K, Bruegel M, Eiber M, et al. Characterization of small (≤10 mm) focal liver lesions: value of respiratory-triggered echo-planar diffusion-weighted MR imaging. Eur J Radiol 2010;76(1):89–95.

37. Sasaki M, Yamada K, Watanabe Y, et al. Variability in absolute apparent diffusion coefficient values across different platforms may be substantial: a multivendor, multi-institutional comparison study. Radiology 2008;249(2):624–30.

38. Braithwaite AC, Dale BM, Boll DT, et al. Short- and midterm reproducibility of apparent diffusion coefficient measurements at 3.0-T diffusion-weighted imaging of the abdomen. Radiology 2009;250(2): 459–65.

39. van Kessel CS, de Boer E, ten Kate FJ, et al. Focal nodular hyperplasia: hepatobiliary enhancement patterns on gadoxetic-acid contrast-enhanced MRI. Abdom Imaging 2013;38(3):490–501.

40. Zech CJ, Grazioli L, Breuer J, et al. Diagnostic performance and description of morphological features of focal nodular hyperplasia in Gd-EOB-DTPA-enhanced liver magnetic resonance imaging: results of a multicenter trial. Invest Radiol 2008; 43(7):504–11.

41. Denecke T, Steffen IG, Agarwal S, et al. Appearance of hepatocellular adenomas on gadoxetic acid-enhanced MRI. Eur Radiol 2012;22(8):1769–75.

Imaging in Patients with Cirrhosis: Current Evidence

Mustafa R. Bashir, MD[a,b,]*, Hero K. Hussain, MD[c]

KEYWORDS

• Cross-sectional imaging • Cirrhosis • Hepatocellular carcinoma • Evidence

KEY POINTS

- There have been major changes in the management and reporting of hepatocellular carcinoma (HCC) in the last decade.
- Cross-sectional imaging is now pivotal in the management of cirrhotic patients, in particular in the diagnosis and staging of HCC.
- Although diagnostic systems have become relatively well developed, approximately one-third of HCC nodules may have an atypical appearance, necessitating ancillary testing, close follow-up, or biopsy.
- The introduction of standardized diagnostic and reporting systems has improved communication between radiologists and clinicians, but there remains substantial disagreement between radiologists in feature assignment and nodule characterization.
- As our understanding of this disease evolves and imaging techniques improve, standardized diagnostic criteria must continue to evolve in order to provide more accurate, early diagnosis.

Cirrhosis is an increasingly common disease. Its sequelae, including portal venous hypertension and hepatocellular carcinoma (HCC), are major causes of morbidity and mortality, with more than half a million new cases of HCC diagnosed every year worldwide.[1] Cross-sectional imaging plays a central role in the care of cirrhotic patients and is used primarily for the detection and treatment planning of HCC. Unlike other types of malignancy, all major guidelines for the management of HCC accept the imaging diagnosis of HCC without requiring tissue confirmation.[2–6] Thus high-quality imaging, interpretation, and communication of findings are central to the care of cirrhotic patients.

SURVEILLANCE

The target population and method for HCC surveillance vary among liver societies.[7] The American Association for the Study of Liver Disease (AASLD) recommends that patients with cirrhosis, regardless of cause, undergo liver ultrasound every 6 months for surveillance.[2] In addition, noncirrhotic hepatitis B virus carriers should undergo ultrasound surveillance if they are of Asian ethnicity (men >40 years old and women >50 years old), black, or have a strong family history of HCC.[2] The European Society for the Study of the Liver (EASL) recommends surveillance ultrasound of all patients with Child-Pugh stage A and B cirrhosis or Child-Pugh stage C cirrhosis awaiting liver transplantation, noncirrhotic hepatitis B carriers with active hepatitis or a family history of HCC, and noncirrhotic patients with chronic hepatitis C infection and stage F3 liver fibrosis.[3] The Japanese Society of Hepatology (JSH) defines 2 at-risk groups: a high-risk group comprising noncirrhotic patients with chronic hepatitis B or C infection and patients with cirrhosis of other causes and a super–high-risk group comprising patients with

[a] Division of Abdominal Imaging, Department of Radiology, Duke University Medical Center, Durham, NC 27710, USA; [b] Department of Radiology, Center for Advanced Magnetic Resonance Development, Duke University Medical Center, Durham, NC 27710, USA; [c] Department of Radiology, University of Michigan Health System, Ann Arbor, MI 48109, USA
* Corresponding author.
E-mail address: mustafa.bashir@duke.edu

Radiol Clin N Am 53 (2015) 919–931
http://dx.doi.org/10.1016/j.rcl.2015.05.006
0033-8389/15/$ – see front matter Published by Elsevier Inc.

hepatitis B– or hepatitis C–related cirrhosis.[4] The JSH includes liver ultrasound, alpha-fetoprotein, and other serum markers in its surveillance algorithm for both groups and dynamic contrast-enhanced computed tomography (CT) or MR imaging for the super–high-risk group.[4]

One of the important issues in imaging surveillance for HCC is the use of ultrasonography. Although all major liver societies agree that ultrasound is the imaging modality of choice for HCC surveillance mainly because of the availability, affordability, simplicity, and reasonable overall sensitivity, it is widely acknowledged that ultrasound has a relatively low sensitivity for detecting early stage HCC (within Milan criteria) (63% in a 2009 meta-analysis); detection of early stage disease is important to the success of any surveillance system.[8] In addition, ultrasonography is highly operator dependent; its performance may be even lower at centers without dedicated liver surveillance programs.[8] However, because the performance of CT and MR imaging have mainly been evaluated in the diagnostic setting rather than that of surveillance, there are currently no data that support their use in routine surveillance.[8] Concerns regarding cost, complexity, false positives, and radiation dose in CT have reduced enthusiasm for their use in general surveillance.

There is, however, good agreement among liver societies regarding diagnostic imaging features for HCC. All major systems allow the definitive diagnosis to be made when classic imaging features are present on multiphasic contrast-enhanced CT or MR imaging; in the JSH guidelines, contrast-enhanced ultrasound features can also be used for the diagnosis of HCC.[4]

COMPUTED TOMOGRAPHY AND MR IMAGING TECHNIQUE

Preferential arterial blood supply is one of the hallmarks of HCC. HCC is typically a highly vascular lesion arising in a highly vascular organ, and visualizing the characteristic features of arterial phase hyperenhancement (APHE) and venous phase hypointensity washout feature requires a high-quality multiphasic contrast-enhanced examination with an accurately timed hepatic arterial phase. All published diagnostic criteria emphasize the importance of multiphase contrast-enhanced imaging.

The US Organ Procurement and Transplant Network's (OPTN) policy on the allocation of livers includes specific technical requirements for both contrast-enhanced CT and MR imaging.[5,9] These requirements include minimum contrast media injection rates (3 mL/s for CT and 2 mL/s for most MR imaging agents), high spatial resolution (5-mm slice thickness or less for dynamic series), and multiple dynamic phases (at least 3 phases for CT and 4 phases for MR imaging). Precontrast imaging is optional for CT because of its relatively low yield and added radiation dose. However, for MR imaging, precontrast T_1-weighted imaging is mandatory because it is needed to assess for APHE in intrinsically hyperintense nodules. Both a portal venous and delayed (>120 seconds after contrast media injection) phase are mandated to optimize sensitivity for the detection of the nodule washout feature.

The ideal hepatic arterial phase is transient, and its timing is variable from patient to patient. Visually, lesional enhancement is typically best seen in the late arterial phase when there is robust enhancement of the hepatic arteries, early enhancement of the portal veins, minimal enhancement of the hepatic parenchyma, and no enhancement of the hepatic veins. Several techniques for attaining a well-timed hepatic arterial phase are currently available, including test bolus technique, automated bolus detection, real-time bolus tracking, and single-breath-hold multi-arterial phase methods.[10–15]

DIAGNOSTIC FEATURES OF HEPATOCELLULAR CARCINOMA
Established Imaging Characteristics

Arterial phase hyperenhancement

Arterial phase hyperenhancement is the single most important imaging feature of HCC. It usually appears diffuse or heterogeneous in tumors with necrosis or varying degrees of cellular dedifferentiation (**Fig. 1**) and sometimes rimlike (**Fig. 2**). This feature alone is highly sensitive for HCC (82%–93%) but not as specific.[16–20] For example, cholangiocarcinoma (CC) often demonstrates rimlike hyperenhancement, and high-grade dysplastic nodules may have homogeneous APHE; thus, APHE alone is not sufficient to make the diagnosis of HCC.

Washout feature

The washout feature has a 2-fold definition under the Liver Imaging-Reporting and Data System (LI-RADS); a nodule must be less enhanced than the surrounding liver parenchyma in a venous phase and less enhanced than it was on a previous dynamic phase (see **Fig. 1**). The washout feature has largely been attributed to the diminished portal venous supply of HCC compared with the surrounding liver, such that although an HCC nodule may appear hyperenhancing in an arterial-dominant phase, the liver appears hyperenhancing (and the nodule hypoenhancing) in a

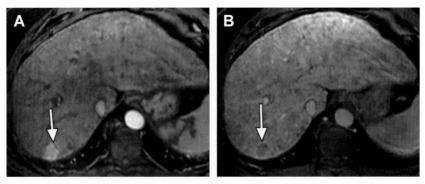

Fig. 1. (*A, B*) A classic 1.2-cm HCC (*arrow*) on MR imaging obtained following extracellular gadolinium-based contrast agent administration in (*A*) the arterial and (*B*) delayed venous phases of enhancement. The HCC hyperenhances relative to liver parenchyma in the arterial phase (*A*), becomes hypointense washout feature, and has a delayed enhancing rim capsular feature in the delayed venous phase (*B*).

venous-dominant phase. Hyperenhancement of the fibrotic liver in the delayed phase is another contributing factor to the washout feature. Although less sensitive (up to 53%) than APHE, the nodule washout feature alone is highly specific for HCC (62%–100%), particularly for APHE nodules larger than 2 cm in diameter (specificity >80%).[18,19,21–25] Also, the washout feature is sometimes more readily detected in delayed venous phases compared with the portal venous phase.[18,26,27]

Capsule feature
A fibrous capsule or pseudocapsule is a well-known feature of HCC (particularly well-differentiated HCC) at histopathology but is a controversial imaging finding. Studies assessing imaging correlates of the histopathological capsule have variably defined it as a hypointense rim at precontrast imaging, a hyperenhancing rim in a venous phase after contrast media administration, or both[18] (see **Fig. 1**). The LI-RADS criteria specifically use the definition based on contrast media enhancement, but there are little data comparing the diagnostic performance of the various imaging definitions. Even assuming a single definition, the utility of the capsule finding is debated. Although the presence of a capsule is generally agreed on as a finding associated with HCC, some studies have found that including a capsule as a criterion for the diagnosis of HCC adds little or no performance to the classic APHE and washout criterion, whereas others have found a diagnostic benefit.[18,24] As a result, some diagnostic guidelines (OPTN and LI-RADS) include a capsule as a major feature of HCC, whereas others (AASLD, EASL, and JSH) do not. In addition, the JSH guidelines include "corona enhancement" (transient perilesional enhancement in the portal venous phase) as a diagnostic criterion, whereas the remainder of the major guidelines do not.[4]

Size and growth
Numerous studies have shown that larger nodules are more likely to be HCC than smaller nodules. Additionally, the classic features of HCC (APHE and washout feature) have better diagnostic performance in nodules larger than 2 cm in diameter than for smaller nodules.[18,21,23,24,28–30] Unfortunately, larger nodules and growing nodules also have a stronger association with microvascular invasion, intrahepatic metastases, and poor treatment outcomes; thus, the detection and characterization of small HCC measuring less than 2 cm remains important.[4,31]

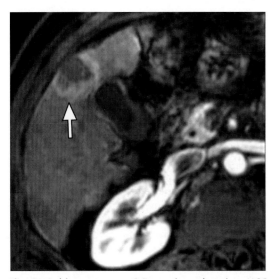

Fig. 2. A biopsy-proven 2.5-cm rim-enhancing HCC (*arrow*) on MR imaging obtained following extracellular gadolinium-based contrast agent administration in the arterial-phase of enhancement.

The AASLD and EASL surveillance guidelines recommend ultrasonographic follow-up of nodules less than 1 cm in size and diagnostic imaging with multiphasic CT or MR imaging for nodules 1 cm in size or larger or nodules that grow at follow-up. The AASLD, EASL, JSH, and recently LI-RADS diagnostic criteria allow the confident diagnosis of HCC to be made for nodules at least 1 cm in size with APHE and washout feature if seen on an antecedent surveillance ultrasound, whereas the OPTN criteria require additional features to be present (capsule and/or growth) in order to ensure a definitive diagnosis of HCC measuring 1 to 2 cm. One reason for this difference is that OPTN does not make the assumption that the nodule was detected on ultrasound and uses only CT and MR imaging features for the diagnosis of HCC.

The definition of growth is another area of debate, particularly because growth has been variably defined (or not specifically defined at all) in the various studies that contribute to consensus criteria. The AASLD and EASL surveillance guidelines use growth as a feature that should prompt diagnostic evaluation of a nodule but do not define growth explicitly. The OPTN and LI-RADS criteria give similar, but slightly different, definitions for growth and consider it to be a major feature of HCC. The OPTN definition of growth is an increase in maximum APHE nodule diameter of at least 50% within 6 months. Such a nodule can be diagnosed as HCC. The LI-RADS further expands this definition by including the requirement for a minimum increase in nodule diameter of 0.5 cm in addition to either at least 50% diameter increase within 6 months (similar to OPTN) or at least 100% diameter increase per year. New lesions measuring at least 1 cm at the time they are first discovered are also given credit for growth under LI-RADS but are not addressed in the OPTN system. Although a major criterion for the diagnosis of HCC by OPTN and LIRADS, the growth feature should be applied judiciously to avoid a false-negative diagnosis of HCC, because well-differentiated HCCs can grow slowly, and to avoid a false-positive diagnosis of HCC, because other lesions, such as dysplastic nodules and cholangiocarcinomas, can grow.

T2-weighted signal hyperintensity

Mild hyperintensity on T2-weighted MR images is another classic imaging feature of malignant or potentially malignant hepatocellular nodules.[20] However, in the cirrhotic liver, the background liver's signal intensity is typically heterogeneous and elevated, reducing the conspicuity of mild nodule signal hyperintensity. In addition, well-differentiated HCC can be isointense or hypointense to the liver on T2-weighted imaging; some nonhepatocellular nodules, such as cholangiocarcinoma, can be hyperintense. Thus, both the sensitivity and specificity of signal hyperintensity on T2-weighted imaging is relatively low for detecting HCC in the cirrhotic liver.[18,19,28,32–34] In addition, it has been shown that T2-weighted signal intensity may add little incremental diagnostic value beyond dynamic vascular features for the detection of HCC.[18,29] As a result, none of the major HCC diagnostic criteria use T2-weighted signal intensity as a primary diagnostic feature; LI-RADS incorporates this feature but only as an ancillary criterion.

Intracellular lipid

The presence of intracellular lipid is a classic feature of HCC. Although an insensitive feature (12%–37% sensitivity), it is a relatively specific feature for HCC (68%–100%).[18,19,28] Like T2-weighted signal intensity, its overall low diagnostic value has prevented the inclusion of this finding into most of the major HCC diagnostic criteria; only LI-RADS incorporates it as an ancillary feature of HCC.

Novel Imaging Characteristics

Hepatobiliary phase hypointensity

Hepatocyte-specific contrast agents are a relatively recent innovation in MR imaging. They are taken up by hepatocellular transporters, concentrated within hepatocytes, and excreted into the biliary system. Nodules whose cells do not express these transporters or express them at a subnormal level, such as high-grade dysplastic nodules and HCC, appear hypointense in the hepatobiliary phase (HBP), thus these agents have shown promise for assessing nodule dedifferentiation in the setting of cirrhosis and, by association, malignant potential.

Although HBP imaging has high sensitivity for HCC (79%–100%), this benefit is reduced by a low specificity for HCC; in addition, reported specificities are highly variable (33%–92%).[19,21,28,35–39] The main challenge in using HBP imaging for the diagnosis of hepatocellular carcinoma is that all nonhepatocellular lesions, such as hemangiomas and cholangiocarcinomas, also demonstrate HBP hypointensity. In addition, some nonmalignant dysplastic nodules downregulate their receptor expression and appear hypointense in the HBP and can be mistaken for HCC. Also, contrast agent uptake by the normal liver parenchyma can be markedly reduced in cirrhosis, reducing sensitivity.[40] Finally, a proportion of HCCs (3%–20%) with some degree of differentiation have been reported to take up these agents, resulting in false negatives,[40–43] especially in the absence of other typical features of HCC, such as APHE.

Of the major HCC diagnostic systems, only the JSH has adopted HPB hypointensity as a major feature of HCC. In that system, hypervascular nodules without washout or corona enhancement, which are HBP hypointense, are considered definitively HCC and can be treated without further workup. The LI-RADS system recognizes HBP hypointensity as an ancillary criterion but does not use it as a feature for the diagnosis of definite HCC. The remaining major systems have not incorporated HBP hypointensity to date.

Diffusion-weighted imaging

Diffusion-weighted imaging (DWI) in MR imaging generates signal according to the degree of impediment of free water motion. By extension, cellular tissues (eg, neoplasms) are expected to impede diffusion to a greater degree than normal tissues because of their closely packed cell membranes and so appear brighter than background tissue on DWI.[44] DWI has shown a benefit in detecting malignant hepatocellular nodules because of the large signal intensity difference between these nodules and the background hepatic parenchyma; however, nodule characterization is more challenging because of the overlap between the diffusion characteristics of benign and malignant nodules. In addition, abnormally impeded diffusion in the background liver caused by cirrhosis can reduce the intrinsic differences between malignant nodules and the hepatic parenchyma.[45] Studies have shown variable degrees of benefit to adding DWI to dynamic contrast-enhanced MR (DCE-MR) imaging for the detection of HCC.[46] To date, only the LI-RADS criteria have incorporated DWI as a diagnostic feature of HCC, and only as an ancillary criterion.

Other Important Imaging Findings

Venous thrombosis

One of the primary microscopic features of advanced HCC is microvascular invasion. Although microvascular invasion is typically occult

at imaging, macrovascular invasion (malignant thrombosis) can often be visualized.[47–49] Malignant thrombosis is a strict contraindication to transplantation.[5] Additionally, patients with HCC and malignant thrombosis have a much higher rate of recurrence following attempts at curative therapies, particularly resection and percutaneous ablation; thus, malignant thrombosis is considered a contraindication to these therapies.[2,50] Both portal and hepatic vein invasion can be seen, though portal vein invasion is more common.

However, because of slow flow through the hepatic circulation in the presence of portal hypertension, bland venous thrombosis is also common in the setting of cirrhosis (Fig. 3). In addition, bland thrombus can arise superimposed on malignant thrombus, further complicating the assessment. Because bland thrombosis is not necessarily a contraindication to potentially curative therapies for HCC, differentiating bland from malignant thrombosis is critical. This differentiation can be difficult; useful features for identifying tumor thrombus include

1. There is contiguity with the instigating HCC.
2. There is arterial-phase hyperenhancement within the thrombus, often appearing thread and streak-like, because of the presence of arterial neovascularity within tumor thrombus (Fig. 4).
3. There is enhancement of the thrombus in any postcontrast phase; enhancement may be subtle, and measuring attenuation values within the thrombus on CT from phase to phase may be helpful. In MR imaging, subtraction images may be useful. Enhancement of tumor thrombus often follows that of the source HCC.
4. Expansion of the vein containing the thrombus is also associated with tumor thrombus.

Non–hepatocellular carcinoma malignancy

Although unusual, non-HCC malignancies can arise in the cirrhotic liver. The most common non-

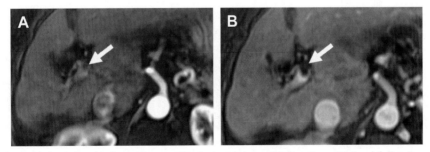

Fig. 3. (*A, B*) Bland thrombus in the main portal vein (*arrow*) on MR imaging obtained following extracellular gadolinium-based contrast agent administration in (*A*) the arterial and (*B*) portal venous (*B*) phases of enhancement. The thrombus does not enhance in the arterial or portal venous phases and does not expand the portal vein.

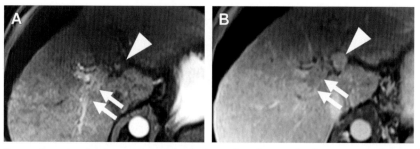

Fig. 4. (*A, B*) Tumor thrombus in the right portal vein (*arrow*) and normal enhancement of the left portal vein (*arrowhead*) on MR imaging obtained following extracellular gadolinium-based contrast agent administration in (*A*) the arterial and (*B*) portal venous phases of enhancement. The thread-and-streak–like enhancement (*arrow*) is caused by the enhancement of neovascularity within the tumor thrombus in the right portal vein.

HCC malignancy encountered in the setting of cirrhosis is CC because the same chronic inflammation and fibrosis that predispose cirrhotic patients to developing HCC are also risk factors for CC.[51,52] Rarely, metastases from extrahepatic primary malignancies, lymphoma, and posttransplant lymphoproliferative disease have been reported.

On arterial-phase imaging, the typical enhancement pattern of CC is that of a peripheral, irregular, continuous rim. However, a subset of HCCs also demonstrates peripheral rim hyperenhancement (see **Fig. 2**). The hallmark feature for differentiating CC from HCC is delayed enhancement (**Fig. 5**). Because of their fibrotic components, most CCs demonstrate progressive enhancement on later-phase imaging, which is often patchy or heterogeneous. Delayed enhancement may be faint but is quite different from the delayed washout characteristic of HCC. Additionally, it is often more readily apparent at MR imaging than CT, thus a 5-minute delayed image set is often adequate in MR imaging, whereas a 10- to 15-minute delayed series may be helpful in CT when CC is suspected.

ATYPICAL HEPATOCELLULAR CARCINOMA

There are extensive data showing that the diagnosis of HCC can be made based on the presence of classic imaging features (APHE with washout feature) with approximately 96% specificity, but this combination of features has a relatively low sensitivity of approximately 58%.[16–18,28] Given the fact that approximately 40% of HCCs may not be correctly diagnosed on initial evaluation using typical criteria, there is a strong interest in other parameters that may improve sensitivity.

The combination of nodule APHE, growth, and large size (at least 2 cm) has been shown to be relatively specific for HCC. Thus both the OPTN and LI-RADS criteria allow for the definitive diagnosis of HCC to be made in these settings. For smaller nodules (1–2 cm), the OPTN and LI-RADS systems allow nodules with the combination of APHE and growth to be considered definite HCC, as described before. However, radiologists must be cautious because small, growing CCs may also demonstrate this combination of APHE and growth. In addition, under the OPTN and LI-RADS criteria, 1 to 2 cm nodules with APHE, washout, and capsule features can also be considered definite HCC. The AASLD and recently LI-RADS allow the combination of APHE and washout feature to be used as diagnostic of HCC in 1 to 2 cm nodules but only if the nodule was detected on an antecedent surveillance ultrasound.

The increase in sensitivity for detecting atypical HCC using these additional criteria (mainly growth) has not been well studied. Other features, such as

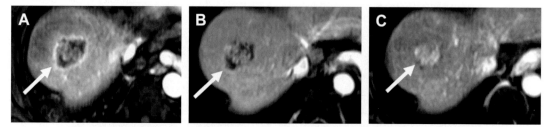

Fig. 5. (*A–C*) A 3-cm CC (*arrow*) in a patient with hepatitis C–related cirrhosis on MR imaging obtained following extracellular gadolinium-based contrast agent administration in (*A*) the arterial, (*B*) portal venous, and (*C*) 5-minute delayed venous phases of enhancement. The CC shows prominent rim enhancement in the arterial phase (*A*), persistent enhancement in the portal venous phase (*B*), and progressive enhancement in the delayed venous phase (*C*).

impeded diffusion and HBP hypointensity, have been shown to increase sensitivity but, in some studies, at the cost of specificity.[19,21,28,38,46] As a result, the constellation of APHE and HBP hypointensity has been incorporated into the JSH criteria as diagnostic features of HCC; however, the other guidelines do not currently allow the definite diagnosis of HCC to be made based on HBP hypointensity unless other major features of HCC are present.

STAGING/TREATMENT

Several staging systems for HCC are used, with the Milan criteria being the most common. The Milan criteria determine eligibility for liver transplantation in the United States and are the basis of the TNM system.[53] Liver transplant eligibility with respect to HCC is based on demonstrating the following extent of disease radiologically:

1. Only liver nodules demonstrating classic enhancement characteristics are considered.
2. The minimum tumor burden for T2 disease includes at least 1 nodule that is at least 2 cm in size or at least 2 nodules each at least 1 cm in size.
3. The maximum tumor burden for T2 disease is a single nodule no more than 5 cm in size or up to 3 nodules each no more than 3 cm in size.
4. There is no imaging evidence of extrahepatic metastatic disease or vascular invasion.

In addition, an extension of the Milan criteria was developed at the University of California, San Francisco (UCSF), known as the UCSF criteria; patients whose disease falls within these criteria have good outcomes with relatively high recurrence-free survival rates.[54–56] In addition, many sites take a downstaging approach to the care of these patients, using percutaneous ablative and embolic therapies to attempt to reduce disease burden to within the Milan criteria. The UCSF criteria include

1. Single nodule no more than 6.5 cm in size
2. Two or 3 nodules, each no more than 4.5 cm in size, and total diameter no more than 8.0 cm

Although these criteria have direct implications for liver transplantation, they do not consider other biochemical and clinical markers of disease and are not used to directly guide other therapies. To this end, the Barcelona Clinic Liver Cancer (BCLC) system was developed to directly link markers of disease with therapeutic modalities.[50] In addition to tumor burden, the BCLC system incorporates Child-Pugh stage, portal venous pressure, and bilirubin into decision making. This system reserves potentially curative treatments (including resection, transplantation, and ablation) for patients with early stage disease and designates palliative modalities (transarterial chemoembolization and chemotherapy) for those with advanced disease. In addition, some centers offer radiation therapy for patients who are poor surgical candidates but have preserved liver function. However, external beam radiation therapy is used sparingly because it carries a substantial risk of post-therapy liver failure caused by the size of the radiation zones needed to treat even small HCCs and the liver's sensitivity to radiation. Focused stereotactic radiation therapy for the management of small HCCs not amenable to surgical or ablative techniques is an area of active research. No single consensus exists for the management of these patients; therapeutic approaches at individual centers rely on a combination of best available data, institutional experience (particularly with newer treatment modalities), and patients' desire for aggressiveness of treatment.

DIAGNOSTIC AND REPORTING SYSTEMS

One of the important potential benefits of using standardized diagnostic reporting systems is to facilitate communication between radiologists interpreting imaging findings and referring physicians who make management decisions. Key components of the major HCC diagnostic systems (OPTN, LIRADS, AASLD) are summarized earlier.

Although there are some areas of disagreement between these systems regarding specific criteria, all systems agree that making the diagnosis of HCC by imaging alone is difficult but essential to successful patient management. As a result, the imaging criteria are highly specific for HCC; it is recommended that all such imaging be interpreted by radiologists experienced in liver imaging, particularly in the diagnosis of HCC. Because OPTN categorization of HCC is required for transplant eligibility in the United States, the OPTN criteria mandate that imaging be interpreted at an OPTN-approved transplantation center for consideration for liver transplant exception points. All guidelines require that scans performed for lesion categorization be multiphasic contrast-enhanced examinations, but both the OPTN and LI-RADS criteria further specify minimum technical requirements as discussed previously.[6,57]

The interpretation of imaging findings is inherently heterogeneous, with relatively poor agreement on important findings such as washout feature and capsule.[58,59] In response, the LI-RADS criteria provide concrete definitions and examples for the major features used for categorizing hepatic nodules, namely arterial phase hyperenhancement, washout, and capsule features. Although there is agreement that the maximal diameter of the nodule should be measured, the OPTN and LI-RADS criteria differ in recommendations regarding how to measure nodule diameter. The OPTN guidelines recommend measurement in the late hepatic-arterial phase. However, because the difficulty in differentiating nodules from surrounding peritumoral enhancement can lead to overestimation of tumor size, the LI-RADS system recommends measurement on phases that are relatively constant over time, such as venous or precontrast phases.

Despite these attempts to standardize the characterization of liver nodules, substantial reader disagreement has been shown for feature assignment, even when the standardized LI-RADS definitions are used,[60,61] likely because of the qualitative nature of these criteria. In particular, readers agree very well with regard to continuous measures (size and change in size, intraclass correlation coefficient (ICC) = 0.95–0.99).[60,61] However, agreement is much lower for arterial-phase hypervascularity (κ = 0.67), washout (κ = 0.48–0.69), and capsule (κ = 0.52–0.59)[60,61] features. These intermediate levels of agreement on features result in relatively low reader agreement in final nodule categorization using various systems (κ = 0.35–0.69).[60,61] Fortunately, reader agreement is higher with regard to eligibility for transplant exception points using the Milan criteria (κ = 0.81).[61]

Despite these differences in reader interpretation and diagnostic criteria, there is relatively strong agreement between the diagnostic systems themselves. Recent work showed near-perfect agreement ($\sim$99%) between the OPTN and LI-RADS systems for the designation of liver nodules as definite HCC and with regard to transplant exception point assignment by the Milan criteria.[61] Therefore, reader disagreement on nodule feature assignment (and not disagreement between systems) seems to be the main driver of discrepancies in HCC diagnosis.

CONTROVERSIES IN CONTRAST AGENT CHOICE

Since the introduction of the first gadolinium-based contrast agent (GBCA) to clinical imaging in the 1980s, GBCAs have played a major role in evaluating tumor vascular and perfusional characteristics (common but off-label usage). These agents traditionally had very similar pharmacokinetic profiles, with gradual distribution between the intravascular and extracellular spaces after intravenous injection, followed by renal clearance.[62] In the 2000s, a new class of GBCA, hepatobiliary contrast agents (gadobenate dimeglumine, gadoxetate disodium), became available for liver imaging. These agents have the added advantage of active hepatocellular uptake capable of producing a so-called HBP wherein the liver appears hyperintense because of hepatocellular uptake and most focal lesions, particularly malignant lesions, appear hypointense relative to the liver.[40] These agents have received considerable attention for the evaluation of HCC, hepatic metastatic disease, differentiation of focal nodule hyperplasia from hepatic adenoma, and other indications.[41,63–65] In particular, some centers have shown a benefit from these agents in characterizing arterially enhancing pseudolesions and risk-stratifying hypovascular liver nodules.[66–68]

However, with growing clinical experience with these agents, several challenges to their use have been discovered. First, the HBP is typically not seen until 1 to 3 hours following contrast injection with gadobenate dimeglumine. As a result of workflow needs, many centers, therefore, do not obtain HBP image sets with this agent but rather use it as though a standard extracellular GBCA. Gadoxetate disodium provides an HBP in most patients by 20 minutes after injection because of the rapid hepatocellular uptake, which leads to more clinically feasible imaging times.

However, because of the same rapid hepatocellular uptake, most patients do not exhibit a traditional interstitial phase at 3 to 5 minutes after gadoxetate injection but rather demonstrate a mixed transitional phase, which has properties of both the interstitial phase and HBP. This mixed transitional phase renders the interpretation of the washout feature more challenging on these phases, and many centers have opted not to use the transitional phase for characterization of hepatocellular nodules because the contrast mechanism is mixed. Because it has been shown that using washout in the interstitial phase (and particularly later interstitial phases) improves reader performance for the diagnosis of HCC, the loss of the true interstitial phase on gadoxetate-enhanced examinations represents a potential loss of diagnostic performance.[27] In addition, the contrast uptake in the interstitial phase, which is characteristic of CC, can be difficult or impossible to detect using gadoxetate.[52] As a result, the ability to differentiate HCC from CC using HBP imaging characteristics may be diminished (**Fig. 6**).

Furthermore, there have been several recent descriptions of transient severe arterial phase motion (TSM) occurring following the injection of gadoxetate disodium.[11,69–72] This phenomenon is characterized by the subjective experience of dyspnea

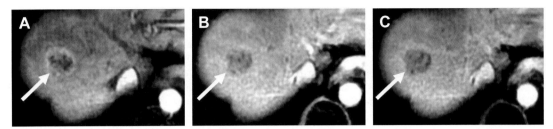

Fig. 6. (A–C) A 3-cm CC (*arrow*) in a patient with hepatitis C–related cirrhosis on MR imaging obtained following gadoxetate disodium administration in (A) the arterial, (B) portal venous, and (C) HBPs of enhancement. The CC shows prominent rim enhancement with central hypointensity in the arterial phase (A), hypointensity in the portal venous phase (B), and hypointensity in the HBP (C) obtained 20 minutes after gadoxetate disodium administration.

and patient motion during the late hepatic-arterial phase, which can severely compromise or render the arterial phase data set nondiagnostic (**Fig. 7**). Although poorly understood, this phenomenon seems to be dose dependent; a single episode of TSM elevates the likelihood of future episodes in the same patient.[69,70] Because the arterial phase image set is so important in lesion detection and characterization, this phenomenon has prompted some centers to either no longer use ga-doxetate in patients who have episodes of TSM or to cease using the agent in cirrhotic patients in general.

Finally, the Food and Drug Administration–approved dose of gadoxetate (0.025 mmol/kg) is substantially lower than that of other contrast agents (0.1 mmol/kg), and the higher T1 relaxivity of gadoxetate does not compensate for the effect of reduced dose. This finding has raised concerns

that arterial-phase enhancement may be less vivid because of the lower peak concentration in liver nodules. In addition, because of artifacts in the arterial phase, several studies have advocated diluting the administered dose of gadoxetate with saline or slowing the injection rate in order to reduce artifacts. These maneuvers further reduce the peak gadolinium concentration in liver nodules and may diminish the intensity of arterial-phase enhancement.[73,74]

For the reasons discussed earlier, the subject of GBCA choice in HCC imaging remains highly controversial. All of the major HCC diagnostic systems allow for the use of either an extracellular or hepatobiliary contrast agent; however, lesion characterization relies entirely on dynamic contrast enhancement features and excludes the HBP appearance as a major criterion for diagnosis. Recently, the LI-RADS system has incorporated HBP hypointensity as an ancillary feature for

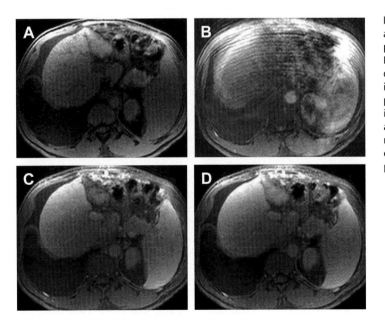

Fig. 7. (A–D) (A) Precontrast, (B) arterial-phase, (C) portal venous phase, and (D) transitional-phase MR images obtained following gadoxetate disodium administration in a patient with a large right pleural effusion and ascites. There is extensive motion artifact in the arterial phase (B) and minimal or no motion artifact on the remainder of the precontrast and postcontrast phases.

the diagnosis of HCC, based on the large body of data showing that including HBP hypointensity can increase sensitivity for the diagnosis at the cost of reduced specificity. The JSH criteria use HBP hypointensity as a secondary test for characterizing atypical, large (>1.5 cm) nodules. The OPTN, AASLD, and EASL guidelines have not incorporated HBP hypointensity as a feature of HCC to date.

SUMMARY

There have been major changes in the management and reporting of HCC in the last decade. Cross-sectional imaging is now pivotal in the management of cirrhotic patients, in particular in the diagnosis and staging of HCC. Although diagnostic systems have become relatively well developed, approximately one-third of HCC nodules may have an atypical appearance, necessitating ancillary testing, close follow-up, or biopsy. The introduction of standardized diagnostic and reporting systems has improved communication between radiologists and clinicians, but there remains substantial disagreement between radiologists in feature assignment and nodule characterization. As our understanding of this disease evolves and imaging techniques improve, standardized diagnostic criteria must continue to evolve in order to provide more accurate, early diagnosis.

REFERENCES

1. Jemal A, Bray F, Center MM, et al. Global cancer statistics. CA Cancer J Clin 2011;61(2):69–90.
2. Bruix J, Sherman M. Management of hepatocellular carcinoma: an update. Hepatology 2011;53(3): 1020–2.
3. European Association for the Study of the Liver, European Organisation for Research and Treatment of Cancer. EASL-EORTC clinical practice guidelines: management of hepatocellular carcinoma. J Hepatol 2012;56(4):908–43.
4. Kudo M, Izumi N, Kokudo N, et al. Management of hepatocellular carcinoma in Japan: consensus-based clinical practice guidelines proposed by the Japan Society of Hepatology (JSH) 2010 updated version. Dig Dis 2011;29(3):339–64.
5. HRSA/OPTN. Policy 3.6 organ distribution: allocation of livers. 2012. Available at: http://optn.transplant.hrsa.gov/policiesAndBylaws/policies.asp. Accessed June 18, 2013.
6. American College of Radiology. Liver imaging reporting and data system version 2013.1. Available at: http://www.acr.org/Quality-Safety/Resources/LIRADS. Accessed January 06, 2014.
7. El-Serag HB, Kanwal F. alpha-Fetoprotein in hepatocellular carcinoma surveillance: mend it but do not end it. Clin Gastroenterol Hepatol 2013;11(4):441–3.
8. Singal A, Volk ML, Waljee A, et al. Meta-analysis: surveillance with ultrasound for early-stage hepatocellular carcinoma in patients with cirrhosis. Aliment Pharmacol Ther 2009;30(1):37–47.
9. Wald C, Russo MW, Heimbach JK, et al. New OPTN/UNOS policy for liver transplant allocation: standardization of liver imaging, diagnosis, classification, and reporting of hepatocellular carcinoma. Radiology 2013;266(2):376–82.
10. Sharma P, Kalb B, Kitajima HD, et al. Optimization of single injection liver arterial phase gadolinium enhanced MRI using bolus track real-time imaging. J Magn Reson Imaging 2011;33(1):110–8.
11. Pietryga JA, Burke LM, Marin D, et al. Respiratory motion artifact affecting hepatic arterial phase imaging with gadoxetate disodium: examination recovery with a multiple arterial phase acquisition. Radiology 2014;271(2):426–34.
12. Earls JP, Rofsky NM, DeCorato DR, et al. Hepatic arterial-phase dynamic gadolinium-enhanced MR imaging: optimization with a test examination and a power injector. Radiology 1997;202(1):268–73.
13. Hussain HK, Londy FJ, Francis IR, et al. Hepatic arterial phase MR imaging with automated bolus-detection three-dimensional fast gradient-recalled-echo sequence: comparison with test-bolus method. Radiology 2003;226(2):558–66.
14. Kanematsu M, Semelka RC, Matsuo M, et al. Gadolinium-enhanced MR imaging of the liver: optimizing imaging delay for hepatic arterial and portal venous phases–a prospective randomized study in patients with chronic liver damage. Radiology 2002;225(2): 407–15.
15. Materne R, Horsmans Y, Jamart J, et al. Gadolinium-enhanced arterial-phase MR imaging of hypervascular liver tumors: comparison between tailored and fixed scanning delays in the same patients. J Magn Reson Imaging 2000;11(3):244–9.
16. Forner A, Vilana R, Ayuso C, et al. Diagnosis of hepatic nodules 20 mm or smaller in cirrhosis: prospective validation of the noninvasive diagnostic criteria for hepatocellular carcinoma. Hepatology 2008;47(1):97–104.
17. Lauenstein TC, Salman K, Morreira R, et al. Gadolinium-enhanced MRI for tumor surveillance before liver transplantation: center-based experience. AJR Am J Roentgenol 2007;189(3):663–70.
18. Rimola J, Forner A, Tremosini S, et al. Non-invasive diagnosis of hepatocellular carcinoma </= 2 cm in cirrhosis. Diagnostic accuracy assessing fat, capsule and signal intensity at dynamic MRI. J Hepatol 2012;56(6):1317–23.
19. Quaia E, De Paoli L, Pizzolato R, et al. Predictors of dysplastic nodule diagnosis in patients with liver

cirrhosis on unenhanced and gadobenate dimeglumine-enhanced MRI with dynamic and hepatobiliary phase. AJR Am J Roentgenol 2013;200(3): 553–62.

20. Kelekis NL, Semelka RC, Worawattanakul S, et al. Hepatocellular carcinoma in North America: a multi-institutional study of appearance on T1-weighted, T2-weighted, and serial gadolinium-enhanced gradient-echo images. AJR Am J Roentgenol 1998; 170(4):1005–13.

21. Rhee H, Kim MJ, Park MS, et al. Differentiation of early hepatocellular carcinoma from benign hepatocellular nodules on gadoxetic acid-enhanced MRI. Br J Radiol 2012;85(1018):e837–44.

22. Carlos RC, Kim HM, Hussain HK, et al. Developing a prediction rule to assess hepatic malignancy in patients with cirrhosis. AJR Am J Roentgenol 2003; 180(4):893–900.

23. Ito K, Fujita T, Shimizu A, et al. Multiarterial phase dynamic MRI of small early enhancing hepatic lesions in cirrhosis or chronic hepatitis: differentiating between hypervascular hepatocellular carcinomas and pseudolesions. AJR Am J Roentgenol 2004; 183(3):699–705.

24. Khan AS, Hussain HK, Johnson TD, et al. Value of delayed hypointensity and delayed enhancing rim in magnetic resonance imaging diagnosis of small hepatocellular carcinoma in the cirrhotic liver. J Magn Reson Imaging 2010;32(2):360–6.

25. Marrero JA, Hussain HK, Nghiem HV, et al. Improving the prediction of hepatocellular carcinoma in cirrhotic patients with an arterially-enhancing liver mass. Liver Transpl 2005;11(3):281–9.

26. Cereser L, Furlan A, Bagatto D, et al. Comparison of portal venous and delayed phases of gadolinium-enhanced magnetic resonance imaging study of cirrhotic liver for the detection of contrast washout of hypervascular hepatocellular carcinoma. J Comput Assist Tomogr 2010;34(5): 706–11.

27. Furlan A, Marin D, Vanzulli A, et al. Hepatocellular carcinoma in cirrhotic patients at multidetector CT: hepatic venous phase versus delayed phase for the detection of tumour washout. Br J Radiol 2011; 84(1001):403–12.

28. Kim TK, Lee KH, Jang HJ, et al. Analysis of gadobenate dimeglumine-enhanced MR findings for characterizing small (1-2-cm) hepatic nodules in patients at high risk for hepatocellular carcinoma. Radiology 2011;259(3):730–8.

29. Hecht EM, Holland AE, Israel GM, et al. Hepatocellular carcinoma in the cirrhotic liver: gadolinium-enhanced 3D T1-weighted MR imaging as a stand-alone sequence for diagnosis. Radiology 2006;239(2):438–47.

30. Sano K, Ichikawa T, Motosugi U, et al. Imaging study of early hepatocellular carcinoma: usefulness of gadoxetic acid-enhanced MR imaging. Radiology 2011;261(3):834–44.

31. Kojiro M. Focus on dysplastic nodules and early hepatocellular carcinoma: an Eastern point of view. Liver Transpl 2004;10(2 Suppl 1):S3–8.

32. Ebara M, Fukuda H, Kojima Y, et al. Small hepatocellular carcinoma: relationship of signal intensity to histopathologic findings and metal content of the tumor and surrounding hepatic parenchyma. Radiology 1999;210(1):81–8.

33. Kadoya M, Matsui O, Takashima T, et al. Hepatocellular carcinoma: correlation of MR imaging and histopathologic findings. Radiology 1992;183(3): 819–25.

34. Yamashita Y, Fan ZM, Yamamoto H, et al. Spin-echo and dynamic gadolinium-enhanced FLASH MR imaging of hepatocellular carcinoma: correlation with histopathologic findings. J Magn Reson Imaging 1994;4(1):83–90.

35. Bartolozzi C, Battaglia V, Bargellini I, et al. Contrast-enhanced magnetic resonance imaging of 102 nodules in cirrhosis: correlation with histological findings on explanted livers. Abdom Imaging 2013;38(2): 290–6.

36. Granito A, Galassi M, Piscaglia F, et al. Impact of gadoxetic acid (Gd-EOB-DTPA)-enhanced magnetic resonance on the non-invasive diagnosis of small hepatocellular carcinoma: a prospective study. Aliment Pharmacol Ther 2013;37(3):355–63.

37. Inoue T, Kudo M, Komuta M, et al. Assessment of Gd-EOB-DTPA-enhanced MRI for HCC and dysplastic nodules and comparison of detection sensitivity versus MDCT. J Gastroenterol 2012;47(9):1036–47.

38. Park MJ, Kim YK, Lee MH, et al. Validation of diagnostic criteria using gadoxetic acid-enhanced and diffusion-weighted MR imaging for small hepatocellular carcinoma (<= 2.0 cm) in patients with hepatitis-induced liver cirrhosis. Acta Radiol 2013; 54(2):127–36.

39. Kogita S, Imai Y, Okada M, et al. Gd-EOB-DTPA-enhanced magnetic resonance images of hepatocellular carcinoma: correlation with histological grading and portal blood flow. Eur Radiol 2010; 20(10):2405–13.

40. Bashir MR, Gupta RT, Davenport MS, et al. Hepatocellular carcinoma in a North American population: does hepatobiliary MR imaging with Gd-EOB-DTPA improve sensitivity and confidence for diagnosis? J Magn Reson Imaging 2013;37(2):398–406.

41. Asayama Y, Tajima T, Nishie A, et al. Uptake of Gd-EOB-DTPA by hepatocellular carcinoma: radiologic-pathologic correlation with special reference to bile production. Eur J Radiol 2011;80(3):e243–8.

42. Tsuda N, Matsui O. Cirrhotic rat liver: reference to transporter activity and morphologic changes in bile canaliculi–gadoxetic acid-enhanced MR imaging. Radiology 2010;256(3):767–73.

43. Tsuboyama T, Onishi H, Kim T, et al. Hepatocellular carcinoma: hepatocyte-selective enhancement at gadoxetic acid-enhanced MR imaging–correlation with expression of sinusoidal and canalicular transporters and bile accumulation. Radiology 2010; 255(3):824–33.

44. Taouli B, Koh DM. Diffusion-weighted MR imaging of the liver. Radiology 2010;254(1):47–66.

45. Park MS, Kim S, Patel J, et al. Hepatocellular carcinoma: detection with diffusion-weighted versus contrast-enhanced magnetic resonance imaging in pretransplant patients. Hepatology 2012;56(1): 140–8.

46. Wu LM, Xu JR, Lu Q, et al. A pooled analysis of diffusion-weighted imaging in the diagnosis of hepatocellular carcinoma in chronic liver diseases. J Gastroenterol Hepatol 2013;28(2):227–34.

47. Chandarana H, Robinson E, Hajdu CH, et al. Microvascular invasion in hepatocellular carcinoma: is it predictable with pretransplant MRI? AJR Am J Roentgenol 2011;196(5):1083–9.

48. Jhaveri KS, Cleary SP, Fischer S, et al. Blood oxygen level-dependent liver MRI: can it predict microvascular invasion in HCC? J Magn Reson Imaging 2013;37(3):692–9.

49. Xu P, Zeng M, Liu K, et al. Microvascular invasion in small hepatocellular carcinoma: is it predictable with preoperative diffusion-weighted imaging? J Gastroenterol Hepatol 2014;29(2):330–6.

50. Llovet JM, Bru C, Bruix J. Prognosis of hepatocellular carcinoma: the BCLC staging classification. Semin Liver Dis 1999;19(3):329–38.

51. Roth CG, Mitchell DG. Hepatocellular carcinoma and other hepatic malignancies: MR imaging. Radiol Clin North Am 2014;52(4):683–707.

52. Barr DC, Hussain HK. Magnetic resonance imaging in cirrhosis: what's new? Top Magn Reson Imaging 2014;23(2):129–49.

53. Mazzaferro V, Regalia E, Doci R, et al. Liver transplantation for the treatment of small hepatocellular carcinomas in patients with cirrhosis. N Engl J Med 1996;334(11):693–9.

54. Herrero JI, Sangro B, Quiroga J, et al. Influence of tumor characteristics on the outcome of liver transplantation among patients with liver cirrhosis and hepatocellular carcinoma. Liver Transpl 2001;7(7): 631–6.

55. Roayaie S, Frischer JS, Emre SH, et al. Long-term results with multimodal adjuvant therapy and liver transplantation for the treatment of hepatocellular carcinomas larger than 5 centimeters. Ann Surg 2002;235(4):533–9.

56. Kneteman NM, Oberholzer J, Al Saghier M, et al. Sirolimus-based immunosuppression for liver transplantation in the presence of extended criteria for hepatocellular carcinoma. Liver Transpl 2004; 10(10):1301–11.

57. OPTN/UNOS policy 3.6 organ distribution: allocation of livers. Available at: http://optn.transplant.hrsa.gov/policiesAndBylaws/policies.asp. Accessed June 18, 2013.

58. Petruzzi N, Mitchell D, Guglielmo F, et al. Hepatocellular carcinoma likelihood on MRI exams: evaluation of a standardized categorization system. Acad Radiol 2013;20(6):694–8.

59. Kushner DC, Lucey LL. Diagnostic radiology reporting and communication: the ACR guideline. J Am Coll Radiol 2005;2(1):15–21.

60. Davenport MS, Khalatbari S, Liu PS, et al. Repeatability of diagnostic features and scoring systems for hepatocellular carcinoma by using MR imaging. Radiology 2014;272(1):132–42.

61. Bashir MR, Huang R, Mayes N, et al. Concordance of hypervascular liver nodule characterization between the organ procurement and transplant network and liver imaging reporting and data system classifications. J Magn Reson Imaging 2015. [Epub ahead of print].

62. Bashir MR. Magnetic resonance contrast agents for liver imaging. Magn Reson Imaging Clin N Am 2014; 22(3):283–93.

63. Kawada N, Ohkawa K, Tanaka S, et al. Improved diagnosis of well-differentiated hepatocellular carcinoma with gadolinium ethoxybenzyl diethylene triamine pentaacetic acid-enhanced magnetic resonance imaging and Sonazoid contrast-enhanced ultrasonography. Hepatol Res 2010; 40(9):930–6.

64. Tamada T, Ito K, Sone T, et al. Gd-EOB-DTPA enhanced MR imaging: evaluation of biliary and renal excretion in normal and cirrhotic livers. Eur J Radiol 2011;80(3):e207–11.

65. Hwang J, Kim SH, Kim YS, et al. Gadoxetic acid-enhanced MRI versus multiphase multidetector row computed tomography for evaluating the viable tumor of hepatocellular carcinomas treated with image-guided tumor therapy. J Magn Reson Imaging 2010;32(3):629–38.

66. Motosugi U, Ichikawa T, Sou H, et al. Distinguishing hypervascular pseudolesions of the liver from hypervascular hepatocellular carcinomas with gadoxetic acid-enhanced MR imaging. Radiology 2010; 256(1):151–8.

67. Komatsu N, Motosugi U, Maekawa S, et al. Hepatocellular carcinoma risk assessment using gadoxetic acid-enhanced hepatocyte phase magnetic resonance imaging. Hepatol Res 2014;44(13):1339–46.

68. Hyodo T, Murakami T, Imai Y, et al. Hypovascular nodules in patients with chronic liver disease: risk factors for development of hypervascular hepatocellular carcinoma. Radiology 2013;266(2):480–90.

69. Bashir MR, Castelli P, Davenport MS, et al. Respiratory motion artifact affecting hepatic arterial phase MR imaging with gadoxetate disodium is more

common in patients with a prior episode of arterial phase motion associated with gadoxetate disodium. Radiology 2015;274(1):141–8.

70. Davenport MS, Bashir MR, Pietryga JA, et al. Dose-toxicity relationship of gadoxetate disodium and transient severe respiratory motion artifact. AJR Am J Roentgenol 2014;203(4):796–802.

71. Davenport MS, Caoili EM, Kaza RK, et al. Matched within-patient cohort study of transient arterial phase respiratory motion-related artifact in MR imaging of the liver: gadoxetate disodium versus gadobenate dimeglumine. Radiology 2014;272(1):123–31.

72. Davenport MS, Viglianti BL, Al-Hawary MM, et al. Comparison of acute transient dyspnea after intravenous administration of gadoxetate disodium and gadobenate dimeglumine: effect on arterial phase image quality. Radiology 2013; 266(2):452–61.

73. Motosugi U, Ichikawa T, Sou H, et al. Dilution method of gadolinium ethoxybenzyl diethylenetriaminepentaacetic acid (Gd-EOB-DTPA)-enhanced magnetic resonance imaging (MRI). J Magn Reson Imaging 2009;30(4):849–54.

74. Tanimoto A, Higuchi N, Ueno A. Reduction of ringing artifacts in the arterial phase of gadoxetic acid-enhanced dynamic MR imaging. Magn Reson Med Sci 2012;11(2):91–7.

Liver Ablation: Best Practice

Shane A. Wells, MD[a,*], J. Louis Hinshaw, MD[a], Meghan G. Lubner, MD[a],
Timothy J. Ziemlewicz, MD[a], Christopher L. Brace, PhD[a,b], Fred T. Lee Jr, MD[a,b]

KEYWORDS

- Tumor ablation • Hepatocellular carcinoma • HCC • Colorectal cancer • Neuroendocrine cancer
- Microwave • Radiofrequency

KEY POINTS

- Percutaneous ablation is considered first-line therapy for very early and early hepatocellular carcinoma and second-line therapy for colorectal carcinoma liver metastases.
- An understanding of the underlying tumor biology is important when weighing the potential benefits of ablation for other primary and secondary liver tumors.
- Achieving a circumferential ablative margin, of at least a 0.5 cm for hepatocellular carcinoma and at least 1.0 cm for liver metastases, decreases the incidence of local tumor progression.
- Surveillance imaging after ablation should be more frequent in the first year, when rates of local tumor progression are the highest.

INTRODUCTION

Tumor ablation is broadly defined as the destruction of focal tumors by direct application of chemicals or energy.[1] Tumor ablation therapies are delivered via needlelike applicators and can be broadly categorized into systems based on chemical (primarily ethanol and acetic acid) and thermal or nonthermal energy. The most widely applied thermal ablation modalities in the liver include radiofrequency (RF), microwave (MW), laser, cryoablation, and high-intensity focused ultrasonography (US). Irreversible electroporation (IRE) is generally classified as a nonthermal ablative modality, although cytotoxic temperatures can be achieved with IRE depending on the parameters used during treatment.[2–4]

Tumor ablation in the liver has evolved to become a well-accepted tool in the management of increasingly complex oncologic patients. Ablative therapies can be used alone, in conjunction with other ablative therapies, or in combination with other oncologic treatment strategies, such as surgery, neoadjuvant and adjuvant chemotherapy, external beam and stereotactic body radiotherapy (SBRT), and arterial liver-directed therapies, including bland embolization, chemoembolization, and/or radioembolization in the treatment of both primary and secondary hepatic malignancies.[5–9]

This image-rich, case-based article introduces some of the considerations that are important for physicians preparing to perform hepatic tumor ablation.

Ablation Modalities

The physical properties of each of the ablation devices are unique and these differences can affect the technical success of ablation procedures. Although an in-depth understanding of the biophysics of each device is not necessary, it is

Disclosures: None (S.A. Wells, M.G. Lubner, T.J. Ziemlewicz); stockholder, member of the Board of Medical Advisors for NeuWave Medical (J.L. Hinshaw); stockholder, consultant for NeuWave Medical (C.L. Brace); patent holder and receives royalties from Covidien, stockholder and member of the Board of Directors for NeuWave Medical (F.T. Lee). This work was supported by grants R01CA142737 and R01CA149379 from the National Institutes of Health.
^a Department of Radiology, University of Wisconsin, 600 Highland Avenue, CSC, Madison, WI 53792, USA;
^b Department of Biomedical Engineering, University of Wisconsin, 600 Highland Avenue, CSC, Madison, WI 53792, USA
* Corresponding author.
E-mail address: swells@uwhealh.org

important to understand the properties of the devices available to your practice. Because operator experience has been correlated with success, it may be beneficial to concentrate experience in a few selected devices rather than dilute experience across multiple technologies.[10,11]

Ethanol

Chemical (nonenergy) ablation with ethanol was the seminal technique for percutaneous ablation. Ethanol induces coagulative necrosis via protein denaturation, cellular dehydration, and chemical occlusion of small tumor vessels. Ethanol injection is well suited for small hepatocellular carcinoma (HCC) because the firm cirrhotic liver surrounding the soft tumor limits diffusion of ethanol into the surrounding liver. Ethanol injection has little utility in the treatment of metastases in which the background liver is normal. Because of the high rate of local tumor progression and the need for repeated treatments, ethanol has largely been replaced with thermal ablation (RF and MW), for which rates of local tumor control and survival have improved.[12–20] Chemical ablation has been used to augment or replace thermal ablation when treating tumors in areas of high perfusion-mediated tissue cooling or tumors in proximity to vulnerable, nontargeted structures, such as bile ducts (**Fig. 1**).[21]

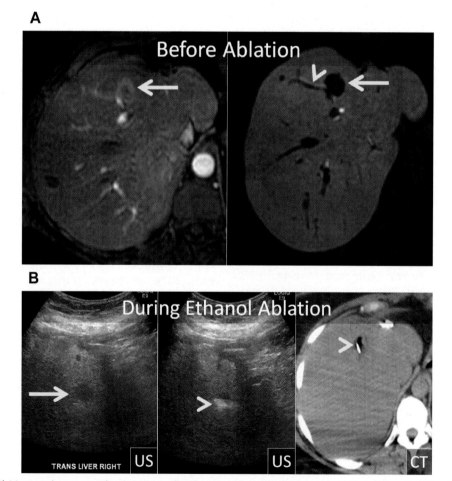

Fig. 1. (*A*) Metastatic neuroendocrine tumor (NET) in the ventral right liver (*arrow*) abutting the bile duct draining Couinaud segment VIII (*arrowhead*). Given prior left hepatectomy and palliative intent of ablation, avoiding a bile duct stricture and further liver volume loss was a priority. (*B*) US and unenhanced computed tomography (CT) images during ethanol ablation. The posterior aspect of the tumor (*arrow*), in proximity to the bile duct, was targeted and 4 mL of 95% ethanol was instilled (*arrowheads*). (*C*) Unenhanced CT and US images after placement of the MW antenna (*arrowhead*) along the anterior aspect of the tumor. When the gas clouds (*arrow*) became confluent the procedure was terminated. (*D*) MR imaging obtained 1 month after combined ethanol and MW ablation. The ablation encompasses the index lesion (*arrow*) and there is no bile duct stricture (*arrowhead*). Because a 1-cm circumferential margin could not be safely obtained, there is a substantial risk for local tumor progress (LTP).

C

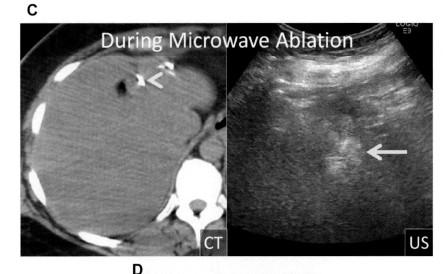

D

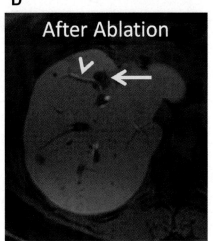

Fig. 1. (*continued*)

Radiofrequency

RF is a heat-based ablation method that creates zones of coagulative necrosis through the application of heat. With RF, an alternating current is conducted through an applicator (electrode) that acts as the cathode of a closed electrical circuit with grounding pads applied to the skin acting as the anode. Ions close to the electrode vibrate rapidly as they attempt to align with the alternating current, resulting in resistive tissue heating (direct heating) that is conducted into adjacent tissues (indirect heating) as a result of the high thermal gradient.[22–24] The final ablation is the result of both direct heating caused by the applied energy, and indirect heating, the result of thermal diffusion into adjacent, cooler tissues. RF is a self-limited process that has limited success in treating large tumors and tumors in regions of high tissue perfusion because of poor conductive heating and limited ability to overcome perfusion-mediated tissue cooling.[23–29] As a result, RF leads to an undesirably high rate of local tumor progress (LTP) in larger tumors (**Figs. 2** and **3**).[30–32]

Microwave

MWs use dielectric hysteresis to produce heat, resulting in coagulative necrosis, and are capable of penetrating tissues that are poor electrical conduits, such as lung, bone, and areas of desiccation/char. Water molecules are forced to align with an oscillating electric field emitted from an antenna, creating kinetic energy that is converted to heat. This method allows direct heating of a volume of tissue around the antenna with less reliance on conductive heating.[25] MW ablation is performed at either 915 MHz or 2.45 GHz.

Compared with RF, MW has more power and can produce larger and hotter ablations. Combined

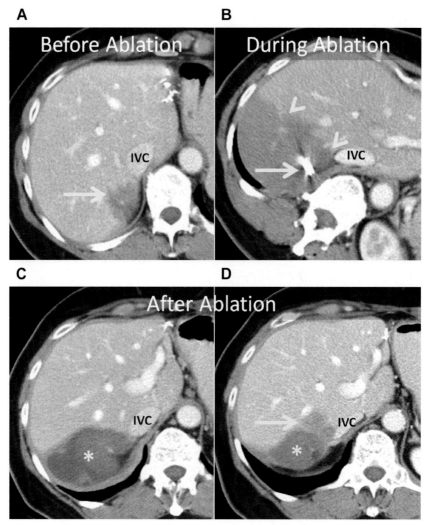

Fig. 2. (A) Enhanced CT shows a CRLM in the medial right liver in proximity to the inferior vena cava (IVC) (arrow). (B) Enhanced CT after placement of RF electrodes (arrow). Segmental hypoenhancement of the dorsal right liver corresponds with the ablation and a hepatic infract (arrowheads). The ablation extends to the margin of the IVC and appears to encompass the index lesion. (C, D) Serial follow-up enhanced CT shows the index ablation (asterisk). (D) The new mass adjacent to the index ablation, in proximity to the IVC (arrow), represents LTP, the result of perfusion-mediated tissue cooling.

with the ability to continuously power multiple antennas simultaneously, MW has improved capacity to overcome perfusion-mediated tissue cooling associated with large vessels (>2 mm) (see **Fig. 3**; **Fig. 4**).[33–35] However, this increased power can result in vascular thrombosis of the portal vein, particularly in cirrhotic patients in whom portal venous flow rate is reduced (**Fig. 5**).[36] Flow velocity within the inferior vena cava (IVC), hepatic arteries, and major hepatic veins is usually sufficient to prevent significant vascular thrombosis (see **Figs. 3** and **4**).[37] MWs generate abundant water vapor, created by tissue out-gassing, which is well seen at both US and computed tomography (CT) (**Figs.**

6–8). This gas cloud seen at US correlates with the size of the ablation zone at immediate postprocedure contrast-enhanced CT and the zone of necrosis at pathology in an animal model (see **Figs. 6** and **8**).[38]

Cryoablation
Modern cryoablation equipment uses the Joule-Thomson principle of thermodynamics. High-pressure argon is forced down a narrow tube within an insulated, hollow cryoprobe; near the tip of the cryoprobe the argon escapes the tube via a small aperture into an expansion chamber, resulting in rapid cooling and formation of an ice

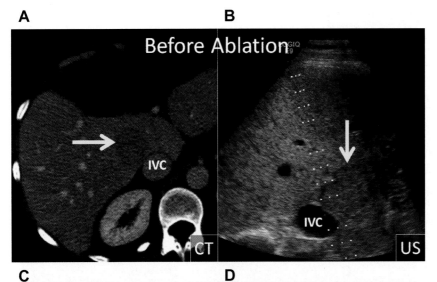

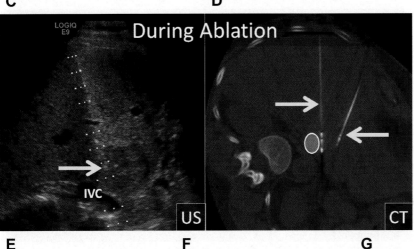

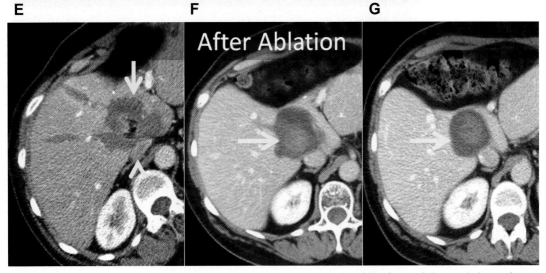

Fig. 3. (*A*, *B*) Enhanced CT and US show a breast metastasis in the caudate lobe (*arrows*), in proximity to the IVC. (*C*, *D*) US and unenhanced CT after placement of the MW antennas (*arrows*). With this approach, the operator placed the MW antennas to mitigate the effect of perfusion-mediated tissue cooling. (*E–G*) Serial follow-up enhanced CT showing the index ablation (*arrows*). The ablation contracts over time and there is no evidence of LTP, despite proximity of the index lesion to the IVC. (*E*) The IVC remained patent without thrombus despite close proximity of MW antenna during ablation (*arrowhead*). Linear low attenuation extending from the index ablation to the liver surface corresponds with ablation of the antenna tracts.

A

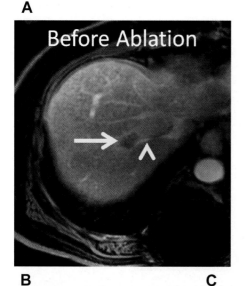

B   **C**   **D**

E

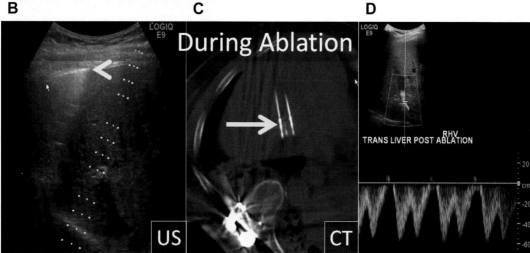

Fig. 4. (*A*) CRLM in Couinaud segment VIII (*arrow*) abutting the right hepatic vein (*arrowhead*). (*B, C*) Three MW antennas were placed with US guidance into the mass and surrounding the right hepatic vein to overcome perfusion-mediated tissue cooling. (*B*) The edge of the lung (*arrowhead*) is easy to see and avoid during applicator placement. (*C*) Unenhanced CT was obtained to confirm precise antenna position (*arrow*). (*D*) Color and spectral Doppler was used intermittently during ablation to confirm patency of the right hepatic vein. (*E*) Axial and coronal enhanced CT immediately following MW ablation. The ablation encompasses the tumor and a margin of greater than 10 mm (*arrow*). The right hepatic vein remained patent (*arrowhead*).

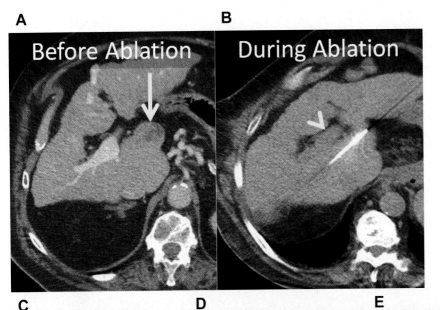

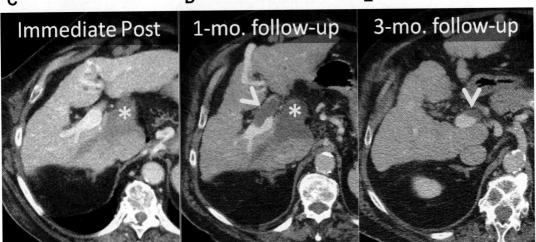

Fig. 5. (*A*) Enhanced CT shows an HCC in the caudate (*arrow*). (*B*) Unenhanced CT after placement of MW antenna. Note the proximity of the main portal vein (*arrowhead*). (*C–E*) Serial follow-up enhanced CT immediately (*C*), 1 month (*D*), and 3 months after MW ablation showing the ablation (*asterisks*) without LTP. (*C*) The main portal vein was patent immediately after ablation. (*D*) At 1-month follow-up, there was thrombosis of the main and right portal veins (*arrowhead*) that (*E*) organized and partially resolved after anticoagulation therapy (*arrowhead*).

ball. When high-pressure helium is forced down the cylinder and allowed to expand within the hollow cryoprobe, the result is rapid heating and subsequent thawing of the ice ball. This combination of rapid cooling followed by thawing brings about the cascade of events leading to cell death that direct cellular injury by formation of intracellular ice crystals and interruption of cellular metabolism and ischemia from vascular thrombosis, resulting in coagulative necrosis and apoptosis.

During cryoablation, the ice ball is readily visible at imaging, allowing assessment of adequacy of ablation and risk to nontargeted anatomy (**Fig. 9**). However, defining the lethal (−20°C and colder) isotherm within the visible ice, which can vary in distance from the ice edge depending on local factors, is not possible with imaging.[31,39] A single cryoprobe ablation creates a very low volume of lethal ice because of perfusion-mediated tissue warming and should not be performed.[40] Multiple cryoprobes can be simultaneously powered to create large ablations; however, this has been associated with an increase in both hepatic and extrahepatic complications, including fracture

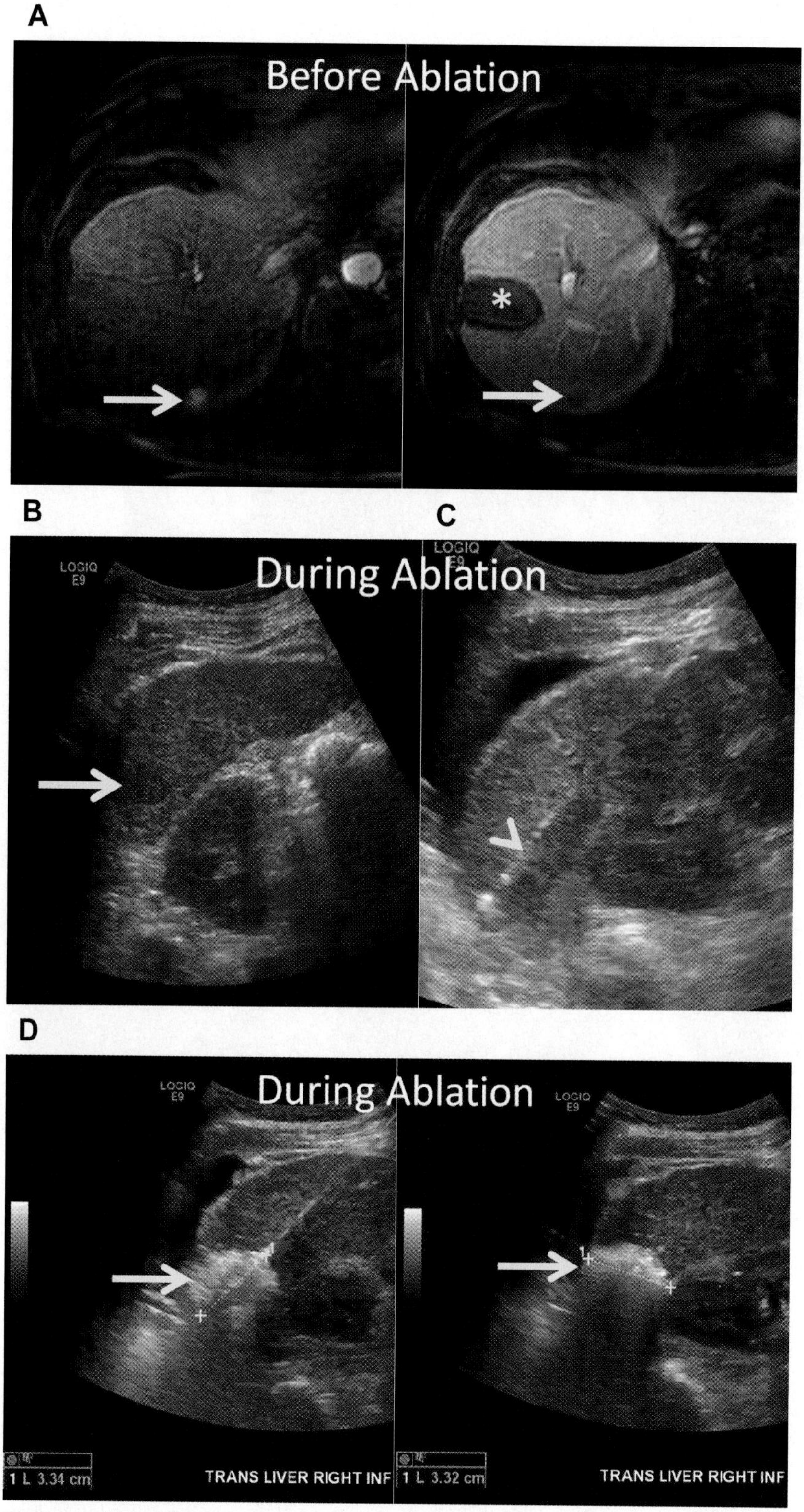

Fig. 6. (*A*) HCC in the inferior right liver (*arrows*). Note the prior ablation in the right midliver (*asterisk*) without LTP. (*B–D*) US before and during ablation with the patient in left decubitus position. (*B*) At US, the HCC is hypoechoic (*arrow*). (*C*) US image after hydrodissection and placement of the MW antenna (*arrowhead*). (*D*) The gas cloud formed during MW ablation can be used to determine adequate coverage of the tumor and margin (arrows). (*E*) Axial and coronal enhanced CT immediately following MW ablation. The 3.3-cm ablation encompasses the index lesion, includes a margin greater than 5 mm, and corresponds with the size of the gas cloud at US (*arrows*).

E

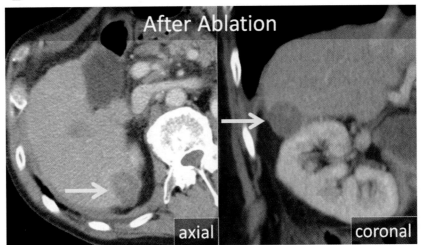

Fig. 6. (*continued*)

of the liver, hemorrhage, and a systemic in-flammatory response (cryoshock) that can lead to thrombocytopenia and coagulopathy, liver fail-ure, acute lung, and kidney injury. These risks may be exacerbated in patients with baseline coagulopathy, and are most frequently reported in patients with cirrhosis.[41–49] Because cry-oablation is associated with minimal pain, it is a viable treatment option for patients who are not candidates for general anesthesia or conscious sedation.

Irreversible electroporation

Irreversible electroporation, the only nonthermal energy-based ablative technology to date, delivers short bursts of high-voltage electrical pulses bet-ween closely approximated electrodes that create nanometer-scale pores in cell membranes, result-ing in cell death.[3,4] Depending on the voltage and duration of electric pulses, very high temperatures (>60 C) can be achieved, resulting in coagulative necrosis.[2] Because the predominant, nonthermal mechanism of cell death allows preservation of

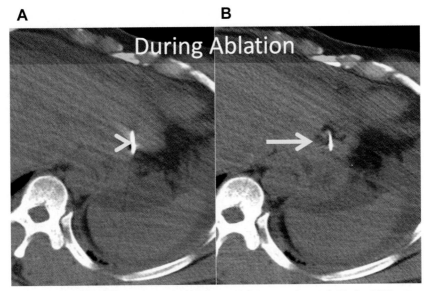

Fig. 7. HCC in a patient with cirrhosis during MW ablation. (*A*) At unenhanced CT, the MW antenna in the left liver is pointed at the stomach (*arrowhead*) and there is artificial ascites in the left upper quadrant. (*B*) The steam generated during MW ablation is also visible at CT (*arrow*).

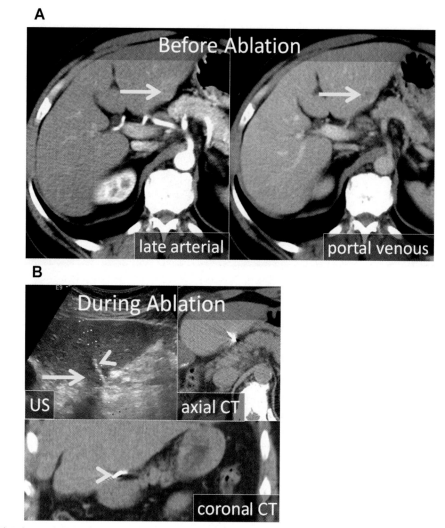

Fig. 8. (*A*) Enhanced CT in the late arterial and portal venous phase shows an exophytic HCC projecting from the inferior left liver (*arrows*). (*B*) At US, the HCC is hypoechoic (*arrow*). The MW antenna is well seen at both US and CT (*arrowhead*). (*C*) Artificial ascites was used to displace the stomach and pancreas; a trocar needle was placed through the left liver and a 2% iohexol-enhanced saline solution was infused (*arrowheads*). At CT, the stomach wall and pancreas were adequately displaced. The gas cloud at US (*arrow*) encompasses the HCC including a margin. (*D*) Enhanced CT in the late arterial (axial) and portal venous phase (coronal reformat) immediately after MW ablation. The ablation encompasses the index lesion including a 5 mm margin (*arrow*) without damage to the stomach or pancreas. The stomach and pancreas remained safely displaced (*arrowhead*) throughout the procedure and were not injured (*arrowhead*).

the extracellular tissue architecture, IRE has a theoretic advantage over thermal ablation, particularly in proximity to at-risk structures such as the biliary tree (**Fig. 10**).[4] In the liver, experience with IRE remains limited and there are no comparison studies with thermal ablation that show equivalent efficacy.

Irreversible electroporation is technically challenging because precise and parallel electrode placement, required to maintain the electric field, is time consuming, generally requires more applicators relative to thermal ablation

and requires the use of CT guidance for applicator placement. General anesthesia with a paralytic and cardiac synchronization is required, otherwise muscle spasms and cardiac dysrhythmias can occur.

INDICATIONS AND PATIENT SELECTION
Hepatocellular Carcinoma

HCC is the most common primary liver cancer, the fourth most common type of cancer overall,

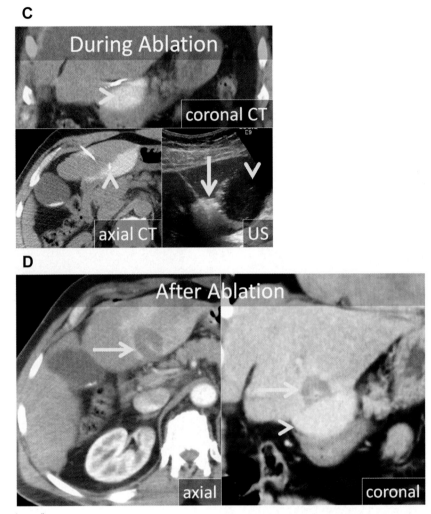

Fig. 8. (*continued*)

and the third most common cause of cancer death worldwide.[50] There are substantial variations in the epidemiology of HCC; globally, the burden of disease is related to hepatitis B virus (HBV) and is largely concentrated in developing countries. In countries where HBV is not endemic, hepatitis C and alcoholic cirrhosis remain the most common risk factors. Nonalcoholic fatty liver disease and nonalcoholic steatohepatitis are other important risk factors for cirrhosis and HCC, particularly in developed countries.[51] In recent years the increased use of surveillance and improved diagnostic and therapeutic modalities have improved patient survival.[52–54] Liver transplantation remains the definitive treatment of patients with both cirrhosis and HCC; however, most patients never receive transplantation because of a lack of organ availability, lack of access to a transplant center, or inability to meet transplant criteria.[55]

Recent advances, such as improved assessment of liver function and tumor burden, have enhanced the management of patients with HCC. Expert panels and consortia, including the European Association for the Study of the Liver and the American Association of the Study of Liver Disease, have generated evidence-based recommendations for the treatment of HCC. The Barcelona Clinic Liver Cancer (BCLC) staging system and treatment strategy incorporates tumor burden, liver function (Child-Pugh classification) and performance status to define prognosis and guide treatment decisions. Treatment options for HCC are stratified by BCLC stage. Transplantation, resection, and ablation are considered curative for very early and early stage HCC (stage 0 and A respectively). Palliative treatment options include transcatheter arterial chemoembolization (TACE) for intermediate stage HCC (stage B), and selective internal radiotherapy (SIRT) and

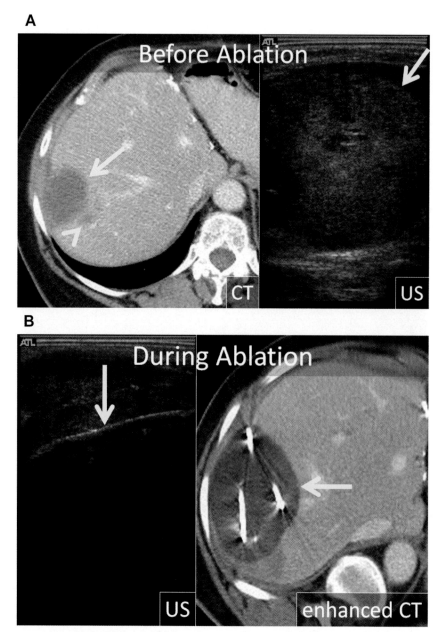

Fig. 9. (A) CRLM in the right liver (arrow) with a dominant satellite tumor along the inferomedial margin (arrowhead). The mass is heterogeneous and echogenic at US. (B) US and enhanced CT during cryoablation. The ice ball is visible at US and CT (arrow); however, shadowing at US precludes evaluation of the deep margin. The distance between the visible ice and the lethal isotherm within the ice ball depends on local factors, including perfusion-mediated tissue warming. (C) Enhanced CT 1 year after cryoablation; there is no evidence of LTP (arrow).

sorafenib for advanced stage HCC (stage C). Best supportive care is reserved for terminal disease (stage D).[56]

Ablation

According to the BCLC criteria, image-guided tumor ablation is recommended for patients with very early and early stage HCC who are not surgical candidates.[57] Very early stage includes patients with Child-Pugh A liver function, an Eastern Cooperative Oncology Group (ECOG) performance status of 0, and a single HCC less than 2 cm. Early stage includes patients with Child-Pugh A-B liver function, an ECOG performance status of 0, and a single HCC up to 5 cm or 3 HCC, each less than 3 cm.

C

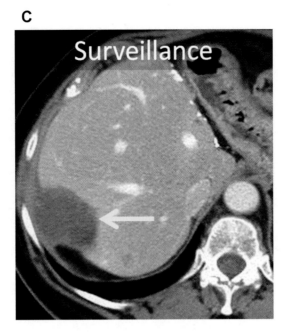

Fig. 9. (*continued*)

RF ablation is considered the reference standard for the ablation of small HCC. Recently, newer generation high-powered MW (915 kHz–2.45 GHz) ablation has emerged as an alternative to RF. Compared with RF, MW systems generate higher tissue temperatures more quickly, and generally create larger ablations that are less susceptible to tissue perfusion from large (>2 mm) vessels.[33–35] Available evidence to date suggests that MW is at least equivalent to RF for the treatment of very early or early stage HCC.[58–67]

RF ablation has been shown to be as effective as surgical resection for very early and early HCC.[68,69] However, it is important to understand that patient characteristics (eg, obesity and portal hypertension) and tumor location (eg, subcapsular location; proximity to the biliary tree, colon, or diaphragm) can influence image-guided ablation results and the occurrence of complications (see **Fig. 5; Fig. 11**).[70–73] In general, heat-based ablation, either RF or MW, should be considered first-line treatment of patients with liver dysfunction who have very early (stage 0) and early (stage A) HCC in favorable locations.

Other ablation devices, such as cryoablation, laser, focused US (high-intensity focused ultrasound [HIFU]), and IRE have been successfully used in the treatment of HCC. Compared with the reference standard (RF), cryoablation is associated with a higher rate of morbidity and mortality. In some studies, the major complication rate for cryoablation exceeds 6% (compared with a major complication rate for RF that is <1%).[49,67,70,74] Major complications of cryoablation include cryoshock, hemorrhage, and liver failure. Laser and HIFU are other heat-based ablation devices that result in coagulative necrosis, similar to RF and MW. From a user standpoint, HIFU and IRE are more technically challenging than RF and MW. In addition, there are limited longitudinal data to accurately determine treatment response and equivalency of these modalities compared with RF.

Combination therapies

Exploiting synergies is the underlying principle for combination therapies. The most widely investigated combinations have been ethanol and RF, and TACE and RF.[6,7,75–92] Ethanol causes coagulative necrosis and thrombosis of tumor vessels, subsequently modifying local tissue perfusion. Chemotherapy combined with embolic particles in TACE induces ischemic necrosis and modifies local tissue perfusion. Ablations with both RF and MW are larger after ethanol and TACE because of decreased perfusion-mediated tissue cooling.[93–100]

Hepatic artery embolization (HAE) therapies such as conventional TACE (cTACE) or TACE with drug-eluding beads (DEB-TACE) combined with ablation seem to improve technical success and decrease the incidence of LTP in select situations.[84,91,101,102] For HCCs larger than 3 cm, those that are poorly encapsulated, or those that have visible satellite tumors, combination therapy

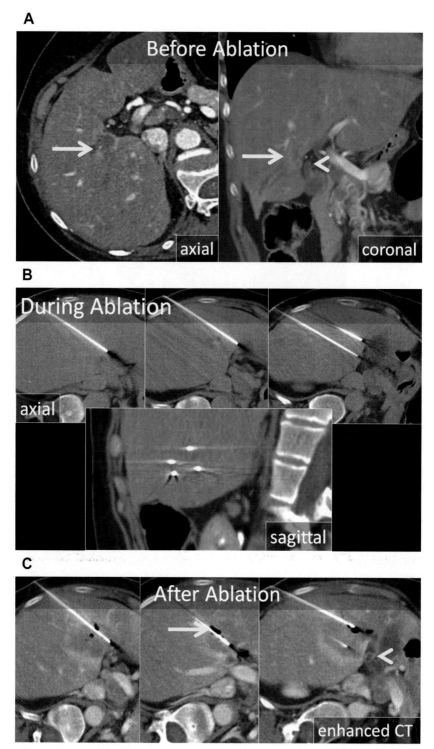

Fig. 10. (*A*) Axial and coronal enhanced CT shows a CRLM in the medial right liver (*arrow*) in proximity to the common duct (*arrowhead*). (*B*) Axial and sagittal unenhanced CT following CT-guided placement of IRE electrodes. The electrodes are nearly parallel with near-equal spacing of 1 to 1.5 cm. Because precise electrode placement is important and a large number of electrodes are generally required for IRE, applicator placement can be time consuming. (*C*) Enhanced CT immediately following IRE. The ablation encompasses the tumor including a 10-mm margin and there is no apparent damage to the bile duct (*arrowhead*). The gas within the ablation zone (*arrow*) suggests that both thermal and nonthermal mechanisms of cell death were present in this case.

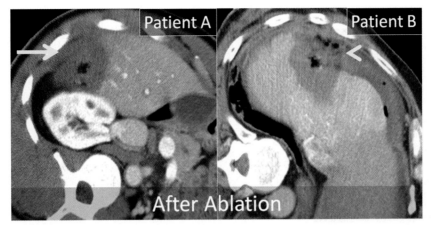

Fig. 11. Enhanced CT immediately following MW ablation in 2 patients. Both patients are in an left posterior oblique (LPO) and received ablation procedures in the subcapsular right liver. Patient A was treated without artificial ascites, whereas patient B was treated after instillation of artificial ascites. In patient A, the ablation extended into the peritoneum and body wall (*arrow*) and resulted in severe postprocedure pain. In patient B, the ablation extended beyond the liver capsule into the extrahepatic fluid and fat but not into the peritoneum or body wall (*arrowhead*). Patient B had minimal postprocedure pain.

should be considered. In addition, HCCs that are in poor anatomic locations, such as Couinaud segment VII and VIII or immediately adjacent to a large vessel (>2 mm), or HCC that are inconspicuous at US, may also be good candidates for combination therapy (see **Fig. 1**). Both RF and MW ablation have been shown to be effective in the treatment of HCC after TACE.[83]

There is no consensus on the optimal timing for intra-arterial therapies and ablation when used in combination. As a result, practice patterns vary widely, with ablation being performed both before and after HAE. The rationale for performing ablation before HAE is the augmented delivery of embolic particles into the hyperemic parenchyma surrounding the ablation, thereby increasing the treatment effect on the heat-damaged cells at the ablative margin; the most common location for LTP.[103] The rationale for performing ablation after HAE is to reduce perfusion-mediated tissue cooling and exploit a chemotherapy-heat synergy. Another reason to perform HAE before ablation is to aid in tumor targeting when CT is used for guidance and when tumors are inconspicuous at US. If ablation is performed after TACE, it is important to treat the entire tumor in addition to at least a 5-mm circumferential margin (**Figs. 12–15**). This technique is well tolerated and has been shown to decrease the incidence of LTP.[104]

Colorectal Cancer Hepatic Metastasis

Colorectal carcinoma (CRC) is the third most common cancer and the second most common cause of cancer-related mortality in the United States.[105] Metastatic disease is present at diagnosis of CRC in 20% and another 30% to 50% develop liver metastasis (colorectal liver metastasis [CRLM]) during treatment. Of those patients with metastatic disease, 25% to 30% have isolated hepatic metastasis.[106] Without treatment, median survival with CRC hepatic metastasis is 6.9 months, with a 5-year survival of 0%.[107,108]

Complete surgical resection confers the best chance for long-term survival; however, only 20% of patients with CRLM are candidates for resection. More effective neoadjuvant chemotherapy regimens and improved surgical techniques have had a significant impact on survival. At present, 5-year survival after hepatic resection for CRLM approaches 50%.[109,110] In comparison, patients with CRLM treated with chemotherapy, but who do not undergo liver resection have a 5-year overall survival (OS) of 10%.[111]

Although OS has improved, approximately 45% of patients experience early recurrence (within 6 months) after liver resection, whereas 75% experience recurrent disease overall. Early recurrence negatively affects prognosis, with an approximately 50% reduction in 5-year OS compared with late recurrence. With repeat resection, OS for early recurrence is similar to patients reresected for late recurrence.[112] Risk factors for recurrence include T3-T4 primary tumor, synchronous liver metastasis, more than 3 liver metastases, largest liver metastasis greater than 5 cm, and a 0-mm resection margin.[112,113] Response to neoadjuvant chemotherapy and administration of

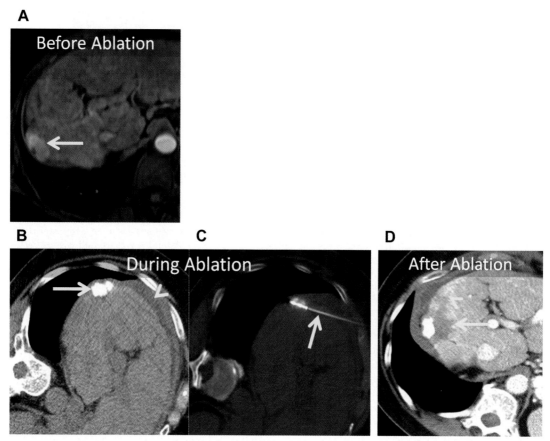

Fig. 12. (*A*) At MR imaging, there is an HCC in the dome of the right liver, near the interface of Couinaud segments VII and VIII (*arrow*). (*B, C*) Because the mass was inconspicuous at US, chemoembolization with ethiodized oil was performed and followed 2 weeks later by CT-guided MW ablation. (*B*) Unenhanced CT with the patient in the left decubitus position. Note ethiodized oil within the index lesion (*arrow*) and artificial ascites interposed between the liver and body wall (*arrowhead*). (*C*) Unenhanced CT after placement of the MW antenna (*arrow*). (*D*) Enhanced CT immediately following MW ablation. The ablation encompasses the index lesion containing ethiodized oil and a 5-mm margin (*arrow*). Linear low attenuation extending from the index ablation corresponds with ablation of the antenna tract (*arrowhead*).

adjuvant chemotherapy reduce early surgical recurrence.[112]

Adjuvant chemotherapy has not been shown to improve OS; however, is still used because of improvement in progression-free survival (PFS).[114–117] A phase II randomized controlled trial comparing systemic therapy alone with RF ablation and adjuvant chemotherapy for CRLM showed improved PFS with adjuvant chemotherapy.[118]

Ablation

The role of percutaneous ablation in the management of CRLM remains in debate; however, ablation is widely accepted for patients with unresectable tumors, those who are not surgical candidates, and in the setting of recurrent disease after liver resection when insufficient liver reserve precludes further resection. Although retrospective

studies have concluded that resection offers better survival than ablation, no randomized controlled trials have been performed to date. Of the studies comparing surgical resection and ablation, patient selection favors surgical resection in virtually all cases.[119,120] Patients in the ablation arm tend to have a greater burden of disease, a higher rate of extrahepatic tumors, and larger tumors, tend to be older, and tend to have more comorbidities. In those studies in which ablation has been used as first-line therapy for patients with resectable CRLM, the 5-year survivals are similar to those of surgical series.[121,122] Other retrospective studies show comparable survival with surgical series when ablation is applied to CRLM less than 3 cm.[123–126]

Small and medium-sized CRLM are suitable for percutaneous ablation, with the most

A

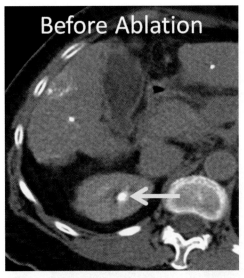

B

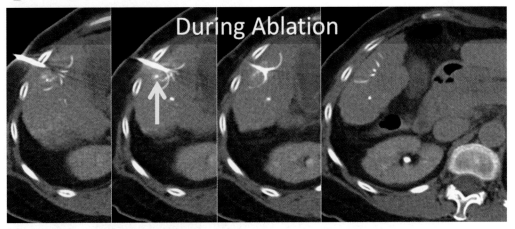

C

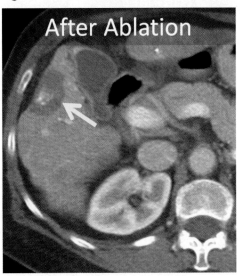

Fig. 13. HCC in a patient with cirrhosis before, during, and after radiofrequency (RF) ablation. (*A, B*) Enhanced CT obtained for ablation planning immediately before RF electrode placement. Note that the contrast has washed out of the liver and is being excreted by the kidneys (*arrow*). (*B*) The only useful guide for placement of the RF electrode was retained ethiodized oil (*arrow*). (*C*) Enhanced CT 1 month after RF ablation. The ablation encompasses the index lesion containing ethiodized oil, including a 5-mm margin (*arrow*).

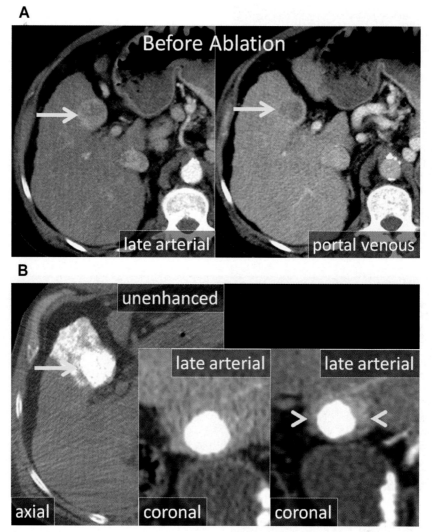

Fig. 14. (*A*) Enhanced CT in the late arterial and portal venous phase shows a large (>3 cm) HCC in the medial left liver in proximity to the gallbladder (*arrow*). (*B*) The HCC was treated with TACE (*arrow*) because of the size and location. Ablation was initially deferred; however, at serial follow-up CT, LTP became apparent (*arrowheads*). (*C*) US during MW antenna placement and ablation. The hypoechoic HCC (*arrow*) becomes encompassed by the gas cloud formed during MW ablation (*arrowhead*). Minimal wall thickening of the gallbladder is the result of thermal injury to the serosa (*curved arrow*). (*D*) Enhanced coronal and sagittal CT immediately after MW ablation. The ablation encompasses the index ethiodized oil-laden lesion including a 5-mm margin (*arrow*). On follow-up images, there was no permanent damage to the gallbladder.

commonly treated tumors measuring up to 3 cm (see **Figs. 2**, **4**, **9**, **10**; **Fig. 16**). Depending on the location of the tumor and the technology, tumors of up to 5 cm can be successfully treated with an acceptable rate of LTP.[121,127–130] Multiple ablations in a single session or repeat ablation can safely be performed for limited disease when there is sufficient hepatic reserve (see **Fig. 16**). As with surgical resection, the best results following liver ablation for CRLM are achieved in the setting of a solitary tumor less than 3 cm.[123,131]

Compared with resection, LTP is more common following ablation and the risk increases for larger tumors.[121,127–130,132] However, these differing rates of LTP have not had an apparent effect on OS.[122,124] One possible explanation for this dichotomy between LTP and OS between patients after ablation and resection may be that patients who have experienced LTP and/or distant intrahepatic tumor progression after ablation are often candidates to undergo repeat ablation (or resection) because ablation spares more healthy liver tissue relative to surgery.

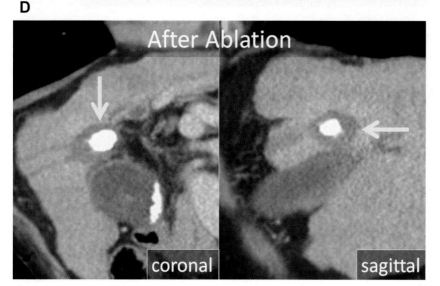

C

During Ablation

D

After Ablation

coronal   sagittal

Fig. 14. (continued)

Neuroendocrine Cancer Hepatic Metastasis

Neuroendocrine tumors (NETs) are a diverse group of malignancies with variable, although often indolent, biological behavior. Clinical behavior and prognosis correlate closely with histologic differentiation and World Health Organization (WHO) grade. For patients with low-grade (G1) or intermediate-grade (G2) histology and metastatic disease, survival is highly variable and can depend on factors unrelated to histology, such as primary tumor location. For example, survival in the setting of advanced carcinoid disease is much worse for patients with the primary tumor arising from the colon and lung (median OS, 7 and 17 months respectively) compared with the small bowel (median OS, 55–65 months). As a result, assessment of comparative benefit among treatment strategies is difficult, given the various natural histories of these malignancies.[133]

Most patients with advanced NET have hepatic metastatic disease. Management of these patients is complex and requires a multidisciplinary team approach, with consideration of age, performance status, clinical symptoms, extent, and biology of disease. Surgical resection provides clear benefit with symptom palliation and favorable long-term survival.[134–138] However, progressive hepatic metastatic disease and recurrent symptoms occur in 85% to 95% of patients. In the setting of limited, isolated liver hepatic metastatic disease, orthotopic liver transplantation (OLT) has been attempted; however, the role of OLT in metastatic NET is not yet established and remains controversial.[139–143]

A

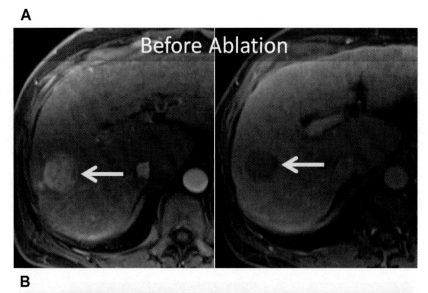

B

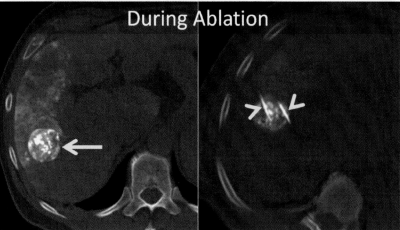

C

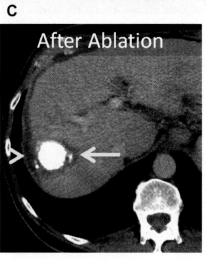

Fig. 15. (*A*) Large (>3 cm) HCC in the right liver (*arrow*). (*B*) Unenhanced CT before and after placement of MW antennas (*arrowheads*). Note the excellent accumulation of ethiodized oil within the tumor (*arrow*) with partial clearance of ethiodized oil from the nontargeted liver in the 2-week interval between TACE and MW ablation. (*C*) Enhanced CT immediately following MW ablation. The ablation encompasses the tumor including a 5-mm margin (*arrow*). Artificial ascites was infused before and during MW ablation (*arrowhead*).

A

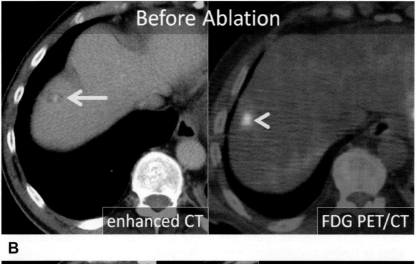

B

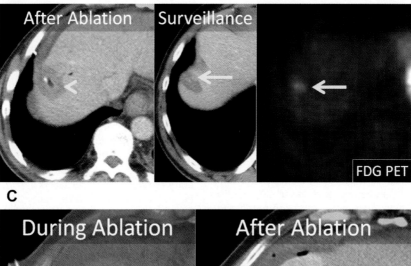

C

Fig. 16. (A) Enhanced CT shows a 1.2-cm CRLM in the right liver, near the dome (*arrow*). The mass is metabolically active on fused 18F-fluorodeoxyglucose (FDG) PET-CT (*arrowhead*). (B) Enhanced CT immediately following MW ablation. The 2.5-cm ablation encompasses the index lesion (*arrowhead*); however, it does not achieve the 1-cm margin needed to mitigate the risk of LTP. At surveillance enhanced CT and FDG PET-CT, there was LTP (*arrows*). (C) On unenhanced CT, 2 MW antennas are positioned within the index lesion with gas surrounding the antennas (*arrowhead*). Artificial ascites was infused before and during MW ablation. Enhanced CT immediately following MW ablation shows a 4.5-cm ablation (*arrow*) covering the prior ablation and a 10-mm margin.

Clinical symptoms depend on a variety of factors, including the site of the primary tumor; the presence of synchronous and metachronous tumors; and the extent and location of local, regional, and distant metastasis. Clinical syndromes are the result of hormone hypersecretion from gastropancreatic NETs or release of vasoactive substances (serotonin) into the systemic circulation from hepatic metastasis. Somatostatin analogues (octreotide or lanreotide) and cytotoxic chemotherapies are useful in controlling both tumor growth and hormone-related symptoms in advanced metastatic disease.[133]

Most patients present with multifocal, bilobar metastatic disease and thus are not surgical candidates and are unlikely to benefit from percutaneous ablation. HAE, alone or as an adjunct to medical therapy, has been a successful palliative technique for patients with liver predominant disease with response rates, as measured by decreased hormone secretion, symptom benefit, and/or radiologic response, generally exceeding 50%. Similar tumor response rates, symptom palliation, and survival have been shown among bland embolization, chemoembolization (cTACE and DEB-TACE), and SIRT.[144–152] Thus, appropriate patient selection is an important consideration to minimize treatment-related side effects among the HAE treatment options.

Ablation

The role of ablation in the management of NET liver metastasis remains undefined, although it is largely accepted as a palliative treatment option in nonsurgical candidates and as an adjunct to surgical resection in patients with oligometastatic disease (see **Fig. 1**). Patients who undergo resection almost always develop new sites of metastatic disease in the liver remnant. Because repeat liver resection may not be feasible because of limited hepatic reserve, percutaneous ablation, in combination with chemotherapy and somatostatin analogues, can provide relief of clinical syndromes and prolong OS.[137,153] Consensus-based guidelines put forth by the National Comprehensive Cancer Network recommend cytoreductive surgery and/or ablation if near-complete eradication of hepatic tumor burden can be achieved.

Most published reports of tumor ablation are small (<40 patients) retrospective case studies. The largest series included 89 patients with hepatic metastatic NET treated with laparoscopic RF.[153] In this cohort, a mean of 6 lesions (and up to 16 lesions) were treated in a single session; most patients (73%) had durable (median, 14 months) symptom relief.

Other Hepatic Tumors

For other hepatic malignancies, either primary or secondary, it is important to understand the underlying disease process and tumor biology. For example, performing tumor ablation if there is rapidly progressing metastatic disease or extensive extrahepatic metastatic disease is unlikely to be beneficial. However, patients with oligometastatic disease who have had a durable response to adjuvant therapies may benefit from liver tumor ablation.[118] The size, location, and number of hepatic tumors and the extent and location of extrahepatic metastases are important considerations.

Breast Cancer Hepatic Metastasis

Breast cancer is the most common malignancy and the leading cause of cancer-related mortality in women.[154] The prognosis remains poor for metastatic breast cancer despite the introduction of modern chemotherapeutic regimens and biologics, with a median OS of 24 to 30 months and a 5-year survival of 23%.[155,156] Both synchronous and metachronous hepatic metastases occur, and usually signify metastatic disease elsewhere; most commonly the lung, bone, nodes, and brain.[157] Isolated hepatic metastasis is uncommon but still portends a poor prognosis, with median OS of approximately 12 months and 5-year survival of 8.5%.[155,158,159] Prognosis has been linked to human epidermal growth factor receptor 2 (HER2) expression in liver metastasis, presence of extrahepatic metastasis, and patient age.[160]

Breast cancer hepatic metastases have typically been treated with chemotherapeutics alone, with surgery reserved for palliation in symptomatic patients.[161] However, more recently several small retrospective series suggest a survival benefit in carefully selected patients even if there is extrahepatic disease.[160,162–164] Alone or combined with surgery, thermal ablation may improve survival. In a small case series of 50 patients, RF ablation of limited hepatic metastatic disease in the setting of stable or limited extrahepatic metastatic disease improved median OS to 43 months (see **Fig. 3**).[160,165]

Benign Hepatic Tumors

Arguably, patients with benign hepatic tumors are the ideal candidates for percutaneous tumor ablation. Because the underlying disorder is benign, complete ablation may not be necessary and there is a wide window of opportunity to obtain a complete ablation, if needed. However, the treatment alternatives generally offered are surgical and are associated with significant morbidity. Thus, a minimally invasive alternative is extremely appealing for these often young and otherwise healthy patients.

There are a variety of benign liver tumors that can be treated, including simple and complex cysts, focal nodular hyperplasia, and hemangiomas and adenomas. Liver cysts and hemangiomas are generally small, follow an indolent course, and require no specific imaging or follow-up. In contrast, adenomas can rupture or infrequently undergo malignant transformation.

Hemangiomas can become large; cause mass effect on local structures, such as the central bile duct, stomach, or duodenum; or stretch the Glisson capsule, resulting in obstructive symptoms, anorexia, weight loss, and abdominal pain. Although surgical resection has been the historic standard of care in symptomatic patients, percutaneous ablation provides a much less invasive option with lower morbidity. Because hemangiomas are benign, complete ablation is not necessary and should be avoided when critical structures, such as central bile ducts, are at risk (**Fig. 17**). There are a few small case series using RF or MW to treat hemangiomas with high technical success, low morbidity, and durable symptom relief.[166–171]

Hepatic adenomas are rare; typically arise in women using oral contraception; and infrequently occur in men, in whom they can be associated with anabolic steroid use. Glycogen storage diseases (type I and III) are associated with multiple adenomas.[172] Compared with other benign tumors, management is more complex because of the risk of hemorrhage and malignant transformation. Active surveillance, surgical resection, embolization, and ablation have all been used. Adenomas larger than 5 cm, those that fail to regress or that grow despite withdrawal of hormones, those that have beta-catenin activation or dysplasia/atypia at biopsy, and adenomas in men should be surgically resected or ablated.[172–174] Even though adenomas are benign, complete ablation should be achieved to avoid delayed complications, such as hemorrhage or malignant transformation (**Fig. 18**).

ABLATION PROCEDURE AND SURVEILLANCE
Local Tumor Progression

The liver surrounding a malignant liver tumor often contains satellites of carcinoma that are invisible at conventional imaging. These tumor satellites are frequently the cause for LTP in technically successful ablations (ie, ablations without imaging evidence of residual tumor on immediate or short-term follow-up; see **Fig. 16**; **Fig. 19**). The extent and distance of the satellites from the index tumor are variable, and depend on factors such as tumor type, size, degree of differentiation, and vascularity. Therefore, the goal of tumor ablation is to encompass both the index tumor and a circumferential margin appropriate for the tumor type.

Ablative margin: hepatocellular carcinoma

The size and degree of differentiation of HCC determine the presence and extent of satellite tumors. Hypervascular HCC is associated with capsular invasion and satellite tumors. As HCC progresses from well to poorly differentiated, the presence and size of satellites increases, and as the index tumor increases in size, the number of satellites increases. However, the size of the index HCC does not affect the distance of the satellite from the index HCC. For HCCs less than 2 cm and HCCs between 2 and 3 cm, the mean distance of the satellite from the index HCC was 5.3 and 4.8 mm, respectively. Nonhypervascular HCC (at CT angiogram) rarely has satellite tumors, regardless of size.[175] For HCCs less than 3 cm, a minimum of a 5-mm circumferential ablative margin must be achieved in order to maximize the odds of complete ablation and reduce the rate of LTP.[175–179]

The overall ablation zone size can easily be underestimated for a particular tumor. For example, a 2-cm HCC should be treated with (at minimum) a 3-cm zone of ablation, provided that the tumor is centered within the ablation. If off center, the zone of ablation should be larger. If an HCC is near or abutting the liver capsule, the ablation should extend to the liver capsule. For HCCs larger than 3 cm, those that lack a capsule, or those that have gross satellites present on conventional imaging, combination therapy and/or larger circumferential margins may be necessary to achieve local tumor control.[180]

Ablative Margin: Colorectal liver metastasis and other hepatic metastases

The biology and perfusion of the tumor relative to the surrounding liver are important factors to consider when planning ablation of hepatic metastases. Relative to the adjacent liver, CRLMs are less well perfused than the surrounding liver. As a result, the index tumor is easier to ablate than the margin of normal liver.[181] Similarly, the water content of metastatic NET relative to adjacent liver parenchyma allows easier ablation of the mass compared with the liver margin. Nevertheless, a minimum of a 1-cm circumferential ablative margin must be achieved in order to maximize the odds of complete ablation and reduce the rate of LTP in CRLM.[132] For example, a 2-cm metastasis should receive (at minimum) a 4-cm zone of ablation, provided the index lesion is centered within the ablation. If off center, the zone of ablation should be larger. If a mass is within 1 cm of the liver capsule, the ablation should extend to the liver capsule. Obtaining at least a 1-cm margin in all directions is particularly important with ill-defined tumors.

A

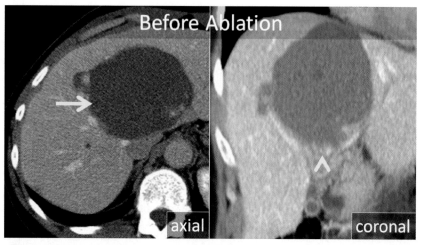

B

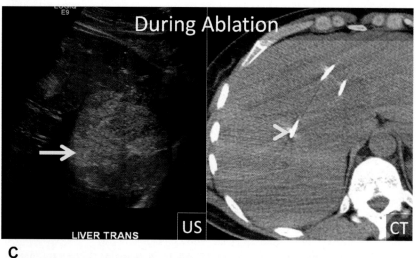

C

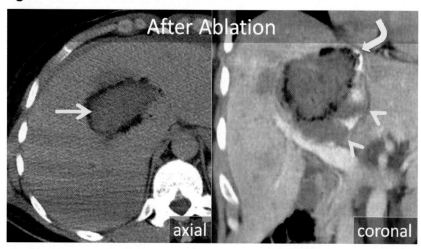

Fig. 17. (*A*) Axial and coronal enhanced CT show a giant cavernous hemangioma centered in the central liver (*arrow*), extending to the hilar plate (*arrowhead*). (*B*) US and unenhanced CT images during MW ablation. The hemangioma is heterogeneous and echogenic at US (*arrow*). Three MW antennas were placed into the mass in a triangular array (*arrowhead*) with approximate spacing of 1.5 cm. (*C*) Enhanced axial and coronal CT immediately after MW ablation. There has been substantial decrease in size of the hemangioma (*arrow*) with resolution of mass effect and stretch of the Glisson capsule at the dome (*curved arrow*). The inferior portion of the mass, near the hilar plate, was purposefully left untreated to avoid injury of the central bile ducts and vasculature (*arrowheads*).

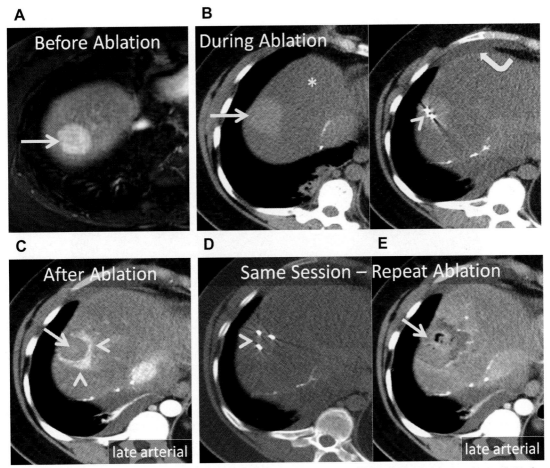

Fig. 18. (*A*) Hepatic adenoma in the dome of the liver, Couinaud segment VIII (*arrow*). (*B*) Unenhanced CT after placement of 2 MW antennas (*arrowhead*). The mass (*arrow*) is conspicuous at unenhanced CT because of severe, diffuse hepatic steatosis (*asterisk*). Note artificial ascites used to protect the body wall and diaphragm (*curved arrow*). (*C*) Enhanced CT immediately following MW ablation. Persistent eccentric avid enhancement (*arrowheads*) surrounding the nonenhancing ablation (*arrow*) is compatible with viable tumor. (*D*) CT image following reinsertion of the 2 antennas and the addition of a third MW antenna (*arrowhead*). (*E*) Enhanced CT immediately following same-session repeat MW ablation. The ablation now encompasses the index lesion (*arrow*).

These tumors tend to have more satellite tumors at distances further from the index tumor.[182,183]

Technique-specific Considerations

Excellent preprocedure imaging, either with contrast-enhanced CT or MR imaging, is necessary for ablation planning. This imaging allows evaluation of the extent of disease within the liver and the proximity of the tumor to major vessels and nontargeted anatomy. When comparison imaging is available, interval change in burden of hepatic and extrahepatic disease can provide insight into tumor biology. For HCC, preprocedure imaging within 1 to 2 months is usually sufficient. However, the doubling rate of CRLM, among other hepatic metastases, is much shorter than that of HCC, so preprocedure imaging should be obtained within 2 weeks of ablation.

Anesthesia

Tumor ablation has been performed with general anesthesia (GA), conscious sedation, and local anesthesia with or without sedation. When combined with a paralytic, GA can render the diaphragm motionless, allowing precise applicator placement. The Valsalva technique can improve tumor conspicuity and access to tumors, particularly those in the dome of the liver. Continuous hemodynamic monitoring by anesthesiology and improved pain control are other advantages of GA.

Relative to GA, deep or conscious sedation reduces procedure time and time between patients and is not associated with the same risks as GA.

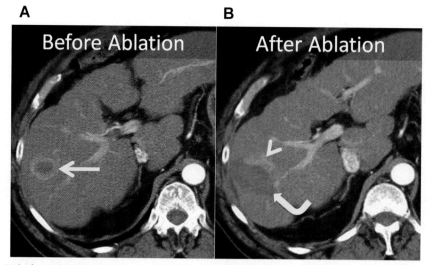

Fig. 19. (*A*) CT before ablation shows an HCC within the right liver (*arrow*). (*B*) At follow-up, eccentric enhancement (*arrowhead*) adjacent to the index ablation (*curved arrow*) is consistent with LTP. Satellite tumors invisible at conventional imaging are generally the cause for LTP, suggesting that an adequate margin was not achieved. For HCC, a minimum of a 5-mm circumferential margin is necessary.

However, shallow tidal volumes can limit tumor conspicuity, particularly for tumors near the dome, and respiratory motion can make applicator placement more challenging. The higher rate of LTP for subcapsular tumors treated under conscious sedation may be partially explained by the fear of inducing pain decreasing treatment time and/or power.[182]

Expected duration of the ablation procedure, number of applicators to be placed, conspicuity of the tumor, expected ease of applicator placement, and the ability of the patient to remain in the preferred position are factors to consider when determining the need for GA.

Nontarget anatomy

A variety of techniques can be used before and/or during ablation to reduce the risk of collateral damage. Patient positioning, instillation of intraperitoneal fluid or gas, insufflation of intraperitoneal balloons, applying traction on applicators, biliary perfusion with chilled fluids, and intentional pneumothorax are techniques that have been used to protect nontargeted anatomy.

Patient positioning A supine position is convenient, safe, and can expedite the procedure. However, nontargeted structures, such as the lung and diaphragm, frequently preclude safe access to liver masses with CT, particularly those near the dome. Even though US provides a greater variety of access points into the liver for tumor ablation, a supine position is frequently suboptimal.

Oblique and lateral decubitus positions allow access to a greater number of hepatic tumors, particularly those near the dome of the liver. These positions can allow nontargeted anatomy to move. In addition, the operator may be able to optimize placement of the applicators so as to protect nontargeted structures while ensuring adequate coverage of the index tumor (see **Figs. 6, 11, 12, 16, 18; Fig. 20**).

Diaphragm Hepatic tumors in proximity to or abutting the liver capsule, particularly those near the dome of the liver, pose unique challenges. Conspicuity of these tumors at US can be suboptimal because of rib shadow, the lung edge, or poor acoustic penetration making applicator placement difficult. As a result, primary effectiveness is reduced, the rate of LTP is higher, and patients experience more postprocedure pain.[184–189] Artificial ascites, directed toward the subdiaphragmatic space, can improve tumor conspicuity at US, reduce the rate of primary failure and LTP, and reduce postprocedural pain (see **Figs. 6, 11, 12, 16, 18, 20**).[190–196]

A transthoracic CT-guided approach to tumors near the dome of the liver, without or following the creation of an artificial pneumothorax or pleural effusion, has been described and can be safe and effective. The most commonly reported complications are pneumothorax and pleural effusion.[100,197–199] Although seeding the pleural space with tumor is a concern, the incidence is likely extremely low and comparable with incidence of seeding the peritoneum.

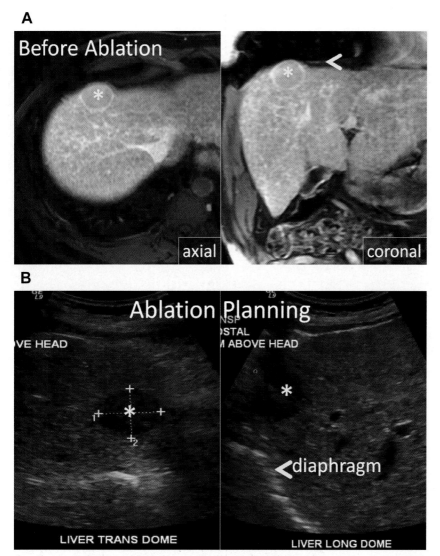

Fig. 20. (*A*) At MR imaging, there is an HCC in Couinaud segment VIII (*asterisks*) abutting the diaphragm (*arrowhead*). (*B*) Shallow LPO improved conspicuity and access to the tumor for US-guided antenna placement (*asterisks*) (*C*) Axial and coronal unenhanced CT with 2 MW antennas (*arrows*) in the mass. The unenhanced CT after applicator placement allows precise localization of the applicator and is particularly useful when evaluating the proximity of nontargeted structures; the diaphragm in this case (*arrowhead*). (*D*) Axial and coronal enhanced CT immediately following MW ablation. The ablation encompasses the index lesion including a margin of greater than 5 mm (*arrow*).

Central bile ducts Extending a zone of ablation to central bile ducts (right and left hepatic ducts, common hepatic and common bile ducts) can result in bile duct stricture and progressive loss of subtended liver parenchyma.[200] Bile leaks, cholangitis, and liver abscesses can subsequently occur, leading to significant morbidity. For patients with metastatic disease, these complications can delay initiation or reinstitution of chemotherapy, potentially resulting in decreased survival. Although high-flow bile duct cooling can be protective, ablation within 1 cm of a central bile duct should be avoided.[201,202] Alternative therapies, such as IRE, ethanol ablation, HAE, and SBRT, should be considered when appropriate for a particular tumor type (see **Figs. 1** and **17**).

Hepatic vasculature Complete ablation of tumors adjacent to high-flow blood vessels larger than 3 mm in diameter is challenging because of perfusion-mediated tissue cooling heat sink (see **Fig. 2**).[23,26,27] Several strategies have been used to combat perfusion-mediated tissue cooling, including increasing power and time of ablations

C

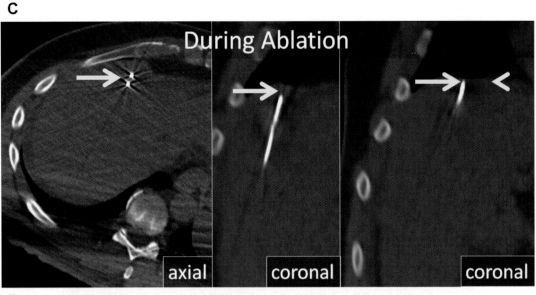

During Ablation

axial | coronal | coronal

D

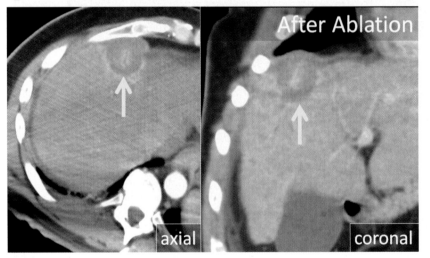

After Ablation

axial | coronal

Fig. 20. (*continued*)

in proximity to major vasculature, targeted placement of applicators closer to vessels, and occlusion of hepatic vasculature with peripherally inserted balloon catheters (see **Figs. 3** and **4**). From a technology perspective, high-powered MW is less susceptible to perfusion-mediated tissue cooling than RF, and IRE may be unaffected by perfusion-mediated cooling (see **Figs. 3** and **4**).[34,203]

In contrast, patients with cirrhosis and slow portal venous flow are at increased risk for portal venous thrombosis (PVT) caused by heat transfer.[29,37] PVT can increase portal vein pressure, leading to decreased liver function, worsening ascites, and increased risk for variceal bleeding. Because of the low incidence with RF and tendency to resolve, historically PVT has been of minimal concern.[204] With the higher temperatures and larger ablations of MW, the risk for PVT may be higher.[34] Anticoagulation therapy generally results in complete or near-complete resolution of PVT (see **Fig. 5**).

Image guidance

Many different tools have been used for imaging guidance, including US, CT, MR imaging, fluoroscopy, and more recently fused PET-CT following the administration of fluorine-18-fluorodeoxyglucose.[205] Each technique has strengths and limitations; the choice of guidance technique should be tailored to the unique situation for each patient.

When technically feasible, US is an excellent guidance tool for applicator placement. The largest published series with the lowest LTP rates following percutaneous ablation almost invariably have used US guidance for applicator placement and ablation monitoring.[36,128,206] Ultrasound offers high soft tissue contrast, simultaneous assessment of the tumor and applicator, fixed guides to assist applicator placement, and the ability to interrogate flow within hepatic vasculature, among other advantages (see **Figs. 1, 3, 4, 6, 8, 14, 20**). However, US is operator dependent and its utility may be compromised by tumor location and body habitus.

CT as a guidance tool allows for evaluation of the entire liver and proximity of non-target anatomy; however, CT is limited by poor soft tissue contrast. Retained ethiodized oil, from prior HAE, can provide a target for CT guidance without compromising the ability to use US (see **Figs. 12–15**). Radiation exposure to the patient and operator is another disadvantage of CT guidance.

Other guidance techniques, such as MR imaging, PET-CT, and fused US/CT-MR imaging, have been used successfully as guidance tools for percutaneous ablation, but are not universally available.[207-218] MR imaging offers superior lesion characterization, relative to CT, and the ability to monitor index ablation temperatures (thermometry); however, not all ablation devices are MR imaging compatible. Small bore sizes can limit applicator placement at MR imaging, particularly in obese patients.

Multiple applicator synergy

Treating large tumors with adequate margins requires the creation of large ablation zones. There are 2 methods to achieve large heat-based ablations: multiple overlapping ablations with a single applicator repositioned to different locations (sequential) and multiple applicator (simultaneous) ablation. Sequential RF and MW ablations result in smaller, less predictable ablations with clefts, whereas simultaneous ablation creates larger, confluent, and more predictable ablations (see **Figs. 3, 7, 9; Fig. 21**).[219,220] There have been no clinical studies directly comparing sequential and simultaneous ablation techniques. However, sequential ablation has been shown to be an independent predictor of primary treatment failure with RF.[221]

Periprocedural monitoring

Monitoring ablations during treatment can facilitate complete ablation.[222] During chemical and thermal ablation, US, CT, and MR imaging can be used to observe the growing ablation and confirm that the tumor and margin are sufficiently covered (see **Figs. 1, 6–9, 14, 16**). Evaluation of the ablation immediately following treatment with contrast-enhanced US, CT, or MR imaging is strongly recommended. If the tumor is inadequately treated, additional ablation should be performed at the same treatment session if possible (see **Fig. 18**).

POSTPROCEDURE SURVEILLANCE

There is no consensus on the optimal interval or frequency of postprocedure imaging. Because LTP is much more common in the first year, most investigators suggest that surveillance imaging in the first year should be more frequent.[223,224] Besides imaging, tumor markers such as alpha-fetoprotein for HCC and carcinoembryonic antigen and/or carbohydrate antigen 19-9 for CRLM, can identify disease progression and provide prognostic information.

Both CT and MR imaging are useful tools in postablation surveillance, each with unique advantages. CT is less prone to artifact compared with MR imaging and has the advantage of complete evaluation of the thorax in the same session. However, contrast-enhanced MR imaging has much better soft tissue characterization, offering improved assessment of the index ablation and progression of hepatic disease. Both CT and MR imaging are useful in the assessment of extrahepatic abdominal metastatic disease. The addition of PET-CT to surveillance in CRLM or breast cancer hepatic metastases is useful in the setting of increasing tumor marker levels if there is negative, equivocal, or indeterminate anatomic imaging (see **Fig. 16**). As a general rule, the postablation imaging modality can be based on the modality that best evaluated the tumor on preablation imaging.

Multiphase postcontrast imaging to include late arterial, portal venous, and delayed (3–5 minutes) phases should be considered after tumor ablation for hypervascular tumors including HCC and NET (see **Figs. 8** and **21**). This technique allows evaluation for both local and regional tumor progression. Growing peripheral nodular enhancement at the ablation margin indicates LTP (see **Figs. 16** and **19**). Dual-energy CT may improve detection of LTP because of improved definition of the ablation zone and higher lesion-to-liver contrast on the iodine map relative to standard blended images. Single-phase postcontrast CT (portal venous phase) is adequate for anatomic surveillance and restaging of CRLM and breast cancer hepatic metastases (see **Figs. 2, 3, 9, 16**). In addition to peripheral nodular enhancement, LTP can also present as enlargement of the index ablation.

A

B

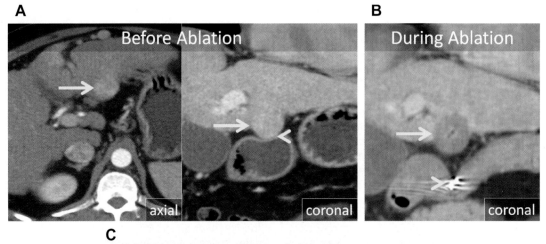

C

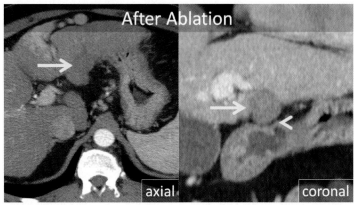

Fig. 21. (*A*) Enhanced CT in the late arterial (axial) and portal venous phase (coronal reformat) shows an exophytic HCC projecting from the inferior left liver (*arrows*), abutting the gastric wall (*arrowhead*). (*B*) Coronal enhanced CT immediately following ablation. Two trocar needles (*arrowhead*) were used as a mechanical lever to displace the stomach from the index ablation (*arrow*). (*C*) Enhanced CT in the late arterial (axial) and portal venous phase (coronal reformat) in follow-up after MW ablation. There is no evidence for LTP (*arrow*) and the gastric wall is normal (*arrowhead*).

With MR imaging, hepatobiliary contrast (gadoxetic acid) is particularly useful in restaging hepatic metastatic disease (see **Fig. 1**).

SUMMARY

Physicians performing ablation should be familiar with the ablation devices they use and the technical aspects of the procedure that can improve primary effectiveness and reduce complications. At present, percutaneous ablation is first-line therapy for very early and early HCC and second-line therapy for CRLM, and is a treatment option for other hepatic tumors on a case-by-case basis. An understanding of the underlying tumor biology is important when weighing the potential benefits of ablation. Achieving a circumferential ablative margin, at least a 0.5 cm for HCC and at least 1.0 cm for liver metastases, decreases LTP.

Surveillance imaging after ablation should be most frequent in the first year, when rates of LTP are the highest.

REFERENCES

1. Ahmed M, Solbiati L, Brace CL, et al. Image-guided tumor ablation: standardization of terminology and reporting criteria–a 10-year update. Radiology 2014;273(1):241–60.
2. Faroja M, Ahmed M, Appelbaum L, et al. Irreversible electroporation ablation: is all the damage nonthermal? Radiology 2013;266(2):462–70.
3. Golberg A, Yarmush ML. Nonthermal irreversible electroporation: fundamentals, applications, and challenges. IEEE Trans Biomed Eng 2013;60(3):707–14.
4. Narayanan G, Hosein PJ, Arora G, et al. Percutaneous irreversible electroporation for

downstaging and control of unresectable pancreatic adenocarcinoma. J Vasc Interv Radiol 2012; 23(12):1613–21.

5. Goldberg SN, Kamel IR, Kruskal JB, et al. Radiofrequency ablation of hepatic tumors: increased tumor destruction with adjuvant liposomal doxorubicin therapy. AJR Am J Roentgenol 2002;179(1): 93–101.

6. Takaki H, Yamakado K, Nakatsuka A, et al. Radiofrequency ablation combined with chemoembolization for the treatment of hepatocellular carcinomas 5 cm or smaller: risk factors for local tumor progression. J Vasc Interv Radiol 2007; 18(7):856–61.

7. Yamakado K, Nakatsuka A, Takaki H, et al. Early-stage hepatocellular carcinoma: radiofrequency ablation combined with chemoembolization versus hepatectomy. Radiology 2008;247(1):260–6.

8. Lewis MA, Hobday TJ. Treatment of neuroendocrine tumor liver metastases. Int J Hepatol 2012; 2012:973946.

9. Huang G, Lin M, Xie X, et al. Combined radiofrequency ablation and ethanol injection with a multipronged needle for the treatment of medium and large hepatocellular carcinoma. Eur Radiol 2014; 24(7):1565–71.

10. Hildebrand P, Leibecke T, Kleemann M, et al. Influence of operator experience in radiofrequency ablation of malignant liver tumours on treatment outcome. Eur J Surg Oncol 2006;32(4):430–4.

11. Poon RT, Ng KK, Lam CM, et al. Learning curve for radiofrequency ablation of liver tumors: prospective analysis of initial 100 patients in a tertiary institution. Ann Surg 2004;239(4):441–9.

12. Lencioni RA, Allgaier HP, Cioni D, et al. Small hepatocellular carcinoma in cirrhosis: randomized comparison of radio-frequency thermal ablation versus percutaneous ethanol injection. Radiology 2003; 228(1):235–40.

13. Lin SM, Lin CJ, Lin CC, et al. Radiofrequency ablation improves prognosis compared with ethanol injection for hepatocellular carcinoma < or =4 cm. Gastroenterology 2004;127(6):1714–23.

14. Shiina S, Teratani T, Obi S, et al. A randomized controlled trial of radiofrequency ablation with ethanol injection for small hepatocellular carcinoma. Gastroenterology 2005;129(1):122–30.

15. Lin SM, Lin CJ, Lin CC, et al. Randomised controlled trial comparing percutaneous radiofrequency thermal ablation, percutaneous ethanol injection, and percutaneous acetic acid injection to treat hepatocellular carcinoma of 3 cm or less. Gut 2005;54(8):1151–6.

16. Brunello F, Veltri A, Carucci P, et al. Radiofrequency ablation versus ethanol injection for early hepatocellular carcinoma: a randomized controlled trial. Scand J Gastroenterol 2008;43(6):727–35.

17. Orlando A, Leandro G, Olivo M, et al. Radiofrequency thermal ablation vs. percutaneous ethanol injection for small hepatocellular carcinoma in cirrhosis: meta-analysis of randomized controlled trials. Am J Gastroenterol 2009;104(2):514–24.

18. Cho YK, Kim JK, Kim MY, et al. Systematic review of randomized trials for hepatocellular carcinoma treated with percutaneous ablation therapies. Hepatology 2009;49(2):453–9.

19. Germani G, Pleguezuelo M, Gurusamy K, et al. Clinical outcomes of radiofrequency ablation, percutaneous alcohol and acetic acid injection for hepatocellular carcinoma: a meta-analysis. J Hepatol 2010;52(3):380–8.

20. Sala M, Llovet JM, Vilana R, et al. Initial response to percutaneous ablation predicts survival in patients with hepatocellular carcinoma. Hepatology 2004; 40(6):1352–60.

21. Lencioni R, Cioni D, Della Pina C, et al. Hepatocellular carcinoma: new options for image-guided ablation. J Hepatobiliary Pancreat Sci 2010;17(4): 399–403.

22. Hong K, Georgiades C. Radiofrequency ablation: mechanism of action and devices. J Vasc Interv Radiol 2010;21(8 Suppl):S179–86.

23. Goldberg SN, Hahn PF, Tanabe KK, et al. Percutaneous radiofrequency tissue ablation: does perfusion-mediated tissue cooling limit coagulation necrosis? J Vasc Interv Radiol 1998;9(1 Pt 1):101–11.

24. Patterson EJ, Scudamore CH, Owen DA, et al. Radiofrequency ablation of porcine liver in vivo: effects of blood flow and treatment time on lesion size. Ann Surg 1998;227(4):559–65.

25. Andreano A, Brace CL. A comparison of direct heating during radiofrequency and microwave ablation in ex vivo liver. Cardiovasc Intervent Radiol 2013;36(2):505–11.

26. Lu DS, Raman SS, Limanond P, et al. Influence of large peritumoral vessels on outcome of radiofrequency ablation of liver tumors. J Vasc Interv Radiol 2003;14(10):1267–74.

27. Lu DS, Raman SS, Vodopich DJ, et al. Effect of vessel size on creation of hepatic radiofrequency lesions in pigs: assessment of the "heat sink" effect. AJR Am J Roentgenol 2002;178(1):47–51.

28. Brace CL. Radiofrequency and microwave ablation of the liver, lung, kidney, and bone: what are the differences? Curr Probl Diagn Radiol 2009; 38(3):135–43.

29. Chiang J, Hynes K, Brace CL. Flow-dependent vascular heat transfer during microwave thermal ablation. Conf Proc IEEE Eng Med Biol Soc 2012; 2012:5582–5.

30. Kim YS, Rhim H, Cho OK, et al. Intrahepatic recurrence after percutaneous radiofrequency ablation of hepatocellular carcinoma: analysis of the pattern and risk factors. Eur J Radiol 2006;59(3):432–41.

31. Bhardwaj N, Strickland AD, Ahmad F, et al. A comparative histological evaluation of the ablations produced by microwave, cryotherapy and radiofrequency in the liver. Pathology 2009;41(2):168–72.

32. Schramm W, Yang D, Wood BJ, et al. Contribution of direct heating, thermal conduction and perfusion during radiofrequency and microwave ablation. Open Biomed Eng J 2007;1:47–52.

33. Lubner MG, Brace CL, Ziemlewicz TJ, et al. Microwave ablation of hepatic malignancy. Semin Intervent Radiol 2013;30(1):56–66.

34. Yu NC, Raman SS, Kim YJ, et al. Microwave liver ablation: influence of hepatic vein size on heat-sink effect in a porcine model. J Vasc Interv Radiol 2008;19(7):1087–92.

35. Huang S, Yu J, Liang P, et al. Percutaneous microwave ablation for hepatocellular carcinoma adjacent to large vessels: a long-term follow-up. Eur J Radiol 2014;83(3):552–8.

36. Livraghi T, Meloni F, Solbiati L, et al. Complications of microwave ablation for liver tumors: results of a multicenter study. Cardiovasc Intervent Radiol 2012;35(4):868–74.

37. Chiang J, Willey BJ, Del Rio AM, et al. Predictors of thrombosis in hepatic vasculature during microwave tumor ablation of an in vivo porcine model. J Vasc Interv Radiol 2014;25(12):1965–71.e2.

38. Jiang J, Brace C, Andreano A, et al. Ultrasound-based relative elastic modulus imaging for visualizing thermal ablation zones in a porcine model. Phys Med Biol 2010;55(8):2281–306.

39. Littrup PJ, Ahmed A, Aoun HD, et al. CT-guided percutaneous cryotherapy of renal masses. J Vasc Interv Radiol 2007;18(3):383–92.

40. Littrup PJ, Jallad B, Vorugu V, et al. Lethal isotherms of cryoablation in a phantom study: effects of heat load, probe size, and number. J Vasc Interv Radiol 2009;20(10):1343–51.

41. Bageacu S, Kaczmarek D, Lacroix M, et al. Cryosurgery for resectable and unresectable hepatic metastases from colorectal cancer. Eur J Surg Oncol 2007;33(5):590–6.

42. Bagia JS, Perera DS, Morris DL. Renal impairment in hepatic cryotherapy. Cryobiology 1998;36(4):263–7.

43. Chapman WC, Debelak JP, Wright Pinson C, et al. Hepatic cryoablation, but not radiofrequency ablation, results in lung inflammation. Ann Surg 2000;231(5):752–61.

44. Dunne RM, Shyn PB, Sung JC, et al. Percutaneous treatment of hepatocellular carcinoma in patients with cirrhosis: a comparison of the safety of cryoablation and radiofrequency ablation. Eur J Radiol 2014;83(4):632–8.

45. Sheen AJ, Poston GJ, Sherlock DJ. Cryotherapeutic ablation of liver tumours. Br J Surg 2002;89(11):1396–401.

46. Sohn RL, Carlin AM, Steffes C, et al. The extent of cryosurgery increases the complication rate after hepatic cryoablation. Am Surg 2003;69(4):317–22 [discussion: 322–3].

47. Washington K, Debelak JP, Gobbell C, et al. Hepatic cryoablation-induced acute lung injury: histopathologic findings. J Surg Res 2001;95(1):1–7.

48. Xu KC, Niu LZ, He WB, et al. Percutaneous cryosurgery for the treatment of hepatic colorectal metastases. World J Gastroenterol 2008;14(9):1430–6.

49. Yang Y, Wang C, Lu Y, et al. Outcomes of ultrasound-guided percutaneous argon-helium cryoablation of hepatocellular carcinoma. J Hepatobiliary Pancreat Sci 2012;19(6):674–84.

50. Ferlay J, Shin HR, Bray F, et al. Estimates of worldwide burden of cancer in 2008: GLOBOCAN 2008. Int J Cancer 2010;127(12):2893–917.

51. Venook AP, Papandreou C, Furuse J, et al. The incidence and epidemiology of hepatocellular carcinoma: a global and regional perspective. Oncologist 2010;15(Suppl 4):5–13.

52. Davila JA, Kramer JR, Duan Z, et al. Referral and receipt of treatment for hepatocellular carcinoma in United States veterans: effect of patient and nonpatient factors. Hepatology 2013;57(5):1858–68.

53. Sangiovanni A, Del Ninno E, Fasani P, et al. Increased survival of cirrhotic patients with a hepatocellular carcinoma detected during surveillance. Gastroenterology 2004;126(4):1005–14.

54. Han KH, Kim do Y, Park JY, et al. Survival of hepatocellular carcinoma patients may be improved in surveillance interval not more than 6 months compared with more than 6 months: a 15-year prospective study. J Clin Gastroenterol 2013;47(6):538–44.

55. Kim WR, Gores GJ, Benson JT, et al. Mortality and hospital utilization for hepatocellular carcinoma in the United States. Gastroenterology 2005;129(2):486–93.

56. Reig M, Darnell A, Forner A, et al. Systemic therapy for hepatocellular carcinoma: the issue of treatment stage migration and registration of progression using the BCLC-refined RECIST. Semin Liver Dis 2014;34(4):444–55.

57. Bruix J, Sherman M. Management of hepatocellular carcinoma. Hepatology 2005;42(5):1208–36.

58. Abdelaziz A, Elbaz T, Shousha HI, et al. Efficacy and survival analysis of percutaneous radiofrequency versus microwave ablation for hepatocellular carcinoma: an Egyptian multidisciplinary clinic experience. Surg Endosc 2014;28(12):3429–34.

59. Ding J, Jing X, Liu J, et al. Comparison of two different thermal techniques for the treatment of hepatocellular carcinoma. Eur J Radiol 2013;82(9):1379–84.

60. Groeschl RT, Pilgrim CH, Hanna EM, et al. Microwave ablation for hepatic malignancies: a multiinstitutional analysis. Ann Surg 2014;259(6):1195–200.

61. Iida H, Aihara T, Ikuta S, et al. A comparative study of therapeutic effect between laparoscopic microwave coagulation and laparoscopic radiofrequency ablation. Hepatogastroenterology 2013; 60(124):662–5.

62. Jiao DC, Zhou Q, Han XW, et al. Microwave ablation treatment of liver cancer with a 2,450-MHz cooled-shaft antenna: pilot study on safety and efficacy. Asian Pac J Cancer Prev 2012;13(2): 737–42.

63. Poggi G, Montagna B, DI Cesare P, et al. Microwave ablation of hepatocellular carcinoma using a new percutaneous device: preliminary results. Anticancer Res 2013;33(3):1221–7.

64. Simo KA, Sereika SE, Newton KN, et al. Laparoscopic-assisted microwave ablation for hepatocellular carcinoma: safety and efficacy in comparison with radiofrequency ablation. J Surg Oncol 2011; 104(7):822–9.

65. Takami Y, Ryu T, Wada Y, et al. Evaluation of intraoperative microwave coagulo-necrotic therapy (MCN) for hepatocellular carcinoma: a single center experience of 719 consecutive cases. J Hepatobiliary Pancreat Sci 2013; 20(3):332–41.

66. Vogl TJ, Farshid P, Naguib NN, et al. Ablation therapy of hepatocellular carcinoma: a comparative study between radiofrequency and microwave ablation. Abdom Imaging 2015. [Epub ahead of print].

67. Ziemlewicz TJ, Hinshaw JL, Lubner MG, et al. Percutaneous microwave ablation of hepatocellular carcinoma with a gas-cooled system: initial clinical results with 107 tumors. J Vasc Interv Radiol 2015; 26(1):62–8.

68. Cho YK, Kim JK, Kim WT, et al. Hepatic resection versus radiofrequency ablation for very early stage hepatocellular carcinoma: a Markov model analysis. Hepatology 2010;51(4):1284–90.

69. Osaki Y, Nishikawa H. Treatment for hepatocellular carcinoma in Japan over the last three decades: our experience and published work review. Hepatol Res 2015;45(1):59–74.

70. Livraghi T, Solbiati L, Meloni MF, et al. Treatment of focal liver tumors with percutaneous radiofrequency ablation: complications encountered in a multicenter study. Radiology 2003;226(2): 441–51.

71. Teratani T, Yoshida H, Shiina S, et al. Radiofrequency ablation for hepatocellular carcinoma in so-called high-risk locations. Hepatology 2006; 43(5):1101–8.

72. Kim SW, Rhim H, Park M, et al. Percutaneous radiofrequency ablation of hepatocellular carcinomas adjacent to the gallbladder with internally cooled electrodes: assessment of safety and therapeutic efficacy. Korean J Radiol 2009;10(4):366–76.

73. Komorizono Y, Oketani M, Sako K, et al. Risk factors for local recurrence of small hepatocellular carcinoma tumors after a single session, single application of percutaneous radiofrequency ablation. Cancer 2003;97(5):1253–62.

74. Song KD, Lim HK, Rhim H, et al. Repeated hepatic resection versus radiofrequency ablation for recurrent hepatocellular carcinoma after hepatic resection: a propensity score matching study. Radiology 2015;275:599–608.

75. Kurokohchi K, Watanabe S, Masaki T, et al. Comparison between combination therapy of percutaneous ethanol injection and radiofrequency ablation and radiofrequency ablation alone for patients with hepatocellular carcinoma. World J Gastroenterol 2005;11(10):1426–32.

76. Lee JM, Lee YH, Kim YK, et al. Combined therapy of radiofrequency ablation and ethanol injection of rabbit liver: an in vivo feasibility study. Cardiovasc Intervent Radiol 2004;27(2):151–7.

77. Ahmed M, Weinstein J, Liu Z, et al. Image-guided percutaneous chemical and radiofrequency tumor ablation in an animal model. J Vasc Interv Radiol 2003;14(8):1045–52.

78. Sakr AA, Saleh AA, Moeaty AA, et al. The combined effect of radiofrequency and ethanol ablation in the management of large hepatocellular carcinoma. Eur J Radiol 2005;54(3):418–25.

79. Gasparini D, Sponza M, Marzio A, et al. Combined treatment, TACE and RF ablation, in HCC: preliminary results. Radiol Med 2002;104(5–6):412–20.

80. Lee MW, Kim YJ, Park SW, et al. Percutaneous radiofrequency ablation of small hepatocellular carcinoma invisible on both ultrasonography and unenhanced CT: a preliminary study of combined treatment with transarterial chemoembolisation. Br J Radiol 2009;82(983):908–15.

81. Peng ZW, Zhang YJ, Liang HH, et al. Recurrent hepatocellular carcinoma treated with sequential transcatheter arterial chemoembolization and RF ablation versus RF ablation alone: a prospective randomized trial. Radiology 2012;262(2):689–700.

82. Hoffmann R, Rempp H, Syha R, et al. Transarterial chemoembolization using drug eluting beads and subsequent percutaneous MR-guided radiofrequency ablation in the therapy of intermediate sized hepatocellular carcinoma. Eur J Radiol 2014;83(10):1793–8.

83. Ginsburg M, Zivin SP, Wroblewski K, et al. Comparison of combination therapies in the management of hepatocellular carcinoma: transarterial chemoembolization with radiofrequency ablation versus microwave ablation. J Vasc Interv Radiol 2015; 26(3):330–41.

84. Peng ZW, Chen MS, Liang HH, et al. A case-control study comparing percutaneous radiofrequency ablation alone or combined with transcatheter

arterial chemoembolization for hepatocellular carcinoma. Eur J Surg Oncol 2010;36(3):257–63.

85. Zhang YJ, Liang HH, Chen MS, et al. Hepatocellular carcinoma treated with radiofrequency ablation with or without ethanol injection: a prospective randomized trial. Radiology 2007;244(2):599–607.

86. Fujimori M, Takaki H, Nakatsuka A, et al. Survival with up to 10-year follow-up after combination therapy of chemoembolization and radiofrequency ablation for the treatment of hepatocellular carcinoma: single-center experience. J Vasc Interv Radiol 2013;24(5):655–66.

87. Fujimori M, Takaki H, Nakatsuka A, et al. Combination therapy of chemoembolization and radiofrequency ablation for the treatment of hepatocellular carcinoma in the caudate lobe. J Vasc Interv Radiol 2012;23(12):1622–8.

88. Kang SG, Yoon CJ, Jeong SH, et al. Single-session combined therapy with chemoembolization and radiofrequency ablation in hepatocellular carcinoma less than or equal to 5 cm: a preliminary study. J Vasc Interv Radiol 2009;20(12):1570–7.

89. Ke S, Ding X, Gao J, et al. Solitary huge hepatocellular carcinomas 10 cm or larger may be completely ablated by repeated radiofrequency ablation combined with chemoembolization: initial experience with 9 patients. Mol Med Rep 2012; 5(3):832–6.

90. Shiraishi R, Yamasaki T, Saeki I, et al. Pilot study of combination therapy with transcatheter arterial infusion chemotherapy using iodized oil and percutaneous radiofrequency ablation during occlusion of hepatic blood flow for hepatocellular carcinoma. Am J Clin Oncol 2008;31(4):311–6.

91. Takaki H, Yamakado K, Uraki J, et al. Radiofrequency ablation combined with chemoembolization for the treatment of hepatocellular carcinomas larger than 5 cm. J Vasc Interv Radiol 2009;20(2):217–24.

92. Kurokohchi K, Watanabe S, Masaki T, et al. Combination therapy of percutaneous ethanol injection and radiofrequency ablation against hepatocellular carcinomas difficult to treat. Int J Oncol 2002;21(3): 611–5.

93. Chung H, Kudo M, Minami Y, et al. Radiofrequency ablation combined with reduction of hepatic blood flow: effect of Lipiodol on coagulation diameter and ablation time in normal pig liver. Hepatogastroenterology 2007;54(75):701–4.

94. Guang C, Kawai N, Sato M, et al. Effect of interval between transcatheter hepatic arterial embolization and radiofrequency ablation on ablated lesion size in a swine model. Jpn J Radiol 2011;29(9): 649–55.

95. Iwamoto T, Kawai N, Sato M, et al. Effectiveness of hepatic arterial embolization on radiofrequency ablation volume in a swine model: relationship to portal venous flow and liver parenchymal pressure. J Vasc Interv Radiol 2008;19(11):1646–51.

96. Morimoto M, Numata K, Nozawa A, et al. Radiofrequency ablation of the liver: extended effect of transcatheter arterial embolization with iodized oil and gelatin sponge on histopathologic changes during follow-up in a pig model. J Vasc Interv Radiol 2010;21(11):1716–24.

97. Mostafa EM, Ganguli S, Faintuch S, et al. Optimal strategies for combining transcatheter arterial chemoembolization and radiofrequency ablation in rabbit VX2 hepatic tumors. J Vasc Interv Radiol 2008;19(12):1740–8.

98. Nakai M, Sato M, Sahara S, et al. Radiofrequency ablation in a porcine liver model: effects of transcatheter arterial embolization with iodized oil on ablation time, maximum output, and coagulation diameter as well as angiographic characteristics. World J Gastroenterol 2007;13(20):2841–5.

99. Yamanaka T, Yamakado K, Takaki H, et al. Ablative zone size created by radiofrequency ablation with and without chemoembolization in small hepatocellular carcinomas. Jpn J Radiol 2012; 30(7):553–9.

100. Toyoda M, Kakizaki S, Horiuchi K, et al. Computed tomography-guided transpulmonary radiofrequency ablation for hepatocellular carcinoma located in hepatic dome. World J Gastroenterol 2006;12(4):608–11.

101. Yamakado K, Nakatsuka A, Ohmori S, et al. Radiofrequency ablation combined with chemoembolization in hepatocellular carcinoma: treatment response based on tumor size and morphology. J Vasc Interv Radiol 2002;13(12):1225–32.

102. Liu HC, Shan EB, Zhou L, et al. Combination of percutaneous radiofrequency ablation with transarterial chemoembolization for hepatocellular carcinoma: observation of clinical effects. Chin J Cancer Res 2014;26(4):471–7.

103. Lencioni R, Crocetti L, Petruzzi P, et al. Doxorubicin-eluting bead-enhanced radiofrequency ablation of hepatocellular carcinoma: a pilot clinical study. J Hepatol 2008;49(2):217–22.

104. Kim JH, Kim PN, Won HJ, et al. Viable hepatocellular carcinoma around retained iodized oil after transarterial chemoembolization: radiofrequency ablation of viable tumor plus retained iodized oil versus viable tumor alone. AJR Am J Roentgenol 2014;203(5):1127–31.

105. Kelly ME, Spolverato G, Lê GN, et al. Synchronous colorectal liver metastasis: a network meta-analysis review comparing classical, combined, and liver-first surgical strategies. J Surg Oncol 2015; 111(3):341–51.

106. Kopetz S, Chang GJ, Overman MJ, et al. Improved survival in metastatic colorectal cancer is associated with adoption of hepatic resection and

improved chemotherapy. J Clin Oncol 2009;27(22): 3677–83.

107. Sharma S, Camci C, Jabbour N. Management of hepatic metastasis from colorectal cancers: an update. J Hepatobiliary Pancreat Surg 2008;15(6): 570–80.

108. Lewis AM, Martin RC. The treatment of hepatic metastases in colorectal carcinoma. Am Surg 2006; 72(6):466–73.

109. Mavros MN, de Jong M, Dogeas E, et al. Impact of complications on long-term survival after resection of colorectal liver metastases. Br J Surg 2013; 100(5):711–8.

110. Tanaka K, Adam R, Shimada H, et al. Role of neo-adjuvant chemotherapy in the treatment of multiple colorectal metastases to the liver. Br J Surg 2003; 90(8):963–9.

111. Sanoff HK, McLeod HL. Predictive factors for response and toxicity in chemotherapy: pharmaco-genomics. Semin Colon Rectal Surg 2008;19(4): 226–30.

112. Vigano L, Capussotti L, Lapointe R, et al. Early recurrence after liver resection for colorectal metastases: risk factors, prognosis, and treatment. A LiverMetSurvey-based study of 6,025 patients. Ann Surg Oncol 2014;21(4):1276–86.

113. Dexiang Z, Li R, Ye W, et al. Outcome of patients with colorectal liver metastasis: analysis of 1,613 consecutive cases. Ann Surg Oncol 2012;19(9): 2860–8.

114. Nordlinger B, Sorbye H, Glimelius B, et al. Periop-erative chemotherapy with FOLFOX4 and surgery versus surgery alone for resectable liver metastases from colorectal cancer (EORTC Intergroup trial 40983): a randomised controlled trial. Lancet 2008; 371(9617):1007–16.

115. Nordlinger B, Sorbye H, Glimelius B, et al. Perioperative FOLFOX4 chemotherapy and surgery versus surgery alone for resectable liver metastases from colorectal cancer (EORTC 40983): long-term results of a randomised, controlled, phase 3 trial. Lancet Oncol 2013; 14(12):1208–15.

116. Mitry E, Fields AL, Bleiberg H, et al. Adjuvant chemotherapy after potentially curative resection of metastases from colorectal cancer: a pooled analysis of two randomized trials. J Clin Oncol 2008;26(30):4906–11.

117. Portier G, Elias D, Bouche O, et al. Multicenter randomized trial of adjuvant fluorouracil and fo-linic acid compared with surgery alone after resection of colorectal liver metastases: FFCD ACHBTH AURC 9002 trial. J Clin Oncol 2006; 24(31):4976–82.

118. Ruers T, Punt C, Van Coevorden F, et al. Radiofre-quency ablation combined with systemic treatment versus systemic treatment alone in patients with non-resectable colorectal liver metastases: a ran-domized EORTC Intergroup phase II study (EORTC 40004). Ann Oncol 2012;23(10):2619–26.

119. Gleisner AL, Choti MA, Assumpcao L, et al. Colo-rectal liver metastases: recurrence and survival following hepatic resection, radiofrequency abla-tion, and combined resection-radiofrequency abla-tion. Arch Surg 2008;143(12):1204–12.

120. Agcaoglu O, Aliyev S, Karabulut K, et al. Comple-mentary use of resection and radiofrequency abla-tion for the treatment of colorectal liver metastases: an analysis of 395 patients. World J Surg 2013; 37(6):1333–9.

121. Hammill CW, Billingsley KG, Cassera MA, et al. Outcome after laparoscopic radiofrequency abla-tion of technically resectable colorectal liver metas-tases. Ann Surg Oncol 2011;18(7):1947–54.

122. Otto G, Düber C, Hoppe-Lotichius M, et al. Radio-frequency ablation as first-line treatment in patients with early colorectal liver metastases amenable to surgery. Ann Surg 2010;251(5):796–803.

123. Kim KH, Yoon YS, Yu CS, et al. Comparative anal-ysis of radiofrequency ablation and surgical resec-tion for colorectal liver metastases. J Korean Surg Soc 2011;81(1):25–34.

124. Reuter NP, Woodall CE, Scoggins CR, et al. Radio-frequency ablation vs. resection for hepatic colo-rectal metastasis: therapeutically equivalent? J Gastrointest Surg 2009;13(3):486–91.

125. Hur H, Ko YT, Min BS, et al. Comparative study of resection and radiofrequency ablation in the treat-ment of solitary colorectal liver metastases. Am J Surg 2009;197(6):728–36.

126. Oshowo A, Gillams A, Harrison E, et al. Compari-son of resection and radiofrequency ablation for treatment of solitary colorectal liver metastases. Br J Surg 2003;90(10):1240–3.

127. Hamada A, Yamakado K, Nakatsuka A, et al. Ra-diofrequency ablation for colorectal liver metasta-ses: prognostic factors in non-surgical candidates. Jpn J Radiol 2012;30(7):567–74.

128. Solbiati L, Ahmed M, Cova L, et al. Small liver colorectal metastases treated with percutaneous radiofrequency ablation: local response rate and long-term survival with up to 10-year follow-up. Radiology 2012;265(3):958–68.

129. Veltri A, Sacchetto P, Tosetti I, et al. Radiofre-quency ablation of colorectal liver metastases: small size favorably predicts technique effective-ness and survival. Cardiovasc Intervent Radiol 2008;31(5):948–56.

130. Nielsen K, van Tilborg AA, Meijerink MR, et al. Inci-dence and treatment of local site recurrences following RFA of colorectal liver metastases. World J Surg 2013;37(6):1340–7.

131. Gillams AR, Lees WR. Five-year survival following radiofrequency ablation of small, solitary, hepatic

colorectal metastases. J Vasc Interv Radiol 2008; 19(5):712–7.

132. Wang X, Sofocleous CT, Erinjeri JP, et al. Margin size is an independent predictor of local tumor progression after ablation of colon cancer liver metastases. Cardiovasc Intervent Radiol 2013;36(1): 166–75.

133. Rind G, Arnold R, Bosman FT, et al. Nomenclature and classification of neuroendocrine neoplasms of the digestive system. In: Bosman TF, Hruban RH, Theise ND, editors. WHO classification of tumours of the digestive system. Lyon (France): International Agency for Research on Cancer (IARC); 2010. p. 13.

134. Chamberlain RS, Canes D, Brown KT, et al. Hepatic neuroendocrine metastases: does intervention alter outcomes? J Am Coll Surg 2000;190(4):432–45.

135. Chen H, Hardacre JM, Uzar A, et al. Isolated liver metastases from neuroendocrine tumors: does resection prolong survival? J Am Coll Surg 1998; 187(1):88–92 [discussion: 92–3].

136. Givi B, Pommier SJ, Thompson AK, et al. Operative resection of primary carcinoid neoplasms in patients with liver metastases yields significantly better survival. Surgery 2006;140(6):891–7 [discussion: 897–8].

137. Mayo SC, de Jong MC, Pulitano C, et al. Surgical management of hepatic neuroendocrine tumor metastasis: results from an international multi-institutional analysis. Ann Surg Oncol 2010; 17(12):3129–36.

138. Glazer ES, Tseng JF, Al-Refaie W, et al. Long-term survival after surgical management of neuroendocrine hepatic metastases. HPB (Oxford) 2010; 12(6):427–33.

139. Gedaly R, Daily MF, Davenport D, et al. Liver transplantation for the treatment of liver metastases from neuroendocrine tumors: an analysis of the UNOS database. Arch Surg 2011;146(8):953–8.

140. Lang H, Oldhafer KJ, Weimann A, et al. Liver transplantation for metastatic neuroendocrine tumors. Ann Surg 1997;225(4):347–54.

141. Le Treut YP, Delpero JR, Dousset B, et al. Results of liver transplantation in the treatment of metastatic neuroendocrine tumors. A 31-case French multicentric report. Ann Surg 1997;225(4):355–64.

142. Marin C, Robles R, Fernández JA, et al. Role of liver transplantation in the management of unresectable neuroendocrine liver metastases. Transplant Proc 2007;39(7):2302–3.

143. van Vilsteren FG, Baskin-Bey ES, Nagorney DM, et al. Liver transplantation for gastroenteropancreatic neuroendocrine cancers: defining selection criteria to improve survival. Liver Transpl 2006; 12(3):448–56.

144. Sward C, Johanson V, Nieveen van Dijkum E, et al. Prolonged survival after hepatic artery embolization in patients with midgut carcinoid syndrome. Br J Surg 2009;96(5):517–21.

145. Christante D, Pommier S, Givi B, et al. Hepatic artery chemoinfusion with chemoembolization for neuroendocrine cancer with progressive hepatic metastases despite octreotide therapy. Surgery 2008;144(6):885–93 [discussion: 893–4].

146. Loewe C, Schindl M, Cejna M, et al. Permanent transarterial embolization of neuroendocrine metastases of the liver using cyanoacrylate and lipiodol: assessment of mid- and long-term results. AJR Am J Roentgenol 2003;180(5):1379–84.

147. de Baere T, Deschamps F, Teriitheau C, et al. Transarterial chemoembolization of liver metastases from well differentiated gastroenteropancreatic endocrine tumors with doxorubicin-eluting beads: preliminary results. J Vasc Interv Radiol 2008;19(6):855–61.

148. Kennedy AS, Dezarn WA, McNeillie P, et al. Radioembolization for unresectable neuroendocrine hepatic metastases using resin 90Y-microspheres: early results in 148 patients. Am J Clin Oncol 2008;31(3):271–9.

149. Kennedy A, Bester L, Salem R, et al. Role of hepatic intra-arterial therapies in metastatic neuroendocrine tumours (NET): guidelines from the NET-liver-metastases consensus conference. HPB (Oxford) 2015;17(1):29–37.

150. Rhee TK, Lewandowski RJ, Liu DM, et al. 90Y Radioembolization for metastatic neuroendocrine liver tumors: preliminary results from a multi-institutional experience. Ann Surg 2008;247(6):1029–35.

151. Gaur SK, Friese JL, Sadow CA, et al. Hepatic arterial chemoembolization using drug-eluting beads in gastrointestinal neuroendocrine tumor metastatic to the liver. Cardiovasc Intervent Radiol 2011;34(3): 566–72.

152. Gupta S, Johnson MM, Murthy R, et al. Hepatic arterial embolization and chemoembolization for the treatment of patients with metastatic neuroendocrine tumors: variables affecting response rates and survival. Cancer 2005;104(8):1590–602.

153. Akyildiz HY, Mitchell J, Milas M, et al. Laparoscopic radiofrequency thermal ablation of neuroendocrine hepatic metastases: long-term follow-up. Surgery 2010;148(6):1288–93 [discussion: 1293].

154. Jemal A, Bray F, Center MM, et al. Global cancer statistics. CA Cancer J Clin 2011;61(2):69–90.

155. Largillier R, Ferrero JM, Doyen J, et al. Prognostic factors in 1,038 women with metastatic breast cancer. Ann Oncol 2008;19(12):2012–9.

156. Chua TC, Saxena A, Liauw W, et al. Hepatic resection for metastatic breast cancer: a systematic review. Eur J Cancer 2011;47(15):2282–90.

157. Singletary SE, Walsh G, Vauthey JN, et al. A role for curative surgery in the treatment of selected patients with metastatic breast cancer. Oncologist 2003;8(3):241–51.

158. Ruiterkamp J, Ernst MF. The role of surgery in metastatic breast cancer. Eur J Cancer 2011;47(Suppl 3):S6–22.

159. Pentheroudakis G, Fountzilas G, Bafaloukos D, et al. Metastatic breast cancer with liver metastases: a registry analysis of clinicopathologic, management and outcome characteristics of 500 women. Breast Cancer Res Treat 2006;97(3): 237–44.

160. Dittmar Y, Altendorf-Hofmann A, Schüle S, et al. Liver resection in selected patients with metastatic breast cancer: a single-centre analysis and review of literature. J Cancer Res Clin Oncol 2013;139(8): 1317–25.

161. O'Rourke TR, Tekkis P, Yeung S, et al. Long-term results of liver resection for non-colorectal, non-neuroendocrine metastases. Ann Surg Oncol 2008;15(1):207–18.

162. Blanchard DK, Shetty PB, Hilsenbeck SG, et al. Association of surgery with improved survival in stage IV breast cancer patients. Ann Surg 2008;247(5): 732–8.

163. Fields RC, Jeffe DB, Trinkaus K, et al. Surgical resection of the primary tumor is associated with increased long-term survival in patients with stage IV breast cancer after controlling for site of metastasis. Ann Surg Oncol 2007;14(12):3345–51.

164. Ruiterkamp J, Ernst MF, van de Poll-Franse LV, et al. Surgical resection of the primary tumour is associated with improved survival in patients with distant metastatic breast cancer at diagnosis. Eur J Surg Oncol 2009;35(11):1146–51.

165. Livraghi T, Goldberg SN, Solbiati L, et al. Percutaneous radio-frequency ablation of liver metastases from breast cancer: initial experience in 24 patients. Radiology 2001;220(1):145–9.

166. Cui Y, Zhou LY, Dong MK, et al. Ultrasonography guided percutaneous radiofrequency ablation for hepatic cavernous hemangioma. World J Gastroenterol 2003;9(9):2132–4.

167. Gao J, Ding X, Ke S, et al. Radiofrequency ablation in the treatment of large hepatic hemangiomas: a comparison of multitined and internally cooled electrodes. J Clin Gastroenterol 2014; 48(6):540–7.

168. Gao J, Ke S, Ding XM, et al. Radiofrequency ablation for large hepatic hemangiomas: initial experience and lessons. Surgery 2013;153(1):78–85.

169. Park SY, Tak WY, Jung MK, et al. Symptomatic-enlarging hepatic hemangiomas are effectively treated by percutaneous ultrasonography-guided radiofrequency ablation. J Hepatol 2011;54(3): 559–65.

170. Tang XY, Wang Z, Wang T, et al. Efficacy, safety and feasibility of ultrasound-guided percutaneous microwave ablation for large hepatic hemangioma. J Dig Dis 2014. [Epub ahead of print].

171. Ziemlewicz TJ, Wells SA, Lubner MA, et al. Microwave ablation of giant hepatic cavernous hemangiomas. Cardiovasc Intervent Radiol 2014;37(5): 1299–305.

172. Liau SS, Qureshi MS, Praseedom R, et al. Molecular pathogenesis of hepatic adenomas and its implications for surgical management. J Gastrointest Surg 2013;17(10):1869–82.

173. Rhim H, Lim HK, Kim YS, et al. Percutaneous radiofrequency ablation of hepatocellular adenoma: initial experience in 10 patients. J Gastroenterol Hepatol 2008;23(8 Pt 2):e422–7.

174. van Vledder MG, van Aalten SM, Terkivatan T, et al. Safety and efficacy of radiofrequency ablation for hepatocellular adenoma. J Vasc Interv Radiol 2011;22(6):787–93.

175. Ikeda K, Seki T, Umehara H, et al. Clinicopathologic study of small hepatocellular carcinoma with microscopic satellite nodules to determine the extent of tumor ablation by local therapy. Int J Oncol 2007;31(3):485–91.

176. Okusaka T, Okada S, Ueno H, et al. Satellite lesions in patients with small hepatocellular carcinoma with reference to clinicopathologic features. Cancer 2002;95(9):1931–7.

177. Maeda T, Takenaka K, Taguchi K, et al. Small hepatocellular carcinoma with minute satellite nodules. Hepatogastroenterology 2000;47(34):1063–6.

178. Nakazawa T, Kokubu S, Shibuya A, et al. Radiofrequency ablation of hepatocellular carcinoma: correlation between local tumor progression after ablation and ablative margin. AJR Am J Roentgenol 2007;188(2):480–8.

179. Liu CH, Arellano RS, Uppot RN, et al. Radiofrequency ablation of hepatic tumours: effect of post-ablation margin on local tumour progression. Eur Radiol 2010;20(4):877–85.

180. Ke S, Ding XM, Qian XJ, et al. Radiofrequency ablation of hepatocellular carcinoma sized >3 and </= 5 cm: is ablative margin of more than 1 cm justified? World J Gastroenterol 2013;19(42): 7389–98.

181. Liu Z, Ahmed M, Sabir A, et al. Computer modeling of the effect of perfusion on heating patterns in radiofrequency tumor ablation. Int J Hyperthermia 2007;23(1):49–58.

182. Mulier S, Ni Y, Jamart J, et al. Local recurrence after hepatic radiofrequency coagulation: multivariate meta-analysis and review of contributing factors. Ann Surg 2005;242(2):158–71.

183. Shirabe K, Takenaka K, Gion T, et al. Analysis of prognostic risk factors in hepatic resection for metastatic colorectal carcinoma with special reference to the surgical margin. Br J Surg 1997; 84(8):1077–80.

184. Smolock AR, Lubner MG, Ziemlewicz TJ, et al. Microwave ablation of hepatic tumors abutting the

diaphragm is safe and effective. AJR Am J Roentgenol 2015;204(1):197–203.

185. Li M, Yu XL, Liang P, et al. Percutaneous microwave ablation for liver cancer adjacent to the diaphragm. Int J Hyperthermia 2012;28(3):218–26.

186. Kim PN, Choi D, Rhim H, et al. Planning ultrasound for percutaneous radiofrequency ablation to treat small (</= 3 cm) hepatocellular carcinomas detected on computed tomography or magnetic resonance imaging: a multicenter prospective study to assess factors affecting ultrasound visibility. J Vasc Interv Radiol 2012;23(5):627–34.

187. Tang Z, Fang H, Kang M, et al. Percutaneous radiofrequency ablation for liver tumors: is it safer and more effective in low-risk areas than in high-risk areas? Hepatol Res 2011;41(7):635–40.

188. Kang TW, Rhim H, Kim EY, et al. Percutaneous radiofrequency ablation for the hepatocellular carcinoma abutting the diaphragm: assessment of safety and therapeutic efficacy. Korean J Radiol 2009;10(1):34–42.

189. Head HW, Dodd GD 3rd, Dalrymple NC, et al. Percutaneous radiofrequency ablation of hepatic tumors against the diaphragm: frequency of diaphragmatic injury. Radiology 2007;243(3):877–84.

190. Hinshaw JL, Laeseke PF, Winter TC 3rd, et al. Radiofrequency ablation of peripheral liver tumors: intraperitoneal 5% dextrose in water decreases postprocedural pain. AJR Am J Roentgenol 2006; 186(5 Suppl):S306–10.

191. Kitchin D, Lubner M, Ziemlewicz T, et al. Microwave ablation of malignant hepatic tumours: intraperitoneal fluid instillation prevents collateral damage and allows more aggressive case selection. Int J Hyperthermia 2014;30(5):299–305.

192. Kang TW, Rhim H, Lee MW, et al. Radiofrequency ablation for hepatocellular carcinoma abutting the diaphragm: comparison of effects of thermal protection and therapeutic efficacy. AJR Am J Roentgenol 2011;196(4):907–13.

193. Song I, Rhim H, Lim HK, et al. Percutaneous radiofrequency ablation of hepatocellular carcinoma abutting the diaphragm and gastrointestinal tracts with the use of artificial ascites: safety and technical efficacy in 143 patients. Eur Radiol 2009; 19(11):2630–40.

194. Rhim H, Lim HK, Kim YS, et al. Percutaneous radiofrequency ablation with artificial ascites for hepatocellular carcinoma in the hepatic dome: initial experience. AJR Am J Roentgenol 2008;190(1): 91–8.

195. Chen MH, Yang W, Yan K, et al. Radiofrequency ablation of problematically located hepatocellular carcinoma: tailored approach. Abdom Imaging 2008;33(4):428–36.

196. Uehara T, Hirooka M, Ishida K, et al. Percutaneous ultrasound-guided radiofrequency ablation of hepatocellular carcinoma with artificially induced pleural effusion and ascites. J Gastroenterol 2007;42(4):306–11.

197. Takaki H, Yamakado K, Nakatsuka A, et al. Frequency of and risk factors for complications after liver radiofrequency ablation under CT fluoroscopic guidance in 1500 sessions: single-center experience. AJR Am J Roentgenol 2013;200(3):658–64.

198. Shibata T, Shibata T, Maetani Y, et al. Transthoracic percutaneous radiofrequency ablation for liver tumors in the hepatic dome. J Vasc Interv Radiol 2004;15(11):1323–7.

199. de Baere T, Dromain C, Lapeyre M, et al. Artificially induced pneumothorax for percutaneous transthoracic radiofrequency ablation of tumors in the hepatic dome: initial experience. Radiology 2005; 236(2):666–70.

200. Marchal F, Elias D, Rauch P, et al. Biliary lesions during radiofrequency ablation in liver. Study on the pig. Eur Surg Res 2004;36(2):88–94.

201. Marchal F, Elias D, Rauch P, et al. Prevention of biliary lesions that may occur during radiofrequency ablation of the liver: study on the pig. Ann Surg 2006;243(1):82–8.

202. Ogawa T, Kawamoto H, Kobayashi Y, et al. Prevention of biliary complication in radiofrequency ablation for hepatocellular carcinoma-Cooling effect by endoscopic nasobiliary drainage tube. Eur J Radiol 2010;73(2):385–90.

203. Kingham TP, Karkar AM, D'Angelica MI, et al. Ablation of perivascular hepatic malignant tumors with irreversible electroporation. J Am Coll Surg 2012; 215(3):379–87.

204. Akahane M, Koga H, Kato N, et al. Complications of percutaneous radiofrequency ablation for hepato-cellular carcinoma: imaging spectrum and management. Radiographics 2005;25(Suppl 1): S57–68.

205. Ryan ER, Sofocleous CT, Schöder H, et al. Split-dose technique for FDG PET/CT-guided percutaneous ablation: a method to facilitate lesion targeting and to provide immediate assessment of treatment effectiveness. Radiology 2013;268(1): 288–95.

206. Liu FY, Yu XL, Liang P, et al. Comparison of percutaneous 915 MHz microwave ablation and 2450 MHz microwave ablation in large hepatocellular carcinoma. Int J Hyperthermia 2010;26(5): 448–55.

207. Krucker J, Xu S, Venkatesan A, et al. Clinical utility of real-time fusion guidance for biopsy and ablation. J Vasc Interv Radiol 2011;22(4):515–24.

208. Venkatesan AM, Kadoury S, Abi-Jaoudeh N, et al. Real-time FDG PET guidance during biopsies and radiofrequency ablation using multimodality fusion with electromagnetic navigation. Radiology 2011; 260(3):848–56.

209. Yu X, Liu F, Liang P, et al. Microwave ablation assisted by a computerised tomography-ultrasonography fusion imaging system for liver lesions: an ex vivo experimental study. Int J Hyperthermia 2011;27(2):172–9.

210. Minami Y, Kudo M. Ultrasound fusion imaging of hepatocellular carcinoma: a review of current evidence. Dig Dis 2014;32(6):690–5.

211. Clasen S, Rempp H, Boss A, et al. MR-guided radiofrequency ablation of hepatocellular carcinoma: long-term effectiveness. J Vasc Interv Radiol 2011;22(6):762–70.

212. Clasen S, Rempp H, Hoffmann R, et al. Image-guided radiofrequency ablation of hepatocellular carcinoma (HCC): is MR guidance more effective than CT guidance? Eur J Radiol 2014;83(1):111–6.

213. Lee MW, Rhim H, Cha DI, et al. Percutaneous radiofrequency ablation of hepatocellular carcinoma: fusion imaging guidance for management of lesions with poor conspicuity at conventional sonography. AJR Am J Roentgenol 2012;198(6):1438–44.

214. Mauri G, Cova L, De Beni S, et al. Real-Time US-CT/MRI image fusion for guidance of thermal ablation of liver tumors undetectable with us: results in 295 cases. Cardiovasc Intervent Radiol 2015;38(1):143–51.

215. Rempp H, Clasen S, Pereira PL. Image-based monitoring of magnetic resonance-guided thermoablative therapies for liver tumors. Cardiovasc Intervent Radiol 2012;35(6):1281–94.

216. Song KD, Lee MW, Rhim H, et al. Fusion imaging-guided radiofrequency ablation for hepatocellular carcinomas not visible on conventional ultrasound. AJR Am J Roentgenol 2013;201(5):1141–7.

217. Terraz S, Cernicanu A, Lepetit-Coiffé M, et al. Radiofrequency ablation of small liver malignancies under magnetic resonance guidance: progress in targeting and preliminary observations with temperature monitoring. Eur Radiol 2010;20(4):886–97.

218. Wu B, Xiao YY, Zhang X, et al. Magnetic resonance imaging-guided percutaneous cryoablation of hepatocellular carcinoma in special regions. Hepatobiliary Pancreat Dis Int 2010;9(4):384–92.

219. Brace CL, Sampson LA, Hinshaw JL, et al. Radiofrequency ablation: simultaneous application of multiple electrodes via switching creates larger, more confluent ablations than sequential application in a large animal model. J Vasc Interv Radiol 2009;20(1):118–24.

220. Lubner MG, Brace CL, Hinshaw JL, et al. Microwave tumor ablation: mechanism of action, clinical results, and devices. J Vasc Interv Radiol 2010;21(8 Suppl):S192–203.

221. Fernandes ML, Lin CC, Lin CJ, et al. Risk of tumour progression in early-stage hepatocellular carcinoma after radiofrequency ablation. Br J Surg 2009;96(7):756–62.

222. Claudon M, Dietrich CF, Choi BI, et al. Guidelines and good clinical practice recommendations for contrast enhanced ultrasound (CEUS) in the liver–update 2012: a WFUMB-EFSUMB initiative in cooperation with representatives of AFSUMB, AIUM, ASUM, FLAUS and ICUS. Ultraschall Med 2013;34(1):11–29.

223. Boas FE, Do B, Louie JD, et al. Optimal imaging surveillance schedules after liver-directed therapy for hepatocellular carcinoma. J Vasc Interv Radiol 2015;26(1):69–73.

224. Liu D, Fong DY, Chan AC, et al. Hepatocellular carcinoma: surveillance CT schedule after hepatectomy based on risk stratification. Radiology 2015;274(1):133–40.

Intra-Arterial Therapies for Liver Masses
Data Distilled

Christopher Molvar, MD[a],*, Robert J. Lewandowski, MD, FSIR[b]

KEYWORDS

- Hepatocellular carcinoma • Colorectal cancer • Liver metastasis • Radioembolization
- Chemoembolization

KEY POINTS

- Staging of hepatocellular carcinoma (HCC) is complex due to cirrhosis, and the Barcelona Clinic Liver Cancer system is commonly utilized.
- Conventional trans arterial chemoembolization (cTACE) has demonstrated a survival benefit for appropriately selected patients with HCC in randomized controlled trials (RCTs).
- Drug-eluting bead trans arterial chemoembolization (DEB TACE) is an evolution of cTACE with an improved pharmacokinetic profile for treatment of HCC and metastatic colorectal cancer (mCRC). However, in an RCT, drug-eluting bead TACE failed to show a response improvement over cTACE for HCC.
- Radioembolization provides selective internal radiation to primary and liver mCRC due to their preferential arterial blood supply. Lack of macroscopic vessel occlusion allows safe treatment of lesions with vascular invasion and limits postembolization syndrome.
- Embolization is a safe and effective alternative treatment for focal nodular hyperplasia and hepatic adenoma.

INTRODUCTION

The liver is a frequent site of metastatic disease, most commonly from a colorectal origin, and also a site of lethal primary malignancy.[1] Hepatocellular carcinoma (HCC) is the most common primary liver tumor and the third most common cause of cancer mortality.[2,3] Colorectal metastatic disease carries utmost prognostic implications, with a median survival of about 2 years in patients with advanced disease treated with chemotherapy.[4] Given the import of liver containing tumor, its treatment draws from multiple cancer specialties, yielding a wide range of treatment options. These include systemic chemotherapy and biologic agents, surgical resection, ablation, and stereotactic body radiation therapy (SBRT); regional therapies include chemoembolization, radioembolization, and chemo infusion. The liver is also affected by benign masses, some of which carry the potential for malignant degeneration. This article presents the current level of evidence on intra-arterial therapies for liver masses, both malignant and benign, including discussions of patient selection, outcomes, and complications.

HEPATOCELLULAR CARCINOMA
Background

HCC develops almost exclusively in a background of cirrhosis, producing 2 disease states in 1 organ. It is the sixth most common cancer, and unlike

Disclosure Statement: The authors have nothing to disclose.
[a] Section of Vascular and Interventional Radiology, Department of Radiology, Loyola University Medical Center, 2160 S 1st Ave, Maywood, IL 60153, USA; [b] Section of Interventional Radiology, Division of Interventional Oncology, Department of Radiology, Northwestern University Feinberg School of Medicine, 676 N St. Clair St #800, Chicago, IL 60611, USA
* Corresponding author.
E-mail address: cmolvar@lumc.edu

0033-8389/15/$ – see front matter © 2015 Elsevier Inc. All rights reserved.

radiologic.theclinics.com

other solid malignancies, the incidence in the United States is on the rise, mostly because of the dissemination of hepatitis C virus.[5] Surveillance programs can achieve an early diagnosis of HCC; however, only about half of the population at risk receives appropriate screening, resulting in frequent disease presentation without curative options.[6]

Noninvasive imaging is the preferred method of HCC diagnosis, where pathognomonic features yield a specificity of greater than 95%.[7,8] Biopsy should be reserved for atypical imaging features, as can be seen with infiltrative disease.[9]

Staging in HCC must account for variables beyond tumor burden, as underlying liver function also affects prognosis.[9] Various staging systems exist, reflecting worldwide patient population differences. The most commonly used system for Western disease is the Barcelona Clinic Liver Cancer (BCLC) classification, and it carries the endorsement of both the American Association for the Study of Liver Diseases (AASLD) and the European Association for the Study of the Liver (EASL).[9,10] This system links the stage of disease with treatment modalities, and subsequently an estimation of life expectancy. The BCLC system separates those patients with early disease, who are eligible for curative therapies, from those with intermediate and advanced disease, who benefit from palliative treatments.[11]

A newly developed prognostic staging system with treatment guidelines, the Hong Kong Liver Cancer Staging (HKLC) classification, produces better survival outcomes when compared with the BCLC system. The HKLC system was developed using data from 3927 patients at a single center in Asia, where about 80% of patients were hepatitis B carriers. Notably, BCLC intermediate and advanced stage patients were further stratified in the HKLC system to receive more aggressive treatment, yielding improved survival. Application of this aggressive treatment schedule outside of Asia requires performance validation in a Western HCC patient population.[12] Nonetheless, the HKLC system reflects an evolution of curative and palliative treatment options for patients with HCC.

Treatment of HCC is complex given the frequent background of cirrhosis, which affects survival and the ability to treat. A multispecialty approach is required, with participation from hepatologists, oncologists, surgeons, radiologists, and pathologists.[9] In deciding on treatment, it is important to recognize that the level of evidence for most therapeutic options is restricted to cohort studies, with a few randomized controlled trials (RCTs), mostly in the setting of advanced disease.[13,14] As such,

patient care is individualized and often reflects opinion, local expertise, and resources.

Potentially curative therapies for HCC are surgical resection, transplantation, and ablation.[13] Palliative therapies include transarterial treatment with chemoembolization, radioembolization, and bland embolization, along with sorafenib, a systemic agent.[9,15] Transarterial therapy for HCC will be explored, with specific attention to evidence and outcomes.

Chemoembolization for Hepatocellular Carcinoma

HCC demonstrates intense neo-angiogenic activity during its progression.[16,17] Chemoembolization produces localized chemotherapy delivery to the tumor, along with tumor ischemia.[16] Chemoembolization is preformed by conventional technique (cTACE) utilizing ethiodized oil (lipidol) or by drug-eluting bead technique (DEB-TACE).

Conventional chemoembolization for hepatocellular carcinoma

Various chemotherapeutic agents have been used in cTACE, including doxorubicin, epirubicin, cisplatin, and mitomycin C. All of these drugs exhibit preferential extraction when delivered intrahepatically and can achieve favorable intratumoral concentrations with lower systemic concentrations.[18] No clear evidence exists to support one or a combination of these agents.[18] Today, the most commonly used agent in the United States is doxorubicin.[18]

Intra-arterial delivery of the aqueous chemotherapy and lipidol emulsion is followed by, or concurrent with, delivery of embolic material in cTACE. Embolization material serves 2 purposes: preventing cytotoxic chemotherapy washout and inducing intratumoral ischemic necrosis[18] (**Fig. 1**).

Patient selection cTACE is used as palliative care, in combination with ablation, or as a bridge to liver transplant. Preserved liver function is essential, as the antitumor effect of chemoembolization can be offset by treatment-induced liver failure.[18] According to the BCLC staging system, cTACE is recommended for those with intermediate stage disease.

Evidence and outcome

The survival benefits of chemoembolization were reported in 2 landmark RCTs in 2002. LLovet and colleagues[19] randomized patients to one of three treatment arms, namely, fixed interval cTACE (doxorubicin), gel foam embolization, or conservative treatment. The trial was stopped when a survival benefit of patients treated with cTACE was identified as compared to conservative treatment.

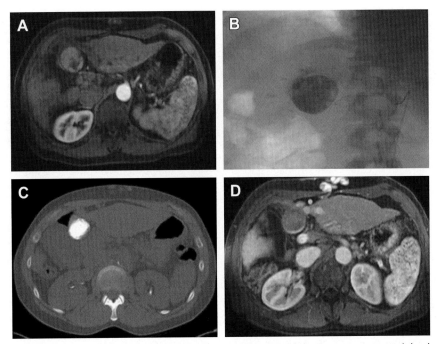

Fig. 1. (A) Gadolinium-enhanced MR imaging shows a cirrhotic liver with heterogeneous arterial enhancing mass in segment 4; venous phase washout consistent with HCC was present. Patient was treated with selective cTACE with dense intratumoral lipidol staining, seen on (B) fluoroscopy and on (C) postprocedure noncontrast-enhanced computed tomography (CT). (D) Follow up MR imaging after 4 weeks shows a complete response by EASL necrosis criteria given lack of nodular arterial enhancement. Noted are subcutaneous paraumbilical vein collaterals indicative of portal hypertension.

Interestingly, no significant survival difference was seen in the gel foam embolization versus the chemoembolization arms.[19] Lo and colleagues[20] randomized patients to cTACE (cisplatin) versus best supportive care. Chemoembolization resulted in significant improvement in 1-, 2-, and 3-year survival rates.[20] A meta-analysis of 18 RCTs clearly demonstrated a 2-year survival benefit of cTACE compared with conservative treatment.[21] Collectively, cTACE was established as the standard of care in appropriately selected patients with unresectable HCC.[18,21]

Complications

Chemoembolization is frequently complicated by postembolization syndrome, specifically, right upper quadrant pain, fever, and nausea. These symptoms tend to reflect the degree of embolization and are self-limited over 1 to 3 days. Complications caused by nontarget embolization can produce necrosis in unwanted arterial distributions including the cystic artery, gut arteries, inferior phrenic arteries, and cutaneous arterial supply.[22,23] Other complications include bile duct injury, liver abscess (in particular, after biliary intervention), vascular injury, and tumor rupture.[22,23]

Drug-Eluting Bead Technique Chemoembolization for Hepatocellular Carcinoma

The ideal TACE platform should allow for maximum and sustained concentration of chemotherapeutic agent within the tumor microenvironment, with minimal systemic exposure.[16] This drug delivery feature, together with calibrated vessel occlusion, underpins the development of drug-eluting microspheres.[16] Through a loading process, the microspheres sequester chemotherapy, which is subsequently released, in a sustained fashion, after intra-arterial administration.[23]

Patient selection

Analogous to cTACE, DEB TACE is a palliative option for patients with unresectable HCC, and can be used as a bridge to liver transplant or in combination with ablation. In accordance with clinical trials, ideal DEB TACE patients should have HCC that can be isolated angiographically, such that sublobar administrations can be performed[23] (**Fig. 2**).

Evidence and outcomes

The rationale for DEB TACE is high intratumoral chemotherapy retention and decreased systemic

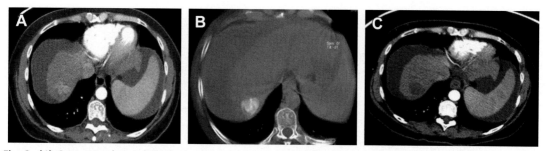

Fig. 2. (*A*) Contrast-enhanced CT demonstrates a heterogeneous arterial enhancing lesion in the dome of the liver compatible with HCC. (*B*) C-arm CT image prior to DEB TACE shows sublobar catheter position with isolated lesion perfusion. (*C*) 1-month follow-up contrast enhanced CT shows a complete response by EASL necrosis criteria.

bioavailability. Several studies have shown an improved pharmacokinetic profile, and fewer adverse effects associated with DEB TACE, as compared to cTACE.[18] Varela and colleagues[24] evaluated the safety, pharmacokinetics, and efficacy of DEB TACE (500–700 μg size) in a 27-patient cohort with Child Pugh A cirrhosis. The pharmacokinetic profile of DEB TACE was compared with matched cTACE controls. DEB TACE demonstrated a favorable profile by sharply decreasing the passage of doxorubicin into the systemic circulation. The objective response rate (complete + partial response) at 6 months was 67% by EASL necrosis criteria for DEB TACE.[24]

Precision V is the only prospective, randomized controlled trail evaluating the efficacy of DEB-TACE compared to cTACE.[25] The primary end point was tumor response (EASL necrosis criteria) at 6 months. DEB TACE failed to show a response improvement over cTACE. However, DEB TACE resulted in a statistically significant reduction in liver toxicity and doxorubicin related adverse events, compared with cTACE. Subset analysis demonstrated an improved DEB TACE objective response rate in select patients with more advanced disease.[25]

Complications

In a 237-patient cohort treated with DEB TACE, overall treatment-related complications (not including postembolization syndrome) occurred in 13% of patients.[26] The Precision V study demonstrated a comparable rate of postembolization syndrome in DEB-TACE and cTACE.[25] However, serious liver toxicity and doxorubicin adverse effects were significantly lower with DEB TACE versus cTACE.[25]

Radioembolization for Hepatocellular Carcinoma

Radioembolization delivers high-dose internal radiation to the liver via the hepatic artery. This technique differs from external beam radiation therapy, where hepatic radiosensitivity limits the amount of radiation that can be delivered before the development radiation-induced liver disease (RILD), especially in cirrhotic livers.[27–29]

Radioembolization is typically performed with small microspheres coated with yttrium-90 (^{90}Y), a beta-emitting isotope. Given the hypervascularity of HCC, ^{90}Y microspheres injected into the hepatic artery are preferentially concentrated in the tumor-containing liver relative to the nontumorous liver.[16] These microspheres emit high-energy, low-penetration radiation (about 2.5 mm) to the tumor while sparing much of the background liver parenchyma. There are 2 commercially available ^{90}Y devices, TheraSphere (BTG International, London, United Kingdom) and SIR-Spheres (Sirtex Medical, Sydney, Australia). TheraSphere is a glass microsphere, 20 to 30 μg size with a high specific activity (2500 Bq) per sphere. SIR-Spheres is a resin microsphere, 20 to 60 μg size with a lower specific activity (50 Bq) per sphere.[16] In distinction to cTACE and DEB TACE, hepatic artery occlusion is not intended with radioembolization.[23] Instead, microspheres lodge in the tumor microenvironment and emit lethal beta radiation, with the formation of reactive oxygen species.[30] The lack of macroscopic vessel occlusions, limits typical postembolization syndrome, and therapy can be administered as an outpatient.[23,27]

Patient selection

The safety of ^{90}Y hepatic radioembolization is documented in several phase 1 and phase 2 investigations.[27,31,32] Patient eligibility parallels criteria for chemoembolization with a few notable exceptions. Patients are not eligible if hepatopulmonary shunting on a macroaggregated albumin (MAA) scan exceeds threshold lung doses or if vascular anatomy is such that spheres would be deposited in the gastrointestinal tract. These absolute contraindications prevent radiation pneumonitis and radiation-induced gut ulceration.[16] The microembolic nature of hepatic radioembolization supports its use in patients with portal vein thrombosis, thus limiting the risk of ischemic hepatitis. A phase 2 study in patients with HCC, with and without portal vein thrombosis (PVT), treated with glass radioembolization, showed a favorable toxicity profile and tumor response rate for branch and lobar PVT.[33]

Evidence and outcome

Cohort and retrospective studies describe the efficacy of radioembolization in the treatment of HCC.[16] Raiz and colleagues[34] reported the correlation between radiologic and pathologic findings in HCC patients treated with radioembolization, prior to resection or transplantation. All target lesions demonstrated some degree of histologic necrosis, and 23 of 38 (61%) lesions showed complete pathologic necrosis. Complete response by EASL necrosis criteria correlated with complete pathologic necrosis in all patients, thus supporting the notion that decreased enhancement of the target lesion corresponds to actual histologic necrosis (**Fig. 3**).

No RCT exists comparing radioembolization with established treatments for HCC.[16] A 2-cohort study compared radioembolization with chemoembolization in patients not eligible for curative therapy. Overall survival was slightly better in the radioembolization group compared with the chemoembolization group (median survival, 11.5 vs 8.5 months; P<.05), yet selection criteria yielded a bias toward milder disease in the radioembolization group.[35] A comparative effectiveness study described treatment outcomes of radioembolization and chemoembolization in a 245-patient cohort with unresectable HCC. Radioembolization resulted in a longer time to progression (TTP) and less toxicity than chemoembolization. However, overall survival did not differ between the 2 techniques, likely because of competing risks of death from HCC and cirrhosis. Posthoc analysis concluded that a sample size of greater than 1000 patients would be needed to establish survival equivalence of radioembolization and chemoembolization.[36]

Complications

Adverse events from radioembolization are different from those of chemoembolization. Postembolization syndrome is rare, and fatigue is common. Serious complications can result from nontarget radiation, including gastrointestinal ulceration, cholecystitis, pancreatitis, and radiation pneumonitis. Radiation-induced liver disease is rare when proper patient selection criteria are utilized.[29,37]

METASTATIC LIVER DISEASE
Background

In patients with cancer, spread to the liver is a common cause of death. Colorectal cancer is the second most commonly diagnosed cancer, and the liver is the most common site of metastatic disease, occurring in 20% to 30% of patients at presentation, with up to 60% developing liver metastatic disease over the course of treatment.[38–40] Most patients with colorectal liver metastases will die because of this disease burden.[41] Complete surgical resection offers the best chance of long-term survival, with 5 year survival rates of about 50%.[42] However, only about 25% of patients with colorectal liver metastases are candidates for resection at presentation.[43] Moreover, for patients who have undergone resection, tumor recurrence rates approach 50%.[44] For unresectable metastatic colorectal cancer (mCRC), systemic chemotherapy is standard first-line treatment. Despite significant advances in systemic chemotherapy and biologic agents, most patients develop progressive disease.[39] As such various interventional approaches exist to increase the number of surgical candidates, provide

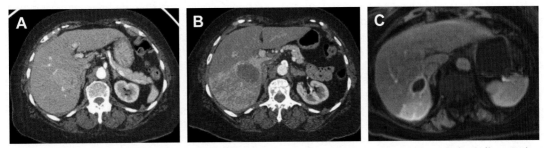

Fig. 3. (A) Contrast-enhanced CT shows arterial enhancing lesion consistent with HCC in a cirrhotic liver. Patient was treated with selective right posterior sector ^{90}Y radioembolization. (B) 1 month follow up contrast-enhanced CT shows a complete response by EASL necrosis criteria. Geographic enhancement in the posterior right lobe is consistent with postradioembolization changes. (C) 6 month after treatment, contrast-enhanced CT demonstrations decreased lesion size with atrophy of the treated posterior sector.

curative therapy, and improve survival in the palliative setting.

Transarterial therapy for liver mCRC is appealing, as nearly all the tumor supply is via the hepatic artery. The nontumorous liver is mostly supplied by the portal vein.[45] Intra-arterial delivery of therapy will preferentially target sites of metastatic disease while sparing the background liver. Chemoembolization, both conventional and drug-eluting bead, and ^{90}Y radioembolization are used to treat liver mCRC.

Patient Selection

Patients considered for chemoembolization and radioembolization therapy have unresectable/unablatable liver dominant mCRC and have often completed standard-of-care chemotherapy.[46,47] Some patients require palliative therapy for painful bulky tumors. Assessment of performance status, liver function and history of chemotherapy, radiation therapy and surgical resection are important factors. Often the decision to proceed with hepatic embolotherapy is made at a multidisciplinary tumor board.

Conventional Chemoembolization for Liver Metastatic Colorectal Cancer

cTACE is the standard of care for BCLC intermediate-stage HCC with a proven survival benefit in RCTs, as discussed earlier. The landscape of cTACE in mCRC is complex due to patient pretreatment with a variety of chemotherapeutic and biologic agents.

Evidence and outcome

Much of the data on cTACE in liver mCRC is retrospective case series from single centers. Vogel and colleagues[48] published a large prospective series, including 463 patients treated with cTACE. The 1-year survival rate after chemoembolization was 62%, and the 2-year survival rate was 28%. Median survival from the time of diagnosis of liver mCRC was 38 months, and from the inception of cTACE, median survival was 14 months. Despite these encouraging results, a recent Cochrane review concluded that hepatic chemoembolization in the metastatic setting cannot be recommended outside of randomized clinical trials.[49] The National Comprehensive Cancer Network (NCCN) version 2.2015 considers chemoembolization a category 3 recommendation (major NCCN disagreement that the intervention is appropriate) in highly selected patients with chemotherapy-refractory liver-dominant disease.

Complications

Postembolization syndrome is commonly seen. Major complications after chemoembolization are present in 2% to 7% of patients. These include hepatic insufficiency or infarction, abscess, biliary necrosis, and nontarget embolization.[50]

Drug-Eluting Bead Technique Chemoembolization for Liver Metastatic Colorectal Cancer

Similar to doxorubicin DEB TACE for HCC, drug-eluting beads loaded with irinotecan (DEBIRI) are used to treat liver mCRC. The principles of sustained drug release with concomitant embolization are the same; however, this product is less tested than doxorubicin DEB TACE. In pharmacokinetic evaluations of DEBIRI, there is minimal systemic exposure to irinotecan, thus allowing for high intratumoral drug delivery.[51]

Evidence and outcome

Fiorentini and colleagues[52] conducted an RCT comparing DEBIRI with systemic chemotherapy, specifically, leucovorin, fluorouracil, and irinotecan (FOLFIRI), in patients with liver mCRC who had failed at least 2 lines of systemic chemotherapy, including the prior FOLFIRI. The primary end point was survival. The median survival of DEBIRI (22 months) was significantly longer than that of FOLFIRI (15 months; $P = .031$). Progression-free survival (PFS) was longer in the DEBIRI arm (7 months) compared with the FOLFIRI arm (4 months; $P = .006$). Notable toxicity differences were identified between the 2 treatment arms. Significantly higher rates of neutropenia, diarrhea, and mucositis were identified in the FOLRIRI group. The only toxicity more common in the DEBIRI group was abdominal pain. In addition, quality-of-life measurements favored DEBIRI over FOLRIRI.

Richardson and colleagues[53] conducted a systematic literature review regarding the use of DEBIRI for the treatment of colorectal liver metastases. They identified a median survival time of 15 to 25 months with DEBIRI, which is roughly equivalent to outcomes achieved with modern systemic chemotherapy. However, the authors note that most patients included in the DEBIRI review had already failed first-line chemotherapy, thus making a favorable comparison to second/third line chemotherapies, where response rates fall to 5% to 25%.[54–56] There are no studies directly comparing DEBIRI and cTACE for mCRC, and as such, the decision is institutional preference (Riemsma, Bala and colleagues 2013).[49]

Complications

Most complications with DEBIRI are grade 1/2, including pain and nausea/vomiting, as is typical with postembolization syndrome.[53] Intra-arterial administration of lidocaine immediately prior to microsphere infusion may abate right upper quadrate pain. Hypertension was the second most common adverse advent in the aforementioned systematic review.[53] This finding may be a consequence of uncontrolled pain, as it coincided with the immediate postembolization period.

Radioembolization for Liver Metastatic Colorectal Cancer

Normal liver parenchyma has a poor tolerance to radiation, thus limiting the use of external beam radiation for liver mCRC. The dose required to treat solid tumors is estimated at about 70 Gy, whereas the tolerance of normal liver tissue is about 30 Gy.[57,58] The heterogeneous distribution of ^{90}Y microspheres, which concentrate in hypervascular tumors, along with a short tissue penetration, results in delivery of greater than 120 Gy to the tumor compartment, without intolerable toxicity to the background liver[59,60] (Fig. 4).

Evidence and outcome

Several randomized studies demonstrate that radioembolization combined with systemic chemotherapy potentiates treatment outcomes compared with systemic chemotherapy alone.[61,62] Van Hazel and colleagues[62] reported results of a randomized trial comparing systemic chemotherapy alone to combination therapy (resin radioembolization together with systemic chemotherapy), as first-line treatment for advanced liver mCRC. Twenty-one patients with unresectable/unablatable liver mCRC were randomized. Median survival was significantly longer for patients receiving combination treatment (29.4 months) versus chemotherapy alone

(12.8 months; $P = .02$). There were more grade 3/4 toxicities in the combination treatment group, yet no significant difference in quality of life.

Several non-randomized cohort studies expound the benefits of radioembolization in advanced mCRC. Lewandowski and colleagues[63] reported prospective data on 214 patients treated with glass radioembolization for unresectable liver mCRC refractory to standard of care therapy. Median overall survival after radioembolization was 10.6 months. On uni/multivariate analysis, independent predictors of survival included prior exposure to no more than 2 cytotoxic agents, thus supporting radioembolization treatment earlier in the course of disease. Most of the clinical toxicities were transient and controlled symptomatically. These results confirmed the safety of glass radioembolization in liver mCRC. A recent large retrospective study of 302 patients reported treatment results with resin radioembolization for unresectable, chemorefractory mCRC, including patients with extrahepatic disease.[64] Median survival was 10.5 months in this heavily pretreated cohort with an advanced burden of disease. Consistent with prior reports, most complications were minor and resolved without intervention. Overall, these results compare favorably with systemic salvage studies, in which median survival has ranged from 3 to 7 months.[65,66] The NCCN version 2.2015 considers radioembolization a category 3 recommendation in select patients with chemotherapy-refractory liver-dominant disease, based on a limited amount of evidence and varying institutional practices.

Further investigation with RCTs is needed to better define the role of radioembolization in the treatment paradigm of mCRC. Ongoing trials to address this need include FOXFIRE, a multicenter randomized controlled trial of FOLFOX (folinic

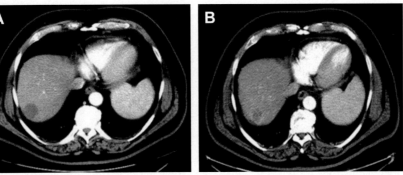

Fig. 4. (A) Contrast-enhanced CT with colorectal metastasis in the dome of the liver refractory to standard of care chemotherapy. At a multidisciplinary tumor board, lesion was deemed unresectable due to comorbidities and decision made to perform hepatic ^{90}Y radioembolization. (B) 9 month after treatment, contrast-enhanced CT demonstrates decreased lesion size; normalization of carcinoembryonic antigen occurred.

acid, fluorouracil, and oxaliplatin) with or without the addition of resin radioembolization, in patients with liver dominant mCRC.[67] The primary outcome is overall survival. Enhanced Peri-Operative Care for High-risk patients (EPOCH) is a multi-institutional RCT evaluating the addition of glass radioembolization to standard-of-care second-line chemotherapy for patients with liver-dominant mCRC. The primary end point is progression-free survival. With these pending clinical trials, the hope of a proven safe and efficacious treatment option for one of the most common causes of cancer death may be on the horizon.

Complications

The most common adverse effect of radioembolization is transient fatigue, with vague influenza-like symptoms, possibly due to low-dose radiation effects on the liver parenchyma. Clinically significant radiation injury to the gallbladder, intestine, or lung is rare. Lymphopenia is a possible sequela of radioembolization, due to the radiation sensitivity of lymphocytes, yet it is usually of no clinical import.[37]

BENIGN LIVER LESIONS
Focal Nodular Hyperplasia

Focal nodular hyperplasia (FNH) is a benign liver tumor predominantly found in healthy women, age 30 to 50 years.[68] FNH is often an incidental finding with no malignant potential.[69] It is usually asymptomatic and may be managed conservatively.[70] However, in up to 30% of patients, FNH produces pain, which may be due to mass effect on the liver capsule.[71,72] Likelihood of symptoms is dependent on size; symptomatic lesions have a mean size of 7.6 cm, while asymptomatic lesions are 4.4 cm.[73] Hepatic resection is the preferred treatment for symptomatic lesions or lesions with rapid growth.[73] When surgery is not feasible, often because of lesion location, embolization is a suitable alternative therapy.[74] Embolization is facile given lesion hypervascularity and presence of a central feeding artery in about 50% of cases[75] (**Fig. 5**).

Embolotherapy for FNH is described primarily in single-institution small case series. In a recent study by Birn and colleagues,[76] 12 patients were treated with bland embolization for symptomatic lesions. After embolization, 7 (58%) patients

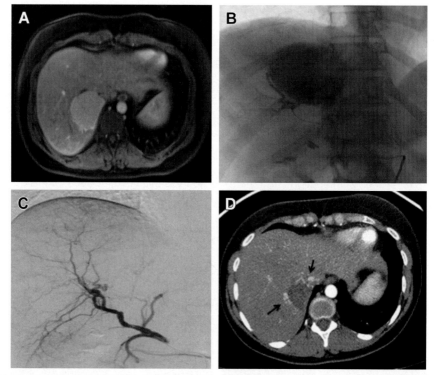

Fig. 5. (*A*) Contrast-enhanced MR imaging with a right hepatic lobe homogenous arterial enhancing lesion consistent with FNH. At multidisciplinary tumor board, decision was made to perform transarterial embolization given increasing size and symptoms, along with patient's desire to avoid surgery. (*B*) Angiogram shows a hypervascular FNH corresponding to MR imaging. (*C*) Postembolization angiogram demonstrates lesion devascularization. (*D*) 5-month follow-up contrast-enhanced CT shows decreased size of FNH with small peripheral foci of residual enhancement (*arrows*). Patient had complete resolution of symptoms, and no further therapy was performed.

had complete resolution of symptoms, and 5 (42%) patients had partial resolution of symptoms. Mean decrease in size of the lesion was 87%. The authors concluded that embolization is a suitable treatment alternative to surgical resection for symptomatic FNH.

Hepatic Adenoma

Hepatic adenomas are rare benign neoplasms that most commonly affect young women with a high estrogen state, including the use of oral contraceptives and fatty liver disease.[77,78] The risk of bleeding from an adenoma, increases with increasing size, subcapsular location and exposure to hormones.[79,80] A multicenter retrospective review identified no ruptured adenoma when the size was less than 5 cm.[79] Hepatic adenomas can undergo malignant transformation. Deneve and colleagues[79] reported a 4% risk of malignancy in resected adenomas, all of which were at least 8 cm in size. Additional risk factors for malignant transformation include male sex and B-catenin mutated subtype hepatic adenoma.[81,82]

Hepatic adenomas can be treated with cessation of oral contraceptives, surgical resection, liver transplant and minimally invasive options of ablation and embolization. Surgical therapy is recommended for hepatic adenomas approaching 4 cm in size and in patients who require long-term hormone treatment.[79] Arterial embolization can be used as an adjunct to surgical resection, or as definitive therapy, in patients not fit for resection. In a retrospective review, Deodhar and colleagues[80] reported the outcome of 8 patients treated with bland embolization, including a patient with ruptured adenoma with active bleeding. Adenoma regression was seen in 81% of lesions. In a follow-up comparative analysis of resection, embolization, and observation, embolization was frequently used to treat multifocal adenomas, whereas resections were mostly preformed for solitary lesions.[82] The local failure rate was similar between resection (4.2%) and embolization (8.1%).[82]

SUMMARY

Intra-arterial therapy, in the form of chemoembolization and radioembolization, are powerful treatment options for primary and metastatic liver disease, along with benign liver lesions. They yield safe and efficacious results, utilizing a minimally invasive treatment platform in patients with often limited therapeutic choices. Much of the data supporting embolotherapy are from retrospective series or noncontrolled prospective studies, with the exception of a demonstrated survival benefit of cTACE for HCC in 2 landmark RCTs. Future studies will continue to refine patient selection criteria, thus minimizing complications and prioritizing quality of life, together with prolonging survival.

REFERENCES

1. Kemeny N, Fata F. Arterial, portal, or systemic chemotherapy for patients with hepatic metastasis of colorectal carcinoma. J Hepatobiliary Pancreat Surg 1999;6(1):39–49.
2. Bosch FX, Ribes J, Diaz M, et al. Primary liver cancer: worldwide incidence and trends. Gastroenterology 2004;127(5 Suppl 1):S5–16.
3. Parkin DM, Bray F, Ferlay J, et al. Global cancer statistics, 2002. CA Cancer J Clin 2005;55(2):74–108.
4. Gallagher DJ, Kemeny N. Metastatic colorectal cancer: from improved survival to potential cure. Oncology 2010;78(3–4):237–48.
5. Davis GL, Alter MJ, El-Serag H, et al. Aging of hepatitis C virus (HCV)-infected persons in the United States: a multiple cohort model of HCV prevalence and disease progression. Gastroenterology 2010; 138:513–21, 521.e1–6.
6. Kim WR, Gores GJ, Benson JT, et al. Mortality and hospital utilization for hepatocellular carcinoma in the United States. Gastroenterology 2005;129(2): 486–93.
7. Forner A, Vilana R, Ayuso C, et al. Diagnosis of hepatic nodules 20 mm or smaller in cirrhosis: prospective validation of the noninvasive diagnostic criteria for hepatocellular carcinoma. Hepatology 2008;47(1):97–104.
8. Marrero JA, Hussain HK, Nghiem HV, et al. Improving the prediction of hepatocellular carcinoma in cirrhotic patients with an arterially-enhancing liver mass. Liver Transpl 2005;11(3):281–9.
9. Bruix J, Sherman M, American Association for the Study of Liver Diseases. Management of hepatocellular carcinoma: an update. Hepatology 2011;53(3): 1020–2.
10. Bruix J, Sherman M, Llovet JM, et al. Clinical management of hepatocellular carcinoma. Conclusions of the Barcelona-2000 EASL conference. European Association for the Study of the Liver. J Hepatol 2001;35(3):421–30.
11. Llovet JM, Bru C, Bruix J. Prognosis of hepatocellular carcinoma: the BCLC staging classification. Semin Liver Dis 1999;19(3):329–38.
12. Yau T, Tang VY, Yao TJ, et al. Development of Hong Kong liver cancer staging system with treatment stratification for patients with hepatocellular carcinoma. Gastroenterology 2014;146(7): 1691–700.e3.

13. Forner A, Reig ME, de Lope CR, et al. Current strategy for staging and treatment: the BCLC update and future prospects. Semin Liver Dis 2010;30(1):61–74.

14. Llovet JM, Bruix J. Systematic review of randomized trials for unresectable hepatocellular carcinoma: chemoembolization improves survival. Hepatology 2003;37(2):429–42.

15. Llovet JM, Ricci S, Mazzaferro V, et al. Sorafenib in advanced hepatocellular carcinoma. N Engl J Med 2008;359(4):378–90.

16. Lencioni R. Loco-regional treatment of hepatocellular carcinoma. Hepatology 2010;52(2):762–73.

17. Kakizoe S, Kojiro M, Nakashima T. Hepatocellular carcinoma with sarcomatous change. Clinicopathologic and immunohistochemical studies of 14 autopsy cases. Cancer 1987;59(2):310–6.

18. Liapi E, Geschwind JF. Intra-arterial therapies for hepatocellular carcinoma: where do we stand? Ann Surg Oncol 2010;17(5):1234–46.

19. Llovet JM, Real MI, Montana X, et al. Arterial embolisation or chemoembolisation versus symptomatic treatment in patients with unresectable hepatocellular carcinoma: a randomised controlled trial. Lancet 2002;359(9319):1734–9.

20. Lo CM, Ngan H, Tso WK, et al. Randomized controlled trial of transarterial lipiodol chemoembolization for unresectable hepatocellular carcinoma. Hepatology 2002;35(5):1164–71.

21. Camma C, Schepis F, Orlando A, et al. Transarterial chemoembolization for unresectable hepatocellular carcinoma: meta-analysis of randomized controlled trials. Radiology 2002;224(1):47–54.

22. Xia J, Ren Z, Ye S, et al. Study of severe and rare complications of transarterial chemoembolization (TACE) for liver cancer. Eur J Radiol 2006;59(3):407–12.

23. Salem R, Lewandowski RJ. Chemoembolization and radioembolization for hepatocellular carcinoma. Clin Gastroenterol Hepatol 2013;11(6):604–11 [quiz: e43–4].

24. Varela M, Real MI, Burrel M, et al. Chemoembolization of hepatocellular carcinoma with drug eluting beads: efficacy and doxorubicin pharmacokinetics. J Hepatol 2007;46(3):474–81.

25. Lammer J, Malagari K, Vogl T, et al. Prospective randomized study of doxorubicin-eluting-bead embolization in the treatment of hepatocellular carcinoma: results of the PRECISION V study. Cardiovasc Intervent Radiol 2010;33(1):41–52.

26. Malagari K, Pomoni M, Spyridopoulos TN, et al. Safety profile of sequential transcatheter chemoembolization with DC Bead: results of 237 hepatocellular carcinoma (HCC) patients. Cardiovasc Intervent Radiol 2011;34(4):774–85.

27. Geschwind JF, Salem R, Carr BI, et al. Yttrium-90 microspheres for the treatment of hepatocellular carcinoma. Gastroenterology 2004;127(5 Suppl 1): S194–205.

28. Ingold JA, Reed GB, Kaplan HS, et al. Radiation hepatitis. Am J Roentgenol Radium Ther Nucl Med 1965;93:200–8.

29. Gil-Alzugaray B, Chopitea A, Inarrairaegui M, et al. Prognostic factors and prevention of radioembolization-induced liver disease. Hepatology 2013;57(3):1078–87.

30. Sato K, Lewandowski RJ, Bui JT, et al. Treatment of unresectable primary and metastatic liver cancer with yttrium-90 microspheres (TheraSphere): assessment of hepatic arterial embolization. Cardiovasc Intervent Radiol 2006;29(4):522–9.

31. Salem R, Lewandowski RJ, Atassi B, et al. Treatment of unresectable hepatocellular carcinoma with use of 90Y microspheres (TheraSphere): safety, tumor response, and survival. J Vasc Interv Radiol 2005; 16(12):1627–39.

32. Sangro B, Bilbao JI, Boan J, et al. Radioembolization using 90Y-resin microspheres for patients with advanced hepatocellular carcinoma. Int J Radiat Oncol Biol Phys 2006;66(3):792–800.

33. Kulik LM, Carr BI, Mulcahy MF, et al. Safety and efficacy of 90Y radiotherapy for hepatocellular carcinoma with and without portal vein thrombosis. Hepatology 2008;47(1):71–81.

34. Riaz A, Kulik L, Lewandowski RJ, et al. Radiologic-pathologic correlation of hepatocellular carcinoma treated with internal radiation using yttrium-90 microspheres. Hepatology 2009;49(4):1185–93.

35. Carr BI, Kondragunta V, Buch SC, et al. Therapeutic equivalence in survival for hepatic arterial chemoembolization and yttrium 90 microsphere treatments in unresectable hepatocellular carcinoma: a two-cohort study. Cancer 2010;116(5):1305–14.

36. Salem R, Lewandowski RJ, Kulik L, et al. Radioembolization results in longer time-to-progression and reduced toxicity compared with chemoembolization in patients with hepatocellular carcinoma. Gastroenterology 2011;140(2):497–507.e2.

37. Riaz A, Lewandowski RJ, Kulik LM, et al. Complications following radioembolization with yttrium-90 microspheres: a comprehensive literature review. J Vasc Interv Radiol 2009;20(9):1121–30 [quiz: 1131].

38. Mahnken AH, Pereira PL, de Baere T. Interventional oncologic approaches to liver metastases. Radiology 2013;266(2):407–30.

39. Wang DS, Louie JD, Sze DY. Intra-arterial therapies for metastatic colorectal cancer. Semin Intervent Radiol 2013;30(1):12–20.

40. Weiss L, Grundmann E, Torhorst J, et al. Haematogenous metastatic patterns in colonic carcinoma: an analysis of 1541 necropsies. J Pathol 1986;150(3): 195–203.

41. Geoghegan JG, Scheele J. Treatment of colorectal liver metastases. Br J Surg 1999;86(2):158–69.

42. Wei AC, Greig PD, Grant D, et al. Survival after hepatic resection for colorectal metastases: a 10-year experience. Ann Surg Oncol 2006;13(5):668–76.

43. Khatri VP, Chee KG, Petrelli NJ. Modern multimodality approach to hepatic colorectal metastases: solutions and controversies. Surg Oncol 2007;16(1):71–83.

44. Bhattacharjya S, Aggarwal R, Davidson BR. Intensive follow-up after liver resection for colorectal liver metastases: results of combined serial tumour marker estimations and computed tomography of the chest and abdomen - a prospective study. Br J Cancer 2006;95(1):21–6.

45. Breedis C, Young G. The blood supply of neoplasms in the liver. Am J Pathol 1954;30(5):969–77.

46. Lewandowski RJ, Thurston KG, Goin JE, et al. 90Y microsphere (TheraSphere) treatment for unresectable colorectal cancer metastases of the liver: response to treatment at targeted doses of 135-150 Gy as measured by [18F]fluorodeoxyglucose positron emission tomography and computed tomographic imaging. J Vasc Interv Radiol 2005;16(12):1641–51.

47. Tellez C, Benson AB 3rd, Lyster MT, et al. Phase II trial of chemoembolization for the treatment of metastatic colorectal carcinoma to the liver and review of the literature. Cancer 1998;82(7):1250–9.

48. Vogl TJ, Gruber T, Balzer JO, et al. Repeated transarterial chemoembolization in the treatment of liver metastases of colorectal cancer: prospective study. Radiology 2009;250(1):281–9.

49. Riemsma RP, Bala MM, Wolff R, et al. Transarterial (chemo)embolisation versus no intervention or placebo intervention for liver metastases. Cochrane Database Syst Rev 2013;(4):CD009498.

50. Geschwind J-FH, Soulen MC. Interventional oncology: principles and practice. Cambridge (UK); New York: Cambridge University Press; 2008.

51. Martin RC 2nd, Scoggins CR, Tomalty D, et al. Irinotecan drug-eluting beads in the treatment of chemonaive unresectable colorectal liver metastasis with concomitant systemic fluorouracil and oxaliplatin: results of pharmacokinetics and phase I trial. J Gastrointest Surg 2012;16(8):1531–8.

52. Fiorentini G, Aliberti C, Tilli M, et al. Intra-arterial infusion of irinotecan-loaded drug-eluting beads (DEBIRI) versus intravenous therapy (FOLFIRI) for hepatic metastases from colorectal cancer: final results of a phase III study. Anticancer Res 2012;32(4):1387–95.

53. Richardson AJ, Laurence JM, Lam VW. Transarterial chemoembolization with irinotecan beads in the treatment of colorectal liver metastases: systematic review. J Vasc Interv Radiol 2013;24(8):1209–17.

54. Kang BW, Kim TW, Lee JL, et al. Bevacizumab plus FOLFIRI or FOLFOX as third-line or later treatment in patients with metastatic colorectal cancer after failure of 5-fluorouracil, irinotecan, and oxaliplatin: a retrospective analysis. Med Oncol 2009;26(1):32–7.

55. Carneiro BA, Ramanathan RK, Fakih MG, et al. Phase II study of irinotecan and cetuximab given every 2 weeks as second-line therapy for advanced colorectal cancer. Clin Colorectal Cancer 2012;11(1):53–9.

56. Cunningham D, Humblet Y, Siena S, et al. Cetuximab monotherapy and cetuximab plus irinotecan in irinotecan-refractory metastatic colorectal cancer. N Engl J Med 2004;351(4):337–45.

57. Dawson LA, McGinn CJ, Normolle D, et al. Escalated focal liver radiation and concurrent hepatic artery fluorodeoxyuridine for unresectable intrahepatic malignancies. J Clin Oncol 2000;18(11):2210–8.

58. Dawson LA, Normolle D, Balter JM, et al. Analysis of radiation-induced liver disease using the Lyman NTCP model. Int J Radiat Oncol Biol Phys 2002;53(4):810–21.

59. Salem R, Mazzaferro V, Sangro B. Yttrium 90 radioembolization for the treatment of hepatocellular carcinoma: biological lessons, current challenges, and clinical perspectives. Hepatology 2013;58(6):2188–97.

60. de Baere T, Deschamps F. Arterial therapies of colorectal cancer metastases to the liver. Abdom Imaging 2011;36(6):661–70.

61. Hendlisz A, Van den Eynde M, Peeters M, et al. Phase III trial comparing protracted intravenous fluorouracil infusion alone or with yttrium-90 resin microspheres radioembolization for liver-limited metastatic colorectal cancer refractory to standard chemotherapy. J Clin Oncol 2010;28(23):3687–94.

62. Van Hazel G, Blackwell A, Anderson J, et al. Randomised phase 2 trial of SIR-Spheres plus fluorouracil/leucovorin chemotherapy versus fluorouracil/leucovorin chemotherapy alone in advanced colorectal cancer. J Surg Oncol 2004;88(2):78–85.

63. Lewandowski RJ, Memon K, Mulcahy MF, et al. Twelve-year experience of radioembolization for colorectal hepatic metastases in 214 patients: survival by era and chemotherapy. Eur J Nucl Med Mol Imaging 2014;41(10):1861–9.

64. Saxena A, Meteling B, Kapoor J, et al. Is Yttrium-90 radioembolization a viable treatment option for unresectable, chemorefractory colorectal cancer liver metastases? A large single-center experience of 302 patients. Ann Surg Oncol 2015;22:794–802.

65. Wasan H, Kennedy A, Coldwell D, et al. Integrating radioembolization with chemotherapy in the treatment paradigm for unresectable colorectal liver metastases. Am J Clin Oncol 2012;35(3):293–301.

66. Seidensticker R, Denecke T, Kraus P, et al. Matched-pair comparison of radioembolization plus best supportive care versus best supportive care alone for chemotherapy refractory liver-dominant colorectal metastases. Cardiovasc Intervent Radiol 2012;35(5):1066–73.

67. Dutton SJ, Kenealy N, Love SB, et al. FOXFIRE protocol: an open-label, randomised, phase III trial of 5-fluorouracil, oxaliplatin and folinic acid (OxMdG)

with or without interventional Selective Internal Radiation Therapy (SIRT) as first-line treatment for patients with unresectable liver-only or liver-dominant metastatic colorectal cancer. BMC Cancer 2014; 14:497.

68. Trotter JF, Everson GT. Benign focal lesions of the liver. Clin Liver Dis 2001;5(1):17–42, v.

69. Bioulac-Sage P, Balabaud C, Wanless IR. Diagnosis of focal nodular hyperplasia: not so easy. Am J Surg Pathol 2001;25(10):1322–5.

70. Nagorney DM. Benign hepatic tumors: focal nodular hyperplasia and hepatocellular adenoma. World J Surg 1995;19(1):13–8.

71. de Rave S, Hussain SM. A liver tumour as an incidental finding: differential diagnosis and treatment. Scand J Gastroenterol Suppl 2002;(236):81–6.

72. Amesur N, Hammond JS, Zajko AB, et al. Management of unresectable symptomatic focal nodular hyperplasia with arterial embolization. J Vasc Interv Radiol 2009;20(4):543–7.

73. Gussick SD, Quebbeman EJ, Rilling WS. Bland embolization of telangiectatic subtype of hepatic focal nodular hyperplasia. J Vasc Interv Radiol 2005;16(11):1535–8.

74. Terkivatan T, Hussain SM, Lameris JS, et al. Transcatheter arterial embolization as a safe and effective treatment for focal nodular hyperplasia of the liver. Cardiovasc Intervent Radiol 2002;25(5):450–3.

75. De Carlis L, Pirotta V, Rondinara GF, et al. Hepatic adenoma and focal nodular hyperplasia: diagnosis and criteria for treatment. Liver Transpl Surg 1997; 3(2):160–5.

76. Birn J, Williams TR, Croteau D, et al. Transarterial embolization of symptomatic focal nodular hyperplasia. J Vasc Interv Radiol 2013;24(11):1647–55.

77. Rooks JB, Ory HW, Ishak KG, et al. Epidemiology of hepatocellular adenoma. The role of oral contraceptive use. JAMA 1979;242(7):644–8.

78. Bunchorntavakul C, Bahirwani R, Drazek D, et al. Clinical features and natural history of hepatocellular adenomas: the impact of obesity. Aliment Pharmacol Ther 2011;34(6):664–74.

79. Deneve JL, Pawlik TM, Cunningham S, et al. Liver cell adenoma: a multicenter analysis of risk factors for rupture and malignancy. Ann Surg Oncol 2009; 16(3):640–8.

80. Deodhar A, Brody LA, Covey AM, et al. Bland embolization in the treatment of hepatic adenomas: preliminary experience. J Vasc Interv Radiol 2011; 22(6):795–9 [quiz: 800].

81. Bioulac-Sage P, Balabaud C, Zucman-Rossi J. Subtype classification of hepatocellular adenoma. Dig Surg 2010;27(1):39–45.

82. Karkar AM, Tang LH, Kashikar ND, et al. Management of hepatocellular adenoma: comparison of resection, embolization and observation. HPB (Oxford) 2013;15(3):235–43.

Renal Masses
Imaging Evaluation

Richard H. Cohan, MD*, James H. Ellis, MD

KEYWORDS

• Cystic renal masses • Solid renal masses • Computed tomography • MR imaging

KEY POINTS

- Cystic renal masses of increasing complexity are more likely to be malignant. Imaging, rather than biopsy, plays a major role in follow-up of cystic renal masses.
- No single imaging feature can be used to distinguish malignant from benign solid renal masses on computed tomography or MR imaging; however, on some occasions, combinations of features can be helpful. Biopsy, rather than imaging, plays a major role in the evaluation of most solid renal masses.
- Renal cancers can be staged with more than 90% accuracy; however, identification of stage T3a disease can be problematic.
- RENAL nephrometry should be performed when evaluating renal masses, because this approach suggests the ease with which partial nephrectomy and, possibly, thermal ablation can be performed (as well as the likelihood of complications).
- Radiologists should be familiar with the posttherapy imaging appearance of renal cancers. This includes the appearance of hemostatic material, which is frequently used during partial nephrectomy, which can last for months after surgery, and which can mimic fluid collections or residual or recurrent tumor masses.
- Metastatic renal cancer often decreases in size following chemotherapy but may become necrotic without substantial size change. Size change can be described using the Response Evaluation Criteria In Solid Tumors (RECIST); however, RECIST alone is not always accurate in patients who respond by developing necrosis within metastases.

INTRODUCTION

After renal mass detection, imaging can sometimes help differentiate benign from malignant renal masses, stage the tumor, and assist surgical planning. In this article, currently used computed tomography (CT) and magnetic resonance (MR) imaging techniques for evaluating renal masses are summarized, with an emphasis on features used to predict whether a cystic or solid renal mass is benign or malignant. When successful in identifying a benign lesion, imaging can prevent the need for biopsy or avoid unnecessary treatment. Also reviewed is the staging of renal cancer as well as the increasingly common use of nephrometry for predicting the likelihood of complications and of success following partial nephrectomy. The post-treatment appearance in patients with renal cancer is also summarized.

RENAL MASS IMAGING TECHNIQUE

Renal masses are frequently detected on ultrasonography, with most identified masses being simple cysts. Ultrasound is effective in determining whether a detected cyst is simple and therefore

Disclosures: None.
Department of Radiology, University of Michigan Hospital, University of Michigan Health System, Room B1-D502, 1500 East Medical Center Drive, Ann Arbor, MI 48109-5030, USA
* Corresponding author.
E-mail address: rcohan@umich.edu

Radiol Clin N Am 53 (2015) 985–1003
http://dx.doi.org/10.1016/j.rcl.2015.05.003

benign. When complex cysts or solid masses are identified with ultrasound, or an indeterminate lesion (ie, pseudolesion vs true mass) is present, CT or MR imaging is usually required for further evaluation (**Table 1**).

When requested to evaluate a patient with a known or suspected renal mass, both CT and MR imaging examinations should include a series of unenhanced and intravenous contrast-enhanced thin-section images, with images reconstructed using no greater than 2.5- to 3.0-mm thickness and 2.5- to 3.0-mm reconstruction intervals. On MR imaging, precontrast images should include T1-weighted and T2-weighted series as well as dual echo gradient echo and diffusion-weighted imaging. Fat suppression is performed to identify macroscopic fat.

Renal enhancement on CT or MR imaging occurs in several phases.[1] During the arterial phase, which normally occurs about 20 seconds after contrast material injection begins, the aorta and renal arteries opacify briskly. There is also bright renal cortical, but little medullary, enhancement. During the portal venous or corticomedullary phase (CMP), which usually peaks at 60 to 70 seconds, the arteries do not enhance as briskly. There is still a pronounced difference in renal cortical and medullary enhancement, with the former remaining of much higher attenuation than the latter. During the nephrographic phase (NP), which usually occurs at 85 to 120 seconds, the renal medulla enhances more intensely and renal cortical enhancement fades, leading to homogeneous renal enhancement. This phase is thought to be most sensitive for renal mass detection.[2] Finally, during the excretory phase (EP), which usually begins at about 180 seconds, the still uniform renal parenchymal enhancement diminishes, while excreted contrast material appears in the renal collecting systems.

Contrast-enhanced images for renal mass CT or MR imaging must include at least one series obtained during the NP or EP, because renal masses are better detected and characterized when delayed enhanced images are acquired (**Fig. 1**). Additional contrast-enhanced series are occasionally required (see **Table 1**). For example, before partial nephrectomy or ablation, arterial phase imaging may be used for detailed assessment of the renal vasculature and its relationship to a renal mass, whereas EP imaging can be used to localize the relationship of a renal mass to the renal collecting system.

DIAGNOSTIC CRITERIA

On noncontrast CT, most of the solid renal neoplasms measure between 20 Hounsfield Units (HU) and 70 HU.[3] Masses that measure less than or greater than this range are most commonly simple or hyperdense cysts, respectively.[4] On noncontrast MR imaging, solid renal neoplasms can have a range of appearances on T1-, T2-, and diffusion-weighted images, with hypointensity on T2-weighted images being investigated as a potentially good prognostic indicator. Marked homogeneous hyperintensity on T2-weighted images is typical of a cyst, whereas marked homogeneous hyperintensity on T1-weighted images is typical of a hemorrhagic or proteinaceous cyst; in both cases, postcontrast imaging is helpful to confirm absent enhancement.

Table 1
Imaging protocols

Goal	CT	MR	Rationale
Renal mass characterization	Nonenhanced Postcontrast NP or EP	T1-weighted T2-weighted Diffusion-weighted Postcontrast NP or EP	Evaluate for macroscopic fat Assess enhancement Characterize tissue parameters (MR) Assess for complexity (cystic masses)
Treatment planning; nephrometry scoring[a]	Postcontrast arterial phase (optional for staging, ablation, nephrometry) Excretory phase	Postcontrast arterial phase (optional for staging, ablation, nephrometry) Excretory phase	Assess arterial vasculature and tumor supply Assess nearness to renal collecting system

All images reconstructed at 3.0 mm thickness or thinner, with contiguous or overlapping slices.
[a] Although EP imaging can be helpful in assessing how close the mass is to the collecting system, nephrometry can be performed without this phase of imaging because nearness to the sinus fat can be used instead.

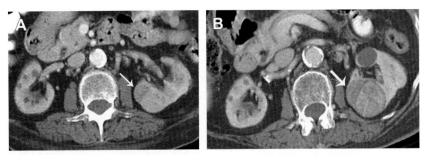

Fig. 1. Increased conspicuity of renal cancer on NP images. (*A*) An axial CMP CT image demonstrates multiple bilateral renal masses. A large renal cancer in the posterior aspect of the mid left kidney (*arrow*) is not well visualized, due in part to the persistent differential cortical and medullary enhancement. (*B*) The cancer is much more easily seen on the NP image (*arrow*).

The primary reason for obtaining both precontrast and delayed postcontrast images on CT or MR imaging is to determine whether a renal mass is enhancing.[5] Any detected measurable nodular enhancement indicates that a renal mass contains solid elements and suggests that the mass is likely a neoplasm. On multidetector CT, many consider an increase in attenuation of any components of a renal mass greater than 20 HU as indicating that solid elements are present. An increase of less than 10 HU is considered proof that there is no enhancement, whereas an increase of 10 to 20 HU is considered equivocal and indicates the need for further evaluation (with follow-up CT or MR imaging).[6] On MR imaging, the optimal way to determine whether a renal mass has any enhancing areas is to obtain subtraction images.

Although measurable nodular enhancement on CT or MR imaging nearly always indicates that a renal mass contains solid elements, the lack of detectable enhancement on CT does not exclude a solid lesion; this is particularly true for papillary renal cancers, which are characteristically hypoenhancing.[7] For this reason, complete CT evaluation of renal masses also should include an assessment of lesion attenuation heterogeneity. Most "nonenhancing" papillary renal cancers will demonstrate heterogeneity on postcontrast CT images. Also, most, if not all, papillary cancers that do not demonstrate enhancement on CT can still be seen to contain solid enhancing areas on subtraction MR images because magnetic resonance (MR) is more sensitive to contrast enhancement than is CT.[7]

Enhancement may occasionally be falsely identified as being present on CT because of volume averaging or pseudoenhancement. Volume averaging, which is a greater problem when renal masses are small (<1.5 cm in diameter), occurs when an axial CT image averages portions of the mass with adjacent enhancing normal renal parenchyma. The measured attenuation on such an image may then erroneously suggest that a cystic mass enhances. The effects of volume averaging can be minimized by ensuring that the CT image thickness does not exceed half the renal mass diameter.

Pseudoenhancement represents artifactual enhancement because of inaccurate correction of beam hardening. Renal mass pseudoenhancement occurs in small masses (<15 mm in maximal diameter) or masses that are centrally located (when a renal mass is completely surrounded by briskly enhancing parenchyma). When present, pseudoenhancement usually results in an increase in attenuation of less than 30 HU.[8] In contrast to volume averaging, pseudoenhancement cannot be eliminated by decreasing CT image thickness. It is also not reduced by use of modern CT reconstruction techniques, such as model-based iterative reconstruction.[9]

Cystic Masses

Simple cysts

Most cystic renal masses are simple cysts that can be definitively diagnosed as such with ultrasonography, CT, or MR imaging. On ultrasound, simple cysts are anechoic, demonstrate increased through transmission, have sharp well-marginated imperceptible walls, and fail to contain septations, nodules, or calcifications. On CT, simple cysts are of homogeneous water attenuation (−5 to +20 HU), have imperceptible walls, no nodules, no septations, and no calcifications, and fail to demonstrate any enhancement.[6] On MR imaging, simple cysts have homogeneous low T1-weighted signal, have high T2-weighted signal, do not have restricted diffusion, and do not have nodules or septations (**Fig. 2**).[6] Simple cysts should not demonstrate any enhancement on subtraction MR images.

Complex cysts and computed tomography

Some cystic renal masses demonstrate features indicating that they are not simple cysts but lesions

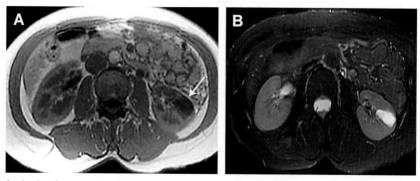

Fig. 2. Endophytic simple cyst seen on MR imaging. (*A*) T1-weighted image demonstrates a large hypointense mass in the mid left kidney (*arrow*). (*B*) The mass has high signal intensity on the T2-weighted fat-saturated images. Subsequent postcontrast images confirmed absent enhancement.

of greater complexity. In general, the more complex a renal cyst is, the more likely it is to be a cystic renal cancer. In 1986, Dr Morton Bosniak created a renal cyst classification system correlating features of complex cysts with the likelihood that the cystic mass will contain malignant cells.[10] The current version of this system,[6,11,12] which was designed to be used with CT, is the most widely used approach for evaluating cystic renal masses today. The system is summarized in **Table 2**, and some examples are provided in **Fig. 3**.

Of the different types of cystic lesions, it is worth commenting briefly on hyperdense cysts, which are cystic lesions that contain hemorrhagic or proteinaceous material. On CT or MR imaging, hyperdense cysts demonstrate all of the features of simple cysts with the exception of their attenuation or signal intensity. On CT, hyperdense cysts measure greater than water attenuation (>20 HU) both before and following contrast material administration. For this reason, most of these lesions cannot be distinguished from solid hypoenhancing renal

Table 2
Bosniak cyst classification system

Category	Features	Likelihood of Malignancy (%)	Management
I	*Simple*	0	No follow-up or treatment needed
II	*Minimally complicated* 1–3 thin/hairline septations Fine calcification Short segment of slightly thickened calcification Hyperdense (if ≤3 cm)	0	No follow-up or treatment needed
IIF	*Slightly more complicated* Hairline thin wall Multiple hairline thin septa Minimal smooth wall thickening or septal thickening Thick or irregular nodular calcification Hyperdense (>3 cm)	10–12	Follow-up imaging needed at 6 and 12 mo and then annually for 5 y
III	*Moderately complex* Thickened walls or septa with measurable enhancement Multiloculated	50–60	Partial or total nephrectomy
IV	*Very complicated* Measurable enhancing soft tissue adjacent to the wall or septa/nodules	100	Partial or total nephrectomy

From Silverman SG, Israel GM, Herts BR, et al. Management of the incidental renal mass. Radiology 2008;249:16–31; Hindman NM, Hecht EM, Bosniak MA. Follow-up for Bosniak category 2F cystic renal lesions. Radiology 2014;272:757–66.

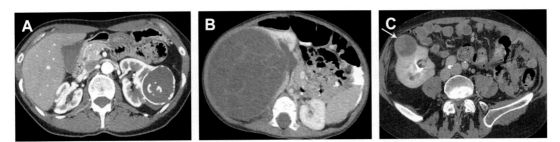

Fig. 3. Complex renal cysts demonstrated on contrast-enhanced CT. (*A*) Bosniak category 2F cyst. There is a large nonenhancing mass in the left kidney containing coarse peripheral and some central calcification. (*B*) Bosniak category 3 cyst. A large multiloculated mass in the right kidney contains multiple internal septations. (*C*) Bosniak category 4 cyst. A cystic right renal mass contains a large enhancing nodular area (*arrow*).

masses when only unenhanced or a single series of contrast-enhanced images are available (because it cannot be determined whether these masses are enhancing under these circumstances). However, it has been shown that nearly all homogeneous renal masses that measure greater than 70 HU on precontrast images are hyperdense cysts.[4] On MR imaging, hyperdense cysts may demonstrate high signal on precontrast T1-weighted images and high or low signal on T2-weighted images (**Fig. 4**). According to the Bosniak system, a hyperdense cyst should be classified as a Bosniak category II lesion if it measures 3 cm or less in size and if it is exophytic; however, once such a lesion exceeds 3 cm or if it is entirely endophytic, it should be considered a category IIF lesion.[11,12]

As seen in **Table 2**, according to Bosniak and others, imaging follow-up is usually recommended only for category IIF lesions to assess these lesions for stability (because category I and II lesions are benign nearly all the time and category III and IV lesions are treated, due to the high risk of malignancy). Follow-up of category IIF lesions is recommended for up to 5 years, because many malignancies grow slowly.[6] When follow-up imaging is performed, renal masses should be assessed primarily for changes in morphology rather than changes in size. Assessing primarily for changes in morphology is done because many benign renal lesions also enlarge over time and there is no evidence that most malignant cystic lesions grow more rapidly than benign lesions.

Complex cysts and ultrasound or MR imaging

Because Dr Bosniak's system was designed for CT, the frequency with which cysts in various categories turn out to be malignancies is likely different on ultrasonography and MR imaging. In one study, 20% of complex cysts had their categories upgraded on MR imaging, sometimes because MR imaging correctly identified complicating features not seen on CT and sometimes as a result of artifacts seen only on MR imaging.[13] The result of this upgrading would be that a smaller percentage of lesions categorized by MR imaging as category IIF, category III, and potentially category IV lesions are malignant in comparison to lesions categorized by CT.

Other considerations with the Bosniak system

Although the Bosniak classification is fairly reproducible in practice, there will not be complete

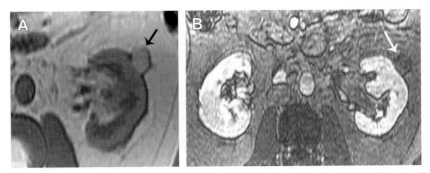

Fig. 4. Bosniak category 2 hyperdense cyst on MR imaging. (*A*) A small exophytic mass in the anterolateral aspect of the left kidney (*arrow*) demonstrates high signal on the T1-weighted image. (*B*) On the gadolinium-enhanced fat-saturated image, there is no enhancement (*arrow*). There is no wall thickening, septation, or nodularity.

agreement on renal mass categorization and management recommendations among radiologists, even among experts.[14] Furthermore, there are exceptions. In rare instances, a few malignant cells may be present in simple or minimally complex-appearing cysts, while some very complex-appearing lesions may be benign.[15]

Biopsy and renal cystic lesions

Percutaneous biopsy of complex cysts is often problematic. This procedure is usually only helpful if malignancy can be diagnosed. A negative biopsy can be confusing, because it is uncertain whether the failure to detect malignant cells indicates that a lesion is truly benign or merely that sparse malignant cells that are present have not been sampled. For this reason, the authors recommend that imaging follow-up alone be considered for category IIF lesions, that treatment or imaging follow-up be considered for category III lesions, and that treatment be considered for Bosniak IV lesions. The decision to treat is complex and based on the patient's age, patient's comorbidities, lesion size, and Bosniak classification. Biopsy of a cystic renal mass should be reserved for patients with higher category lesions who have comorbidities that may preclude definitive treatment.

Solid Renal Masses

Most solid renal masses are malignant,[16] with the most common malignancy being renal cancer, followed by urothelial cancer, and then lymphoma. It is estimated that approximately 20% of solid renal masses measuring 4 cm or less in diameter are benign,[16] with the most common benign renal masses being angiomyolipomas (AMLs) and oncocytomas.[17]

Angiomyolipomas

AMLs are benign neoplasms most often encountered as isolated lesions in middle-aged or elderly women, or in patients with tuberous sclerosis. AMLs can bleed, especially when large (>4 cm in diameter), and the hemorrhage can be life-threatening.

Most AMLs contain macroscopic fat, a characteristic that allows these masses to be identified with a high degree of certainty on imaging studies. AMLs that contain macroscopic fat possess internal areas that measure less than −10 HU on CT,[18] that demonstrate signal loss on fat-suppressed MR pulse sequences, and that exhibit "India ink" artifact at interfaces between the intratumoral fat and adjacent water-containing soft tissue on opposed-phase chemical shift MR (**Figs. 5** and **6**).[12,19] In the vast majority of cases, small areas of macroscopic fat in a solid renal mass are sufficient to allow for a diagnosis of AML to be made, with no need for biopsy confirmation.

Because AMLs are benign and small AMLs are unlikely to bleed, there is no need for treatment of small renal masses that contain macroscopic fat. There are, however, case-reportable exceptions to this rule. A small minority of fat-containing AMLs exhibit aggressive behavior and are considered malignancies. These aggressive AMLs, which represent a subset of the epithelioid AML group, do not appear to have any distinctive imaging characteristics to allow them to be differentiated from other AMLs[20]; however, they are so uncommon that it is generally agreed that daily practice should not be affected by the existence of these variants. In addition, a tiny number of renal cancers contain areas of macroscopic fat (**Fig. 7**).[21,22] As with aggressive epithelioid AMLs, given the rarity of macroscopic fat-containing renal cancers, their existence should not alter clinical practice, unless both fat and calcification are detected in the same mass (a feature extremely uncommon in AMLs, but more typical of at least some of the rare fat-containing renal cancers).

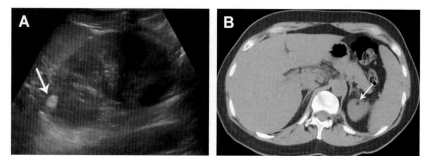

Fig. 5. AML on ultrasound and CT. (*A*) Sagittal ultrasound image in a 41-year-old woman demonstrates a tiny echogenic focus in the upper pole of the right kidney (*arrow*). There is no identifiable posterior shadowing. (*B*) Noncontrast CT shows that the mass is of very low attenuation (*arrow*). Region of interest measurements demonstrated a mean attenuation of −22 HU, diagnostic of AML.

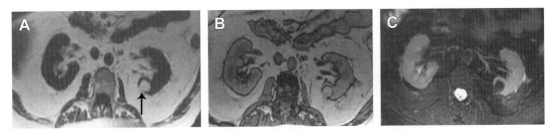

Fig. 6. AML on MR imaging. (*A*) T1-weighted image shows a high signal intensity mass in the left kidney (*arrow*). (*B*) The mass does not lose signal on opposed-phase images and there is a dark line ("India ink" artifact) between the mass and the adjacent renal parenchyma (at a fat–water interface). (*C*) The mass loses signal on fat-suppressed images.

Diagnosis of AML is more problematic on ultrasonography. The vast majority of these neoplasms are echogenic (see **Fig. 5**A); however, many small renal cancers are also echogenic, so assessment of solid renal mass echogenicity alone is not helpful. Some AMLs and very few renal cancers demonstrate posterior acoustic shadowing.[23] Some renal cancers, and very few, if any, AMLs demonstrate a hypoechoic peripheral halo.[23,24] Thus, some ultrasonographers are willing to make definitive diagnoses when either of these features is encountered in the setting of an echogenic renal mass. Unfortunately, most echogenic renal masses possess neither of these features,[23,24] and the safest approach is to perform a CT or MR imaging for additional assessment of all echogenic solid renal masses detected by ultrasound.[25]

Rarely, AMLs can be markedly exophytic and difficult to distinguish from perinephric liposarcomas. Differentiation between these 2 entities is important, because the former, if large, may require treatment with angioembolization or partial nephrectomy, while the latter may require extensive surgical resection, usually including ipsilateral nephrectomy. Several imaging features may allow for AMLs to be more strongly suggested, including identification of a renal parenchymal defect adjacent to the fatty mass, and tumor hypervascularity (**Fig. 8**).[26] If the diagnosis is uncertain, percutaneous biopsy with immunohistochemical staining (including human melanoma, black [HMB]-45) can usually make a definitive diagnosis.

Solid renal masses that do not contain macroscopic fat

Imaging is of limited utility in distinguishing among the many types of solid renal masses that do not contain macroscopic fat. Features that have been evaluated on hundreds of prior CT studies include noncontrast CT attenuation, pixel distribution and histogram analysis to detect tiny foci of macroscopic fat in minimal fat-containing AMLs,[27,28] degree of enhancement with contrast material, rate of enhancement, differential enhancement within a mass, enhancement washout,[29–31] and the presence of central areas

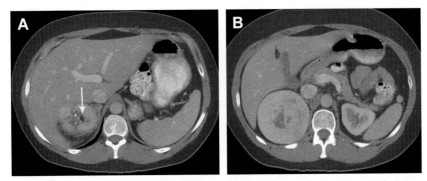

Fig. 7. Renal cancer containing macroscopic fat. (*A*) The cephalic aspect of a large mass demonstrates areas of both calcification and macroscopic fat (*arrow*). (*B*) More caudally, the mass is heterogeneous, but no other areas containing macroscopic fat are identified. At surgery, this lesion was diagnosed as a renal cell cancer with osseous metaplasia. The presence of fat within a solid renal mass is diagnostic of an AML in almost all cases; presence of calcification in addition to macroscopic fat makes atypical RCC more likely.

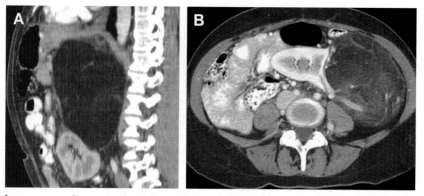

Fig. 8. Large fatty masses adjacent to the kidney. (A) On a sagittal reconstructed image, a large liposarcoma compresses the left kidney, but does not extend into the renal parenchyma. (B) In comparison, a large AML adjacent to the left kidney in another patient is associated with a defect in the kidney.

of low attenuation. These studies have led to the identification of several tendencies, some of which are summarized here:

1. Both minimal fat-containing AMLs and papillary renal cancers tend to have higher noncontrast CT attenuation than normal renal parenchyma or other neoplasms.[32]
2. Although clear cell renal cancers, AMLs, and oncocytomas demonstrate brisk enhancement in comparison to most papillary renal cancers (which enhance less avidly and on a more delayed basis), clear cell cancers demonstrate the highest attenuation among this group on CMP images.[30,31,33]
3. Only clear cell cancers (due to extensive intracellular lipid) and minimal fat-containing AMLs will demonstrate nonlinear signal loss on opposed-phase gradient echo images.
4. The central scar commonly associated with oncocytomas is often indistinguishable from the necrosis frequently seen in renal cancers and therefore is not a helpful diagnostic criterion.[34]
5. Segmental enhancement inversion, whereby initially briskly enhancing components of a renal mass subsequently become lower in attenuation than initially hypoenhancing components, has been described in oncocytomas,[35,36] but has been found to be uncommon in some studies, and therefore, not very helpful for distinguishing oncocytoma from renal cell carcinoma (RCC).[35]

Features previously evaluated on MR imaging include T1 and T2 signal intensity, chemical shift imaging, diffusion characteristics,[37] degree of contrast enhancement, rate of enhancement,[38,39] as well as other techniques.[40] Several MR observations have also been made, some of which are summarized here.

1. Unlike other renal tumors, most minimal fat-containing AMLs and papillary renal cancers have low T2-signal intensity.[41]
2. As with CT, although most solid renal neoplasms enhance briskly, papillary renal cancers tend to enhance to a lesser and more delayed extent than do other renal tumors.[7,38]

In the authors' opinion, no single imaging characteristic is definitive in allowing for a benign renal mass without macroscopic fat to be distinguished from a malignant one in most instances. The authors agree with the recent statement by Kang and colleagues[19] that, in many patients, "despite extensive study of morphologic and quantitative criteria at conventional imaging, no single CT or MR imaging techniques can reliably distinguish solid benign tumors, such as oncocytoma and lipid-poor angiomyolipoma, from malignant renal tumors."

Certain combinations of features may occasionally be strongly suggestive, however. If a mass demonstrates high noncontrast CT attenuation AND is hypoenhancing after contrast material administration, papillary renal cancer is the most likely diagnosis (Fig. 9). If a mass demonstrates low T2 MR signal intensity AND is hypoenhancing after contrast material administration, papillary renal cancer is the most likely diagnosis (Fig. 10). If a mass demonstrates opposed-phase chemical shift signal loss in the absence of an "India ink" artifact and is relatively hyperintense to cortex on T2-weighted imaging, then clear cell renal cancer is the most likely diagnosis (Fig. 11).

Centrally located solid renal masses

Some renal masses have a central location, with their epicenter in the renal sinus. The differential diagnosis of these lesions includes centrally located renal cancer, including the more aggressive collecting duct and medullary renal cancers (Fig. 12). Other centrally located renal masses

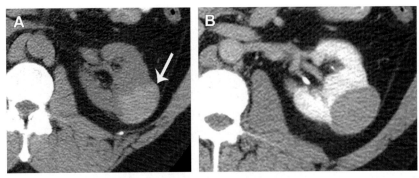

Fig. 9. Papillary renal cancer. (*A*) Unenhanced axial CT image demonstrates a renal mass that is of higher attenuation than normal renal parenchyma (*arrow*). The most common renal masses to display this feature are hyperdense cysts, minimal fat-containing AMLs, and papillary renal cancers. (*B*) The mass demonstrates enhancement on EP images (from 43 to 67 HU), which excludes the diagnosis of hyperdense cyst. It is not hypervascular, which makes AML less likely.

include urothelial cancer and lymphoma. Differentiation of urothelial from centrally located renal cancers can be difficult; however, urothelial cancer is more likely to be centered in the renal collecting system, to produce collecting system filling defects, to preserve the normal renal contour, to fail to demonstrate any cystic or necrotic areas, and to enhance homogeneously.[42]

On rare occasions, renal artery aneurysms can mimic enhancing hypervascular solid masses on CT (**Fig. 13**). Renal artery aneurysms usually, but not always, demonstrate some peripheral curvilinear calcification. This confusion does not occur as often with Doppler or color Doppler ultrasonography or MR imaging, where the vascular nature of these lesions can be identified more readily.

18-Fluorodeoxyglucose-PET
PET with 18-fluorodeoxyglucose (FDG) has mixed efficacy in evaluating patients with renal cancer. Although most renal cancers are very FDG-avid, others are only mildly so. Because FDG is excreted

by the urinary tract, differentiation of RCC from normal parenchyma can be difficult. When PET is combined with CT, however, sensitivity has exceeded 90%.[43] FDG uptake within a renal mass can help confirm that the mass is solid and not a cyst. Unfortunately, benign solid renal masses, such as some oncocytomas, and some benign cystic renal masses, such as calyceal diverticula, can also be FDG-avid,[44] leading to potential false positive diagnoses. FDG-PET may be more effective in detecting metastatic renal cancer (**Fig. 14**).[44]

Assessing growth of solid renal lesions on follow-up imaging studies
Most benign and malignant renal masses grow slowly with a linear growth curve (**Fig. 15**).[34,45–48] Although it has been suggested that rapid growth of a renal mass (of 5 mm or more within a 12 months) indicates an aggressive cancer is likely present,[49] studies have demonstrated that most malignant and benign solid renal masses grow at

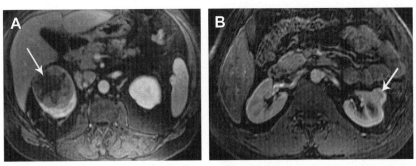

Fig. 10. Central areas of low T1-signal within solid renal masses. (*A*) A large area of low signal intensity seen on a fat-saturated gadolinium-enhanced T1-weighted MR image within a right renal clear cell carcinoma (*arrow*) represents an area of necrosis. This cannot be distinguished from a central scar seen in an oncocytoma. (*B*) A left renal mass in another patient contains a small area of low signal intensity on a gadolinium-enhanced T1-weighted MR image (*arrow*). This represents a central scar in an oncocytoma.

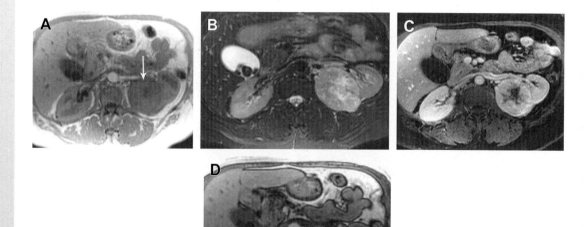

Fig. 11. Clear cell renal cancer. (*A*) T1-weighted MR image demonstrates a large mass in the left kidney, which has comparable signal intensity to the normal left renal parenchyma (*arrow*). (*B*) The mass contains central, likely necrotic, areas of bright signal intensity on the T2-weighted fat-saturated image. (*C*) The mass enhances briskly and heterogeneously after gadolinium-based contrast material administration. (*D*) On the opposed-phase T1-weighted unenhanced image, the mass demonstrates signal loss, but no "India ink" artifact. The MR imaging features are most consistent with a clear cell renal cancer.

comparable rates.[35,46,47] Therefore, rapid growth is only helpful for differentiation when it is present.

Biopsy and solid renal lesions

The only way in which many benign and malignant solid renal masses can be differentiated from one another is by tissue sampling, with either percutaneous biopsy or surgical resection. The risk of needle track seeding from following biopsy of a renal cancer is extremely low. Although biopsy of cortical renal masses is often easily undertaken,

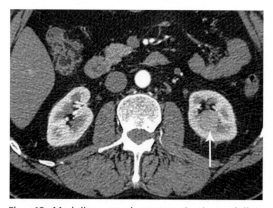

Fig. 12. Medullary renal cancer. Corticomedullary phase contrast-enhanced CT image demonstrates a small centrally located solid mass in the lower pole of the left kidney (*arrow*).

biopsy of centrally located renal masses should be performed with more caution, because the chances of tumor tract seeding is thought to be greater with urothelial cancer than renal cancer. Also, it is crucial to be sure that a centrally located mass identified on CT and referred for biopsy does not represent a renal artery aneurysm.

Assessment of a Solid Renal Mass Before Presumed Treatment

Suspected or known renal cancers should be staged according to the TNM system with CT or MR imaging and also assessed using a nephrometry scoring system.

Staging of renal cancer

CT and MR imaging are more than 90% accurate in staging renal cancers (**Fig. 16, Table 3**).[50,51] Renal mass size is easily evaluated. Thrombus can be detected easily in the renal vein and inferior vena cava (see **Fig. 16**B). Adjacent organ invasion is rare, but, when present, is usually obvious. Involved lymph nodes are frequently identified by their enlargement. Distant metastases, which are commonly seen in the adrenal gland, liver, lungs, pancreas, and bones, are usually well visualized. It is worth emphasizing the proclivity that renal cancer has to metastasize to the pancreas. In one study of pancreatic metastases,[52] renal

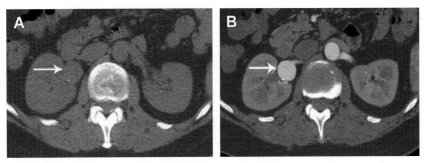

Fig. 13. Renal artery aneurysm. (*A*) Unenhanced and (*B*) arterial phase enhanced CT image demonstrates a briskly enhancing soft tissue attenuation structure in the right renal sinus (*arrow*). This lesion could be misdiagnosed as a centrally located hypervascular renal cancer. A minimal amount of peripheral curvilinear calcification is noted along the posterior aspect of the mass, and there is comparable enhancement to the aorta, consistent with the correct diagnosis.

cancer was much more likely to spread to this organ than any other primary neoplasm (**Fig. 17**). Pancreatic metastases may be better seen on arterial phase images.[53]

The most frequently encountered limitation of CT and MR imaging in staging of renal cancer concerns the occasional inability of these modalities to accurately identify tumor extension through the capsule into the perinephric space. Linear soft tissue attenuation or signal intensity structures are frequently seen in the perinephric space on CT and can be caused by edema, collateral vessels, or infiltrative tumor. Microscopic capsular invasion will also be undetected. One study[54] showed that identification of perinephric fat stranding and increased vascularity in the perinephric space was only 36% respectively and 56% specific for diagnosing capsular invasion (stage T3a disease).

RENAL mass scoring (RENAL nephrometry and PADUA classification systems)

Although some patients with renal masses must undergo total nephrectomy, the preferred method of treatment of small renal malignancies

(measuring 4 cm or less in maximal diameter) is now partial nephrectomy or, in cases in which patients are considered to be poor operative candidates, thermal ablation. Imaging evaluation can assist the urologist in determining the least invasive treatment that can be performed without major complications. Several systems have been promulgated to aid in treatment planning. RENAL nephrometry scoring[55] is most commonly used and is summarized in **Table 4**. In this system, the word "RENAL" is an acronym for the 5 graded components of this system: (1) *R*enal size, (2) *E*xophyticity, (3) *N*earness to the collecting system or renal sinus, (4) *A*nterior or posterior location, and (5) *L*ocation with respect to the renal poles (as determined by polar lines drawn on coronal images at the level where the medial lip of the kidney is interrupted by renal sinus fat). In this system, each component (except for anterior or posterior location) is assigned points on a scale of 1 to 3 and summed to derive the total score. Patients with masses whose RENAL nephrometry scores are low (4–6) have fewer complications after partial nephrectomy[56,57] or thermal ablation[58] than do patients whose

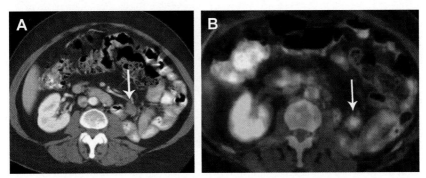

Fig. 14. A patient presented with back pain 4 years following left nephrectomy for renal cancer. (*A*) The contrast-enhanced CT image reveals a small soft tissue nodule just anterior to the left renal fossa (*arrow*), which could represent fibrosis, unopacified bowel, or recurrent tumor. (*B*) On the PET-CT fusion image, this nodule, which was subsequently confirmed to represent recurrent tumor, has avid FDG uptake (*arrow*).

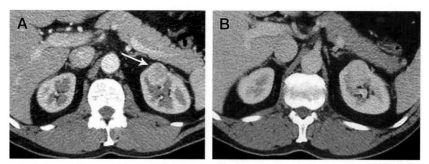

Fig. 15. Slow growth of renal cancer. (*A*) A small solid renal mass was detected incidentally on a contrast-enhanced CT (*arrow*). The patient was lost to follow-up. (*B*) A repeat CT performed 4 years later demonstrates that the mass enlarged only slightly. This mass, which was subsequently determined to be a renal cancer and is typical of most malignant renal masses, demonstrates a similar growth rate to that of benign renal neoplasms.

RENAL nephrometry scores are high (10–12). An example for renal mass scoring with the RENAL nephrometry system is provided in **Fig. 18**.

Another mass assessment system is the PADUA classification, where PADUA is an acronym for *P*reoperative *A*spects and *D*imensions *U*sed for *A*natomical classification.[59] This system, which is summarized in **Table 4**, differs only slightly from the RENAL nephrometry scoring system in that masses are assessed for nearness to the renal collecting systems and renal sinus separately (rather than together) and the polar location of masses is determined by a "renal sinus line" drawn at the first (for the upper pole) or last (for the lower pole) axial level where pericollecting system fat is seen entirely within the kidney.

Treatment of Renal Masses

Traditionally, renal cancers are treated with surgery, with nephron-sparing partial nephrectomy preferred. It is usually reserved for patients whose renal masses have lower nephrometry scores. Thermal ablation has been used in patients who are not good operative candidates. Both of these approaches have very high success rates. Recently, it has been suggested that some patients with biopsy-proven renal cancers can be managed alternatively with active surveillance. This alternative management is used because some patients, particularly those who are elderly and who have small renal cancers, are more likely to die with, rather than of their cancers. At some institutions, including the authors' institution, active surveillance is being performed in patients who have small masses ($\leq$4 cm in size) that have favorable histologic prognosis, as determined by percutaneous biopsy (low-grade papillary neoplasms and some chromophobe cancers, for example).[60,61] Active surveillance in these patients consists of periodic imaging, with no intervention performed unless the mass eventually exceeds

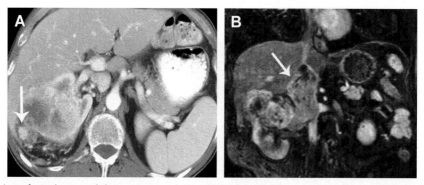

Fig. 16. Staging of renal cancer. (*A*) A contrast-enhanced CT image demonstrates a tumor nodule in the perinephric fat, confirming the presence of stage T3a disease (*arrow*). Although such a finding is very specific for capsular invasion, the much more commonly encountered finding of increased perinephric linear stranding or vascularity is not specific and could represent either tumor or merely edema and collateral vessels. (*B*) A contrast-enhanced fat-saturated T1-weighted coronal image in another patient demonstrates tumor invasion of the right renal vein and infradiaphragmatic inferior vena cava (*arrow*), confirming the presence of stage T3b disease.

Table 3
Computed tomography and MR imaging tumor, nodes, metastasis staging of renal cancer

T1a	≤4 cm in maximal diameter
T1b	>4–7 cm in maximal diameter
T2a	>7–10 cm in maximal diameter
T2b	>10 cm maximal diameter
T3a	Grossly extends into renal vein or its branches or invades perirenal space or renal sinus
T3b	Grossly extends into infradiaphragmatic inferior vena cava
T3c	Grossly extends into supradiaphragmatic inferior vena cava
T4	Direct invasion through perinephric fascia or ipsilateral adrenal gland
N0	No enlarged lymph nodes
N1	Enlarged regional lymph nodes
M0	No distant metastases
M1	Distant metastases

4 cm in maximal diameter or if the mass demonstrates rapid growth (increasing in size by 5 mm or more in 12 months). Using this algorithm, many patients with renal cancers have been followed effectively, with no development of metastatic disease and no change in patient prognosis.[60]

Unfortunately, accurate assessment of renal mass growth can be problematic. Intraobserver measurement variability (which is usually only about 2 mm[62]) may lead to the erroneous identification of growth or lack of growth on sequential examinations. Rapid growth of 5 mm or more can be identified erroneously about 5% of the time when NP images are used and about 25% of the time when CMP images are used.[63]

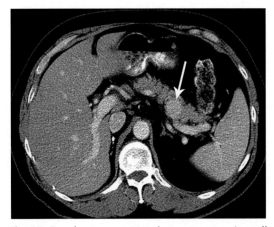

Fig. 17. Renal cancer metastatic to pancreas. A small homogeneous hypervascular mass is identified in the body of the pancreas (*arrow*) on this contrast-enhanced axial CT image obtained on a patient with renal cancer. Differential diagnosis includes pancreatic neuroendocrine tumor.

RENAL IMAGING AFTER RENAL MASS TREATMENT

Imagers are frequently called on to assess patients who have been treated for renal cancer, following either partial nephrectomy or thermal ablation. In both instances, imaging studies are performed to assess patients for locally recurrent disease, metachronous renal cancers, and regional or distant metastatic disease.[64]

After Partial or Total Nephrectomy

The American Urological Association (AUA) has recommended that following partial or total nephrectomy, patients should undergo baseline abdominal CT or MR imaging evaluation at 3 to 12 months.[65] Patients with T1N0 or T1Nx (with the "x" indicating the degree of lymph node involvement is unknown) disease should then undergo imaging with abdominal CT or MR imaging and chest radiography on an annual basis for 3 years. Additional follow-up is usually not necessary. For patients with T2-4N0 or Nx or patients with stage N1 tumors, thoracic and abdominal CT or MR imaging is recommended within 3 to 6 months of surgery, with follow-up imaging performed every 6 months for 3 years and then annually for an additional 2 years. Routine imaging with FDG-PET is not recommended.

In most patients, following partial nephrectomy, there is initially increased soft tissue inflammation at the surgical site, which is associated with a renal parenchymal defect and surgical staples. Hemostatic packing material is often placed at the surgical site, which can have an appearance similar to that of either a postoperative fluid collection or a residual mass.[66] These postoperative collections or masses can contain gas bubbles for prolonged

Table 4
Renal mass scoring systems

	RENAL Nephrometry			PADUA Classification		
	1 Point	2 Points	3 Points	1 Point	2 Points	3 Points
Renal mass size (cm)	≤4	>4–7	>7	≤4	>4–7	>7
Exophyticity (%)	≥50	<50	Endophytic	≥50	<50	Endophytic
Renal collecting system invasion	—	—	—	**Absent**	**Present**	—
Renal sinus fat invasion	—	—	—	**Absent**	**Present**	—
Nearness to collecting system or renal sinus (mm)	≥7	>4–<7	≤4	—	—	—
Anterior or posterior	No points given. Anterior = "a", posterior = "p", and neither = "x"					
Location with respect to polar lines (coronal images)	**Entirely above or below**	**Crosses**	**>50% across, across axial renal midline, or entirely between**	—		—
Location with respect to renal sinus lines (first or last axial image on which renal sinus fat is seen within the kidney)	—	—	—	**Superior or inferior**	**Mid kidney (between)**	—

Note: Differences between the 2 systems are set in bold.

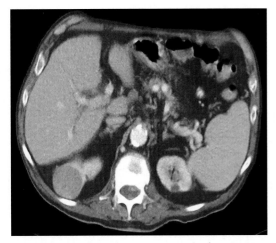

Fig. 18. RENAL nephrometry. A single contrast-enhanced CT image demonstrates a 3-cm (1 point), greater than 50% exophytic (1 point), posteriorly located ("p"), polar (1 point) renal cancer in the right kidney. On other images, the lesion was confirmed to lie more than 7 mm from the renal collecting system (1 point). Total nephrometry score for this lesion was 4p, indicating a low likelihood of complication following partial nephrectomy.

periods of time (**Fig. 19**). In one recent series,[67] nearly three-quarters of patients had postoperative fluid collections following laparoscopic partial nephrectomy, most of which were due to hemostatic material, with some of these lasting up to a year after surgery. Obviously, these collections could be mistaken for abscesses (especially when they contain gas) or recurrent or residual tumor. Unlike abscesses and tumor masses, these postoperative collections will gradually decrease in size and eventually resolve over time.

The major reason for routinely imaging patients after partial or total nephrectomy is to detect recurrent or metastatic tumor. In most instances, locally recurrent tumor is easily identified as an enhancing nodule at the surgical site, although it may occasionally be difficult to differentiate it from postoperative granulation tissue.[68] On some occasions, recurrent tumor may develop in adjacent inflammatory or fibrotic tissue in the perinephric space, or, even more rarely, along the tracts used for laparoscopic ports (**Fig. 20**).[69] Recurrent tumor nodules enlarge over time, whereas granulation tissue will be stable or decrease, so if there is any question about locally recurrent disease, short-term follow-up imaging may be warranted.

In rare instances, imaging may be performed to assess patients for surgical complications. Renal-collecting pseudoaneurysms and leaks, which can sometimes develop after partial nephrectomy, are usually easily detected[68]; however, arterial phase images most easily identify the former, and EP images are required to confirm the latter (**Fig. 21**).

After Thermal Ablation

The AUA recommends that patients who undergo thermal ablation should be imaged with CT or MR imaging at 3 and 6 months following the procedure to determine whether there is any evidence of residual or recurrent tumor.[65] Thereafter, annual

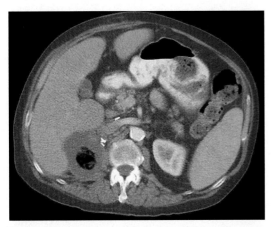

Fig. 19. Hemostatic material at partial nephrectomy site. A postoperative contrast-enhanced CT demonstrates a collection of gas and fluid attenuation material at the operative site following right partial nephrectomy, which could be confused for an infected fluid collection.

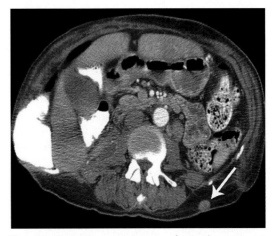

Fig. 20. Port site recurrence of renal cancer. A contrast-enhanced CT image demonstrates a new subcutaneous nodule in the left back (*arrow*) of this patient, who had undergone a laparoscopic nephrectomy for renal cancer. This represents a tumor nodule at a port site.

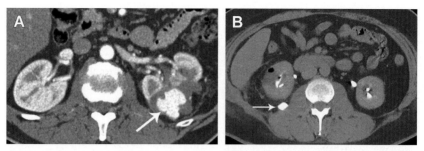

Fig. 21. Complications after partial nephrectomy seen on contrast-enhanced CT. (*A*) A large arterially enhancing structure at the site of surgery in the left kidney (*arrow*) is a pseudoaneurysm. (*B*) An EP image in another patient demonstrates excreted contrast material outside of the renal collecting system (*arrow*) consistent with a urine leak.

imaging with CT or MR imaging is recommended for a total of 5 years.

Often after renal mass thermal ablation, the ablation bed, as seen on CT or MR imaging, is initially much larger in size than the originally treated renal neoplasm, particularly when the treated mass was small. The ablation bed then decreases in size, albeit slowly.[70,71] In one study, ablation beds were, on average, relatively similar in size to the original treated renal mass at 1 to 2 years.[71] Other normally encountered findings in ablation beds on CT or MR imaging include increased perinephric stranding, gradual invagination of perinephric fat into the defect at the site of the ablated tumor, such that the ablation cavity can mimic an AML, and a halo of soft tissue attenuation surrounding the invaginated fat.[71] A thin rim of peripheral enhancement may also be seen normally, especially within 2 to 6 weeks following the procedure.[70,72] This phenomenon has been detected more frequently on MR imaging examinations.[71]

Follow-up imaging in patients after thermal ablation is primarily performed to detect residual or recurrent local neoplasm. Residual or recurrent neoplasm can be suspected when there are persistent areas of enhancement noted more than 2 weeks after the ablation, particularly if the enhancing components are nodular or crescent-shaped.[73] Recurrent or residual tumor may be best seen on arterial phase images. It is most commonly detected at the interface between the ablation bed and the normal renal parenchyma (**Fig. 22**). Residual tumor must also be suspected when the ablation bed is enlarging (rather than slowly decreasing in size), regardless of whether enhancing areas are detected.

Follow-up imaging occasionally detects rare procedural complications, including collecting system injury (which can lead to leaks or strictures), hematomas, pseudoaneurysms, renal infarction, bowel perforation, and chyluria

(resulting from postprocedure communication between the renal collecting system and the lymphatics). Of these, chyluria is the most common and the least concerning, manifesting as a fat-fluid level within the urinary bladder.

After Chemotherapy

Patients who develop regional or distant metastases from renal cancer are treated with chemotherapeutic agents, with multikinase inhibitors used frequently. Although, in the past, response to treatment has been assessed by evaluating changes in tumor size (eg, RECIST 1.1 [response evaluation criteria in solid tumors]), it has become apparent that the new chemotherapeutic agents frequently produce tumor necrosis as the tumor responds, with or without a decrease in tumor size (**Fig. 23**). For this reason, metastatic foci

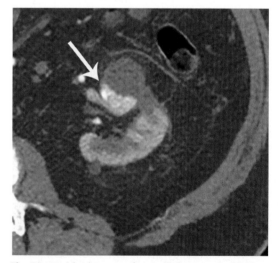

Fig. 22. Residual tumor after radiofrequency ablation. A large crescent of enhancing tissue between the ablation bed and the normal renal parenchyma (*arrow*) represents residual tumor. This was treated successfully with a repeat ablation.

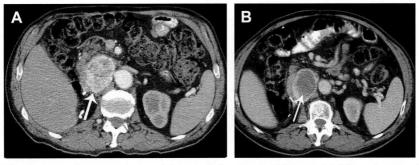

Fig. 23. Partial response of metastatic renal cancer following multikinase inhibitor therapy. (*A*) Contrast-enhanced axial CT image demonstrates a large hypervascular metastatic right aortocaval lymph node in this patient who had previously undergone right nephrectomy for renal cancer (*arrow*). (*B*) Ten months after the institution of therapy, the tumor mass has not decreased in size; however, it is of much lower attenuation (*arrow*), indicating extensive tumor necrosis.

evaluated on follow-up imaging should be assessed for changes in the degree of enhancement as well as changes in size.

SUMMARY

Although imaging continues to be relied on to categorize solid and cystic renal masses, it is often not possible to provide a definitive malignant or benign diagnosis by imaging despite recent advances in the field. As a result, percutaneous biopsy has emerged as a primary method for providing a definitive diagnosis for non-fat-containing solid renal masses. When a patient with a suspected or known renal cancer is imaged with CT or MR imaging, radiologists should stage the tumor and perform nephrometry scoring to determine the likelihood of success or complications from partial nephrectomy or ablation. Finally, following treatment, it is imperative that the radiologist be familiar with the normal appearance of a partial nephrectomy site or an ablation cavity, the appearance of occasionally encountered complications, and the measures of treatment response to systemic therapy.

REFERENCES

1. Yuh BI, Cohan RH. Different phases of renal enhancement: role in detecting and characterizing renal masses during helical CT. AJR Am J Roentgenol 1999;173:747–55.
2. Cohan RH, Sherman LS, Korobkin M, et al. Renal masses: assessment of corticomedullary-phase and nephrographic-phase CT scans. Radiology 1995;196:445–51.
3. Pooler BD, Pickhardt PJ, O'Connor SD, et al. Renal cell carcinoma: attenuation values on unenhanced CT. AJR Am J Roentgenol 2012;198:1115–20.
4. Jonisch AI, Rubinowitz AN, Mutalik PG, et al. Can high-attenuation renal cysts be differentiated from renal cell carcinoma at unenhanced CT. Radiology 2007;243:445–50.
5. Hecht EM, Israel GM, Krinsky GA, et al. Renal masses: quantitative analysis of enhancement with signal intensity measurements versus qualitative analysis of enhancement with image subtraction for diagnosing malignancy at MR imaging. Radiology 2004;232:373–8.
6. Silverman SG, Israel GM, Herts BR, et al. Management of the incidental renal mass. Radiology 2008; 249:16–31.
7. Egbert ND, Caoili EM, Cohan RH, et al. Differentiation of papillary renal cell carcinoma subtypes on CT and MRI. AJR Am J Roentgenol 2013;201: 347–55.
8. Tappouni R, Kissane J, Sarwani N, et al. Pseudoenhancement of renal cysts: influence of lesion size, lesion location, slice thickness, and number of MDCT detectors. AJR Am J Roentgenol 2012;198: 133–7.
9. Shampain KL, Davenport MS, Cohan RH, et al. Effect of model-based iterative reconstruction on CT number measurements within small (10-29 mm) low-attenuation renal masses. AJR Am J Roentgenol 2015.
10. Bosniak MA. The current radiological approach to renal cysts. Radiology 1986;158:1–10.
11. Israel GM, Hindman N, Bosniak MA. Evaluation of cystic renal masses: comparison of CT and MR imaging by using the Bosniak classification system. Radiology 2004;231:365–71.
12. Israel GM, Bosniak MA. How I do it: evaluating renal masses. Radiology 2005;236:441–50.
13. Hindman NM, Hecht EM, Bosniak MA. Follow-up for Bosniak category 2F cystic renal lesions. Radiology 2014;272:757–66.
14. Siegel CL, McFarland EG, Brink JA, et al. CT of cystic renal masses: analysis of diagnostic

performance and interobserver variation. AJR Am J Roentgenol 1997;169:813–8.

15. Hartman DS, Weatherby E, Laskin WB, et al. Cystic renal carcinoma: CT findings simulating a benign hyperdense cyst. AJR Am J Roentgenol 1992;159: 1235–7.

16. Frank I, Blute ML, Cheville JC, et al. Solid renal tumors: an analysis of pathological features related to tumor size. J Urol 2003;170:2217–20.

17. Thompson RH, Kurta JM, Kaag M, et al. Tumor size is associated with malignant potential in renal cell carcinoma cases. J Urol 2009;181:2033–6.

18. Davenport MS, Neville AM, Ellis JH, et al. Diagnosis of renal angiomyolipoma with hounsfield unit thresholds: effect of size and region of interest and nephrographic phase imaging. Radiology 2011;260:158–65.

19. Kang SK, Huang WC, Panharipande PV, et al. Solid renal masses: what the numbers tell us. AJR Am J Roentgenol 2014;202:1196–206.

20. Ryan MJ, Francis IR, Cohan RH, et al. Imaging appearance of renal epithelioid angiomyolipomas. J Comput Assist Tomogr 2013;37:957–61.

21. Helenon O, Merran S, Paraf F, et al. Unusual fat-containing tumors of the kidney: a diagnostic dilemma. Radiographics 1997;17:129–44.

22. Wasser EJ, Shyn PB, Riveros-Angel M, et al. Renal cell carcinoma containing abundant non-calcified fat. Abdom Imaging 2013;38:598–602.

23. Siegel CL, Middleton WD, Teefy SA, et al. Angiomyolipoma and renal cell carcinoma: US differentiation. Radiology 1996;198:789–93.

24. Yamashita Y, Ueno S, Makita O, et al. Hyperechoic renal tumors: anechoic rim and intratumoral cysts in US differentiation of renal cell carcinoma from angiomyolipoma. Radiology 1993;188:179–92.

25. Farrelly C, Delaney H, McDermott R, et al. Do all non-calcified echogenic renal lesions found on ultrasound need further evaluation with CT? Abdom Imaging 2008;33:44–7.

26. Israel GM, Bosniak MA, Slywotzky CM, et al. CT differentiation of large exophytic renal angiomyolipomas and perirenal liposarcomas. AJR Am J Roentgenol 2005;179:769–73.

27. Catalano OA, Samir AE, Sahani DV, et al. Pixel distribution analysis: can it be used to distinguish clear cell carcinomas from angiomyolipomas with minimal fat? Radiology 2008;247:738–46.

28. Simpfendorfer C, Herts BR, Motta-Ramirez GA, et al. Angiomyolipoma with minimal fat on MDCT: can counts of negative attenuation pixels aid diagnosis? AJR Am J Roentgenol 2009;192:438–43.

29. Bird VG, Kanagarajah P, Morillo G, et al. Differentiation of oncocytoma and renal cell carcinoma in small renal masses (<4 cm): the role of 4-phase computerized tomography. World J Urol 2011;29:787–92.

30. Pierorazio PM, Hyams ES, Tsai S, et al. Multiphase enhancement patterns of small renal masses (<4 cm) on preoperative computed tomography: utility for distinguishing subtypes of renal cell carcinoma, angiomyolipoma, and oncocytoma. Urology 2013;81:1265–72.

31. Young JR, Margolis D, Sauk S, et al. Clear cell renal cell carcinoma: discrimination from other renal cell carcinoma subtypes and oncocytoma at multiphasic multidetector CT. Radiology 2013;267:444–53.

32. Zhang YY, Luo S, Liu Y, et al. Angiomyolipoma with minimal fat: differentiation from papillary renal cell carcinoma by helical CT. Clin Radiol 2013;68: 365–70.

33. Kim MH, Lee JB, Cho G, et al. MDCT-based scoring system for differentiating angiomyolipoma with minimal fat from renal cell carcinoma. Acta Radiol 2013; 54:1201–9.

34. Choudhary S, Rajesh A, Mayer NJ, et al. Renal oncocytoma: CT features cannot reliably distinguish oncocytoma from other renal neoplasms. Clin Radiol 2009;64:517–22.

35. O' Malley ME, Tran P, Hanbidge A, et al. Small renal oncocytomas: is segmental enhancement inversion a characteristic finding at biphasic MDCT? AJR Am J Roentgenol 2012;199:1312–5.

36. Woo S, Cho JY, Kim SY, et al. Segmental enhancement inversion of small renal oncocytoma: differences in prevalence according to tumor size. AJR Am J Roentgenol 2013;200:1054–9.

37. Sevcenco S, Heinz-Peer G, Ponhold L, et al. Utility and limitations of 3-Tesla diffusion-weighted magnetic resonance imaging for differentiation of renal tumors. Eur J Radiol 2014;83:909–13.

38. Sun MRM, Ngo L, Genega EM, et al. Renal cell carcinoma: dynamic contrast-enhanced MR imaging for differentiation of tumor subtypes—correlation with pathologic findings. Radiology 2009;250:793–802.

39. Kim JH, Bae JH, Lee KW, et al. Predicting the histology of small renal masses using preoperative dynamic contrast-enhanced magnetic resonance imaging. Urology 2012;80:872–6.

40. Kim JK, Kim HS, Jang YJ, et al. Renal angiomyolipoma with minimal fat: differentiation from other neoplasms at double-echo chemical shift FLASH MR imaging. Radiology 2006;239:274–80.

41. Oliva MR, Glickman JN, Zou KH, et al. Renal cell carcinoma: T1 and T2 signal intensity characteristics of papillary and clear cell types correlated with pathology. AJR Am J Roentgenol 2009;192:1524–30.

42. Raza SA, Sohaib SA, Sahdev A, et al. Centrally infiltrating renal masses on CT: differentiating intrarenal transitional cell carcinoma from centrally located renal cell carcinoma. AJR Am J Roentgenol 2012; 198:846–53.

43. Wang HY, Ding HJ, Chen JH, et al. Meta-analysis of the diagnostic performance of [18F]FDG-PET and PET/CT in renal cell carcinoma. Cancer Imaging 2012;12:464–74.

44. Zukotynski K, Lewis A, O'Regan K, et al. PET/CT and renal pathology: a blind spot for radiologists? Part I, primary pathology. AJR Am J Roentgenol 2012;199: W163–7.

45. Bosniak MA, Birnbaum BA, Krinsky GA, et al. Small renal parenchymal neoplasms: further observations on growth. Radiology 1995;197:589–97.

46. Zhang J, Kang SK, Wang L, et al. Distribution of renal tumor growth rates determined by using serial volumetric CT measurements. Radiology 2009;250:137–44.

47. Kawaguchi S, Fernandes KA, Finelli FA, et al. Most oncocytomas appear to grow: observations of tumor kinetics with active surveillance. J Urol 2011;186: 1218–22.

48. Choi SJ, Jim HS, Ahn SJ, et al. Differentiating radiological features of rapid- and slow-growing renal cell carcinoma using multidetector computed tomography. J Comput Assist Tomogr 2012;36:313–8.

49. Pierorazio PM, Hyams ES, Mullens JK, et al. Active surveillance of small renal masses. Rev Urol 2012; 14:13–9.

50. Johnson CD, Dunnick NR, Cohan RH, et al. Renal adenocarcinoma: CT staging of 100 tumors. AJR Am J Roentgenol 1987;148:59–63.

51. Spero M, Brkljacic B, Kolaric B, et al. Preoperative staging of renal cell carcinoma using magnetic resonance imaging: comparison with pathological staging. Clin Imaging 2010;34:441–7.

52. Palmowski M, Hacke N, Satzl S, et al. Metastases to the pancreas: characterization by morphology and contrast enhancement features on CT and MRI. Pancreatology 2008;9:199–203.

53. Corwin MT, Lamba R, Wilson M, et al. Renal cell carcinoma metastases to the pancreas: value of arterial imaging. Acta Radiol 2013;54:349–54.

54. Tsili AC, Goussia AC, Baltogiannis D, et al. Perirenal fat invasion on renal cell carcinoma: evaluation with multidetector computed tomography, a multivariate analysis. J Comput Assist Tomogr 2013; 37:450–7.

55. Kutikov A, Uzzo RG. The R.E.N.A.L. nephrometry score: a comprehensive standardized system for quantitating renal tumor size, location and depth. J Urol 2009;182:844–53.

56. Ellison JS, Montgomery JS, Hafez KS, et al. Association of RENAL nephrometry score with outcomes of minimally invasive partial nephrectomy. Int J Urol 2013;20:564–70.

57. Liu ZW, Olweny EO, Yin G, et al. Prediction of perioperative outcomes following minimally invasive partial nephrectomy: role of R.E.N.A.L. nephrometry score. World J Urol 2013;31:1183–90.

58. Schmitt GD, Thompson RH, Kuruo AN, et al. Usefulness of R.E.N.A.L. nephrometry scoring system for predicting outcomes and complications of percutaneous ablation of 751 renal tumors. J Urol 2013;189:30–5.

59. Ficarra V, Novara G, Secco S, et al. Preoperative aspects and dimensions used for an anatomical (PADUA) classification of renal tumours in patients who are candidates for nephron-sparing surgery. Eur Urol 2009;56:786–93.

60. Haramis G, Mues AC, Rosales JC, et al. Natural history of renal cortical neoplasms during active surveillance with follow-up longer than 5 years. Urology 2011;77:787–91.

61. Halverson SJ, Kunju LP, Bhalla R, et al. Accuracy of determining small renal mass management with risk stratified biopsies: confirmation by final pathology. J Urol 2013;189:441–6.

62. Punnen S, Haider MA, Lockwood G, et al. Variability in size measurement of renal masses smaller than 4 cm on computerized tomography. J Urol 2006;176: 2386–90.

63. Orton LP, Cohan RH, Davenport MS, et al. Variability in computed tomography diameter measurements of solid renal masses. Abdom Imaging 2014;39:533–42.

64. Ng CS, Wood CG, Silverman PM, et al. Renal cell carcinoma: diagnosis, staging, and surveillance. AJR Am J Roentgenol 2008;191:1220–32.

65. Donat SM, Diaz M, Bishoff JT, et al. Follow-up for clinically localized renal neoplasms: AUA guideline. J Urol 2013;190:407–16.

66. Pai D, Willatt JM, Korobkin M, et al. CT appearances following laparoscopic partial nephrectomy for renal cell carcinoma using a rolled cellulose bolster. Cancer Imaging 2010;10:161–8.

67. Hecht EM, Bennett GL, Brown KW, et al. Laparoscopic and open partial nephrectomy: frequency and long-term follow-up of postoperative collections. Radiology 2010;255:476–84.

68. Lall CG, Patel HP, Fujimoto S, et al. Making sense of postoperative CT imaging following laparoscopic partial nephrectomy. Clin Radiol 2012;67:675–86.

69. Ramirez PT, Wolf JK, Levenback C. Laparoscopic port-site metastases: etiology and prevention. Gynecol Oncol 2003;91:179–89.

70. Rutherford EE, Cast JEI, Breen DJ. Immediate and long-term CT appearances following radiofrequency ablation of renal tumours. Clin Radiol 2008;63:220–30.

71. Davenport M, Caoili EM, Cohan RH, et al. MR and CT characteristics of successfully ablated renal masses status-post radiofrequency ablation. AJR Am J Roentgenol 2009;192:1571–8.

72. Tsivian M, Kim CY, Caso JR, et al. Contrast enhancement on computed tomography after renal cryoablation: an evidence of treatment failure? J Endourol 2012;26:330–5.

73. Kawamoto S, Solomon SB, Bluemke DA, et al. Computed tomography and magnetic resonance imaging appearance of renal neoplasms after radiofrequency ablation and cryoablation. Semin Ultrasound CT MR 2009;30:67–77.

Image-Guided Renal Intervention

Gregory T. Frey, MD, MPH[a], David M. Sella, MD[a], Thomas D. Atwell, MD[b],*

KEYWORDS

- Renal ablation • Embolization • Radiofrequency ablation • Cryoablation • Microwave ablation
- Complications

KEY POINTS

- The increasing incidence of small renal cell carcinomas (RCCs), particularly in older patients, has led to the expanding role of renal ablation in tumor management.
- Radiofrequency ablation (RFA) and cryoablation have proven efficacy in managing small renal masses.
- Adjunctive procedural techniques can be used to assist in successful tumor treatment.

BACKGROUND

RCC is the most common malignant renal tumor, accounting for an estimated 2% to 3% of all malignancies in the United States.[1] The American Cancer Society predicted that an estimated 63,920 new cases of kidney (renal) cancer would be diagnosed in the United States in 2014.[2] The incidence has plateaued in North America and Europe in recent years but is increasing in developing countries.[3]

The classic symptoms associated with RCC include hematuria, flank pain, and a palpable mass. However, patients with these symptoms usually have advanced-stage disease.[4] The survival profile for patients with localized disease is significantly better than that for those with regional or distant metastasis, emphasizing the importance of early detection.

Known risk factors in the development of RCC include smoking, hypertension, and obesity. Hereditary syndromes, including von Hippel-Lindau disease, hereditary papillary RCC, hereditary leiomyomatosis and RCC, and Birt-Hogg-Dube syndrome, are also risk factors. Widespread use of computed tomography (CT) and ultrasonography (US) for evaluation of nonspecific symptoms and other abdominal disease has led to an increased amount of incidentally diagnosed RCCs. These tumors are commonly of a smaller and lower stage.[4]

STAGING OF RENAL CELL CARCINOMA

The staging systems for RCC have gradually evolved from the Robson classification to the TNM system as defined by International Union Against Cancer and the American Joint Committee on Cancer. The TNM system was most recently revised in 2010.[5] The T stage consists of 5 stages: T0 to T4. Stages T1 and T2 and their subdivisions are defined based on size alone, while stages T3 and T4 are defined based on the degree of locoregional extension, which includes characteristics such as invasion of the renal vein, inferior vena cava, Gerota fascia, or the ipsilateral adrenal gland. T1a tumors are less than 4 cm, and T1b tumors are between 4 and 7 cm.

The Fuhrman nuclear grade classification system is the most commonly found histologic classification system.[4] The World Health Organization

None of the authors have any disclosures or conflicts of interest.

[a] Department of Radiology, Mayo Clinic College of Medicine, 4500 San Pablo Road, Jacksonville, FL 32224, USA; [b] Department of Radiology, Mayo Clinic College of Medicine, 200 1st Street Southwest, Rochester, MN 55905, USA

* Corresponding author.

E-mail address: Atwell.Thomas@Mayo.edu

radiologic.theclinics.com

defines 3 histologic RCC types: clear cell RCC (80%–90%), papillary RCC (10%–15%), and chromophobe RCC (4%–5%). Four Fuhrman nuclear grades are then assigned according to increasing nuclear size, irregularity, and nuclear prominence.

CURRENT TREATMENT GUIDELINES

The increased incidence of the incidentally detected renal mass along with the development of various nephron-sparing strategies has greatly affected the management of RCC. Both the American Urological Association (AUA) and the European Association of Urology (EAU) have published extensive guidelines regarding the treatment of localized RCC, local treatment of metastatic RCC, systemic therapy for metastatic RCC, and follow-up after radical nephrectomy (RN) or partial nephrectomy (PN) or ablative therapies for RCC.

The AUA management algorithm for the T1 renal mass incorporates the presence of major comorbidities, increased surgical risk, and tumor size. This algorithm essentially defines PN or RN as a standard therapy with ablative therapy or active surveillance as a recommendation only for those patients with a T1a renal mass and major comorbidities or at increased surgical risk.[6]

The EAU summary of the current evidence suggests that localized renal cancers are best managed by PN rather than RN, regardless of the surgical approach.[4] The EUA makes no recommendation on RFA and cryoablation because of the low quality of the available data. In the elderly and/or comorbid patients with small renal masses and limited life expectancy, active surveillance, RFA, and cryoablation can be offered.

STANDARD OF CARE: SURGICAL OUTCOMES FOR T1 RENAL MASSES

Over the past several decades, the surgical management of T1 renal masses (<7 cm) has evolved almost entirely to PN, including open, laparoscopic, and robotic approaches. PN has the proven benefit of preserving renal parenchyma and thus renal function with equivalent oncologic outcomes.[6–8]

Equal oncological outcomes have been demonstrated in several studies for patients with T1a (up to 4 cm) tumors treated with PN versus RN, citing a 5-year disease-specific survival up to 96%.[7,9] Population-based analysis comparing outcomes of RN and PN for T1a tumors demonstrate a disease-specific survival for PN of 97.5%.[10] In addition, there are growing data supporting equal oncologic outcomes for select T1b (4–7 cm) tumors reporting a 5-year disease-specific survival

rate of 98%; this is with the added benefit of preserving kidney function, therefore preventing secondary causes of morbidity and mortality.[11–13]

ROLE OF SURVEILLANCE

Active surveillance has gained support in the past several years, based on the fact that despite earlier detection and treatment of small RCCs, disease-specific mortality has continued to increase.[14,15] The increase in mortality is attributed to tumors larger than 4 cm, suggesting that smaller tumors have an indolent course. In fact, the average rate of small renal mass growth while under surveillance is 3 mm per year,[16] and 1 in 4 tumors do not grow while under surveillance.[17]

Certain groups, including elderly patients, those with significant comorbidities, or those with limited life expectancy, have been managed safely with surveillance in several trials.[18,19] There are no standardized active surveillance protocols addressing items such as patient selection; role of percutaneous renal mass biopsy; timing, type, or frequency of imaging follow-up; and growth rate thresholds at which to initiate intervention.

The AUA has published clinical guidelines pertaining to percutaneous biopsy and follow-up imaging.[20] These guidelines suggest that imaging follow-up take place with MR imaging or CT initially within 6 months of diagnosis to establish a growth rate. Following this, yearly follow-up is adequate unless the morphology of the mass changes or the growth rates increase.[20]

EMBOLIZATION OF RENAL CELL CARCINOMA

Renal artery embolization (RAE) is currently used for several indications in the setting of both primary renal tumors and metastatic RCC, including preoperative embolization before nephrectomy, treatment of angiomyolipoma, as an adjunctive therapy for RCC ablation, and for palliation of advanced-stage RCC.[21]

Preoperative embolization in RCC has numerous proposed benefits including decrease in perioperative blood loss, creation of a tissue plane of edema facilitating dissection, and reduction in tumor bulk.[21] Observational and retrospective studies demonstrate a wide variation in the achievement of desired results of reduction in intraoperative blood loss, transfusion requirements, surgical procedure time, surgical complications, and survival outcomes.[22–25] There is no consensus on the appropriate timing of preoperative embolization and resection, and this in combination with the varied results have limited the use to local practice patterns.

RAE can be used as a palliative method for patients who are not eligible for definitive therapy. There are several small series that have focused on embolization for palliation of hematuria and/or flank pain with promising results.[26–29] Onishi and colleagues[29] demonstrated a statistically significant median survival benefit of 229 days in an RAE group versus 116 days for a matched historical control group. This finding suggests a possible improvement in outcome that may be through a cytoreductive effect or via immunomodulation.[21,29]

A few case reports and case series have been published demonstrating the safety or feasibility of combined transarterial embolization and ablation in the management of RCC.[30–34] This approach may have a particular advantage when treating T1b tumors in an effort to minimize periprocedural blood loss (**Fig. 1**). There are various methods of combination therapy with regard to the type of ablation, type of embolic material, and sequential order of the procedures that have been described.[35]

The primary role for embolization in the setting of metastatic RCC is to achieve preoperative devascularization to minimize blood loss before resection or in combination with soft tissue ablation for palliative purposes.

ABLATION MODALITIES
Radiofrequency Ablation

A radiofrequency (RF) electrode acts as a cathode. Alternating current is applied to the RF electrode, changing the direction of the current. Water molecules and other dipoles attempt to align with the changing current, and this causes vibration and friction with adjacent molecules. The friction results in energy deposition in the form of heat.[36] At a temperature of 55 C, cell death occurs in 2 seconds. Effective thermal ablation using heat typically occurs at temperatures between 60°C and 100°C. At temperatures greater than 100°C, water evaporates. Cell death is instantaneous at this temperature, but because of the desiccating effect and the tissue charring that occurs, the RF

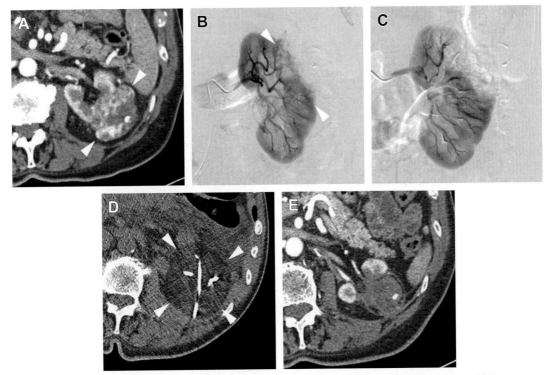

Fig. 1. Prophylactic embolization before definitive cryoablation of large clear cell RCC. (*A*) CT with intravenous contrast shows a 6-cm vascular mass in the left kidney (*arrowheads*). (*B*) Selective left renal artery angiogram shows a vascular RCC arising from the mid and upper left kidney (*arrowheads*). (*C*) Selective left renal artery angiogram after embolization of the mass with 150- to 250-μm polyvinyl alcohol particles shows lack of perfusion within the mass. (*D*) CT without intravenous contrast after the placement of 7 cryoprobes of 2.4 mm outer diameter shows a large iceball encompassing the mass (*arrowheads*). (*E*) CT with intravenous contrast 3 years after treatment shows an involuting mass without recurrence.

electrode becomes insulated and tissue penetration is limited.[37]

There are multiple RF electrode designs including single- and multitine designs. Electrode design affects the size of the ablation. It is important to refer to and understand the probe design and the ensuing size limitations of the RF probe in the case planning process.

RFA can be affected by large blood vessels dispersing heat from the ablation area, the so-called heat-sink effect.[38] RF electrodes require placement of grounding pads for the procedure. Skin burns associated with grounding pad placement have been reported.[39] RFA is associated with increased risks in central lesions.[38]

Microwave Ablation

Microwaves are another form of electromagnetic radiation. The mechanism of action is similar to that described for RF, although energy is emitted as a field rather than being propagated from the electrode. The frequency of microwave energy ranges from 900 to 2450 MHz (2.4 GHz). At these frequencies, directional changes of water molecules occur 2 to 5 billion times a second.[40]

Microwave is a relatively fast and efficient way to produce temperature increase in renal tissue.[41] Microwave does not have the same size limitations as seen in RFA. Because of the increased power of microwave, it is less affected by a vascular heat-sink effect.[42] Grounding pads are not needed with the use of microwave ablation (MWA).

Cryoablation

Cryoablation has been used in clinical medicine for over 50 years.[43] The objective of cryoablation is temperature reduction that produces cell death. Universal cell death in kidney parenchyma occurs at -19°C.[44] Cryoablation takes advantage of the Joule-Thompson effect in creating lethal cold temperatures at the end of the cryoprobe. With a drop in argon gas pressure, temperatures below -100°C are generated with secondary evolution of a lethal iceball from the distal shaft of the cryoprobe. Alternating freeze-thaw cycles ultimately lead to cellular dehydration, cell membrane rupture, and vascular thrombosis.[45]

In contrast to the heat-based techniques, the lethal iceball created during cryoablation is visible with US, CT, and MR imaging. The leading edge of the iceball corresponds to 0°C.[46] In normal kidney parenchyma, one study showed that a target lethal temperature of -20°C was 3 mm inside the edge of the visualized iceball.[47] Manufacturers provide isotherm diagrams that provide information regarding the expected size of the iceball

and relative ablation sizes that can be obtained with specific probes.

Other Ablative Technologies

Other modalities including irreversible electroporation (IRE) and laser ablation have been used in renal cell cancer. IRE units apply high-voltage current across a cellular membrane, which creates small pores and destabilizes the cellular membrane.[48] Early results have demonstrated efficacy in RCC. However, additional data are needed. IRE typically requires general anesthesia and complete muscle relaxation.

Laser ablation, high-intensity focused US, and stereotactic radiotherapy are also being investigated for treatment of RCC. Data is currently limited for each of these modalities.

PROCEDURAL CONSIDERATIONS
Patient-Specific Considerations

Percutaneous ablation can be performed as either an inpatient or an outpatient procedure.[49] Postprocedural evaluation is necessary, and overnight hospitalization may be needed. The method of anesthesia used during the case depends on patient factors and operator preference. Ablation is feasible using general anesthesia, deep sedation with an anesthetist, or moderate sedation.

Despite the rather significant effect of the ablation on the renal tumor, the ablation itself is minimally invasive and well tolerated by most patients. In those patients with preexisting anemia and/or patients at increased risk of bleeding (eg, owing to planned treatment of a large renal mass), blood typing and cross-matching may be considered if a transfusion is needed.

Placement of a urinary bladder catheter in patients with a solitary kidney can be helpful to confidently measure urine output, particularly allowing one to discriminate between urine retention following anesthesia and renal obstruction or failure. Similarly, prophylactic placement of a ureteral stent in patients with a solitary kidney and increased risk of obstructive hematuria may be reasonable.

Tumor-Specific Considerations

The AUA consensus guidelines recommend tumor biopsy, preferably core biopsy, before treatment; the timing of such biopsy was not specified, recognizing that some will allow biopsy to guide management, whereas others will proceed with ablation despite the biopsy result.[6] Arguments have been made both for and against biopsy.[50,51] The Society of Interventional Radiology Standard of Practice documentation supports biopsy when possible.[52]

When considering the different ablation modalities, tumor size and location should be accounted for in the triage process. Particularly with the heat-based ablation modalities, T1a lesions are more likely to be completely ablated than larger T1b lesions.[53–55] Tumors that extend centrally toward the renal sinus may be difficult to treat with heat-based techniques, likely related to greater heat-sink effects.[56]

Larger and central tumors can be effectively treated with cryoablation, although procedure times are longer and the complication rate is higher.[57–61] In patients with larger tumors, prophylactic selective arterial embolization can be considered to decrease the risk of bleeding.[33]

Intraprocedural Considerations

Historically, proximity to the central collecting system, bowel, and adrenal gland were regarded as relative contraindications to percutaneous therapy because of increased risk of nontarget ablation.[52] Adjunctive techniques can be used to mitigate these risks.

Retrograde irrigation of the collecting system via an externalized ureteral stent has been described and successfully used in the ablation of renal masses adjacent the ureter.[62] In addition to the creation of a beneficial thermal sink, the presence of the stent allows confident identification of the ureter during the course of treatment (**Fig. 2**).

Fluid can be directly injected along the margin of the index renal mass in order to displace viscera at risk of thermal injury, notably bowel (**Fig. 3**).[63–65] For RFA, nonionic fluid such as dextrose 5% in water should be used because of concerns of conductivity of energy within the fluid.

Collateral thermal injury to the adrenal gland may result in marked fluctuations of the patient's blood pressure and has been reported following

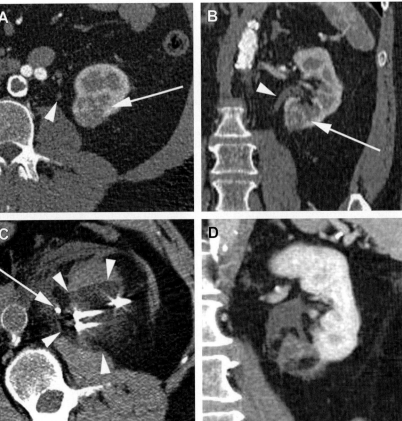

Fig. 2. Ureteral stent placement to allow cryoablation of a mass in proximity to the ureter. Axial (*A*) and coronal (*B*) CT angiogram show a 2.8-cm enhancing mass in the lower part of the left kidney (*arrow*) in close proximity to the ureter (*arrowhead*). (*C*) CT without intravenous contrast obtained after placement of a left ureteral stent and during cryoablation shows the opaque stent (*arrow*) with iceball (*arrowheads*) encompassing the tumor and encroaching on the stent. (*D*) Coronal CT with intravenous contrast 42 months after treatment shows involuting ablation defect with no recurrent tumor and no urinary obstruction.

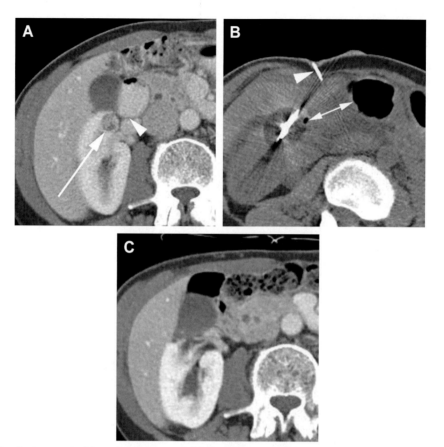

Fig. 3. Hydrodisplacement of bowel during renal ablation. (*A*) CT with intravenous contrast shows a 1.2-cm mass in the anterior hilar lip of the right kidney (*arrow*), directly adjacent to the duodenum (*arrowhead*). (*B*) CT without intravenous contrast obtained during cryoablation shows displacement of the duodenum from the ice-ball (*double arrow*) following infusion of fluid via a 19-gauge needle (*arrowhead*). (*C*) CT with intravenous contrast 5 years after ablation shows a renal parenchymal defect at the former ablation site and no recurrence.

hepatic ablation.[66] In patients in whom injury to the adrenal gland may occur, arterial blood pressure monitoring may be reasonable.

IMAGING FOLLOW-UP

Multiple recommendations have been made regarding imaging follow-up after percutaneous ablation. In general, follow-up intervals are short for the first year, with annual follow-ups for at least 5 years if no residual or recurrent disease is noted. The AUA recommends CT or MR imaging of the abdomen with and without intravenous contrast at 3 and 6 months after ablation. If stable, annual scanning is recommended for 5 years. After 5 years, imaging is optional and should be tailored to individual risk factors.[20]

ABLATION OUTCOMES
Radiofrequency Ablation

In the era of percutaneous renal ablation, RFA has the longest duration of follow-up and perhaps the

greatest volume of published experience (**Table 1**); this has provided several important observations regarding the best role for RFA in the ablation of renal tumors.

First, and perhaps most importantly, RFA is highly effective in the treatment of small renal masses. Many studies have shown RFA to be more than 95% effective in the local control of renal masses smaller than 3 cm (**Fig. 4**).[38,55,59,67–69] Best and colleagues[70] showed improved disease-free survival (DFS) at 5 years in those with tumors less than 3.0 cm in size (95%) compared with those with tumors measuring 3.0 cm or larger (79%).

Some investigators have shown reasonable success in the ablation of renal tumors measuring up to 4 cm. In 2 studies with a mean follow-up of approximately 5 years, 100% local tumor control was achieved in the RFA of tumors measuring less than 4 cm.[55,71] Veltri and colleagues[72] demonstrated significantly improved DFS in those with tumors measuring 4 cm or less compared with those with larger masses.

Table 1
Contemporary outcomes following renal RFA

Author, y	# Tumors	% RCC	Size (Median or Mean)	Mean f/u (mo)	Technical Success (%)	Technique Success (%)	RFS (%)	DFS (%)	CSS (%)	Technique
del Cura et al,[89] 2010	65	70.7	3.1 cm	26	—	91	—	—	—	Perc
Zagoria et al,[55] 2011	48	100	2.6 cm	56	100	88[a]	88 @ 5 y	83 @ 5 y	—	Perc
Best et al,[70] 2012	119	61.3	<3 cm	54	99.2	100[b]	—	95 @ 5 y	—	Perc/Lap
	40	87.5	≥3 cm	48	95.0	88.2	—	79 @ 5 y	—	
Psutka et al, 2013[53]	143	100	T1a	77	94.4	95.8	96.1 @ 5 y	91.5 @ 5 y	100 @ 5 y	Perc
	42	100	T1b		80.9	85.7	91.9 @ 5 y	74.5 @ 5 y	97.3 @ 5 y	
Balageas et al,[67] 2013	71	100[c]	2.3 cm	39	95.2	96.8	—	88 @ 3 y	—	Perc
Karam et al,[90] 2013	150	72	2.6 cm	27	—	96.7	—	—	100	Perc/lap
Veltri et al,[72] 2014	203	92	≤3 cm	39	100	93	—	86	100	Perc
			≤4 cm			89	—	83	100	
Wah et al,[68] 2014	133	91	≤3 cm	48	100	97.5	93.5 @ 5 y	—	97.9 @ 5 y	Perc
	67		>3 cm		95.5					
Lorber et al,[91] 2014	53	100	T1a	66	—	92.5	—	—	100% @ 5 y	Perc/lap
Takaki et al,[92] 2014	21	100	T1b	41	81.0	100	—	88 @ 5 y	94 @ 5 y	Perc
McClure et al,[93] 2014	100	100	2.3 cm	24	99.1	95	86 @ 2.1 y	—	100	Perc
Thompson et al,[86] 2015	166	55	T1a	35	100	—	98% @ 3 y	—	—	Perc

Abbreviations: CSS, cancer-specific survival; DFS, disease-free survival; f/u, follow-up; lap, laparoscopic; perc, percutaneous; RFS, recurrence-free survival.
[a] No recurrences in tumors measuring smaller than 4.0 cm.
[b] Single suspected recurrence shown to be giant cell reaction at surgery.
[c] Almost 10% tumors were Bosniak 4 cystic masses and presumed malignant.

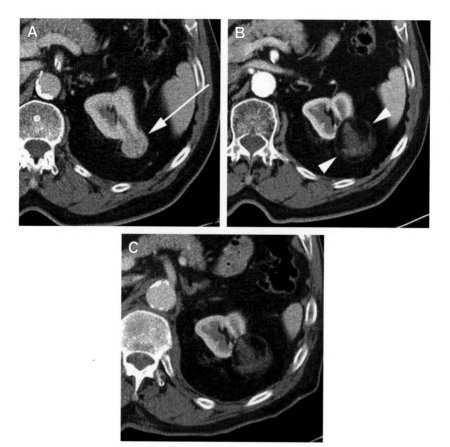

Fig. 4. Long-term follow-up after RFA of a 2.8-cm clear cell RCC in the left kidney. (*A*) CT with intravenous contrast shows an exophytic enhancing solid mass in the upper part of the left kidney laterally (*arrow*). (*B*) CT 3 years after RFA shows a generous ablation defect delineated by the rim of fat necrosis with retracting ablated tumor centrally (*arrowheads*). (*C*) CT shows slight retraction of the ablation site at 6 years without recurrent tumor.

Likely related to inherent limitations of RFA devices[73] and technical challenges in generating effective overlapping ablations,[74] outcomes in the RFA of larger renal masses have been less impressive. Combined incomplete treatment and local progression rates of over 20% have been reported following RFA of tumors measuring over 3 to 4 cm.[53,67,70] Similarly, central thermal sink effects can limit the efficacy of RFA in treating centrally located renal masses.[38,68,72]

Cryoablation

While the body of experience in the percutaneous application of renal cryoablation was slow to emerge following its initial description in 1995,[75] small series in the mid-2000s showed technical feasibility, an acceptable safety profile, and favorable short-term outcomes (**Table 2**).[76–80] In 2 early studies using MR imaging guidance, cryoablation achieved primary local tumor control rates of 95% and 88% at a mean follow-up of 9 and 14 months, respectively .[79,80] Subsequent studies using CT monitoring showed local tumor control rates of 92% to 97% at 6 to 19 months of follow-up.[76,77,81]

More recent experience has slowly proved the durability of percutaneous cryoablation. Schmit and colleagues[82] described 99% technical and technique success in the treatment of 116 patients with sporadic RCCs at a mean follow-up of 21 months. In their treatment of 134 RCCs, Georgiades and Rodriguez[83] found only 2 locally recurrent tumors following percutaneous cryoablation, yielding a 97% recurrence-free survival at 5 years.

A potential advantage of cryoablation over the heat-based modalities is the ability to effectively treat larger renal masses (**Fig. 5**). In one study, 97% local tumor control was achieved in the treatment of 108 tumors measuring 3.0 cm or larger at a mean follow-up of 15 months.[84] In the treatment of 139 renal tumors measuring up to 6.5 cm, Blute

Table 2
Outcomes following percutaneous renal cryoablation

Author, y	# Tumors	% RCC	Size (Median or Mean)	Months f/u (Median or Mean)	Technical Success (%)	Technique Success (%)	RFS (%)	DFS (%)	CSS (%)	Technique
Blute et al,[61] 2012	139	87	2.4 cm	24	—	93	—	—	—	Perc
Breen et al,[94] 2013	62	100	3.3 cm	18	—	98	—	—	—	Perc
Buy et al, 2013[95]	100	80	T1a	28	98	—	—	96 @ 12 mo	—	Perc
	20		T1b		75					
Kim et al,[96] 2013	129	—[a]	2.7 cm	30	—	87	—	85% @ 3 y	100	Perc
Georgiades & Rodriguez,[83] 2014	134	100	2.8 cm	—	—	98.5	97.0 @ 5 y	—	100 @ 5 y	Perc
Thompson et al,[86] 2015	174	62	T1a	17	100	—	98 @ 3 y	—	—	Perc
	48	69	T1b	23	98		97 @ 3 y			

Abbreviations: CSS, cancer-specific survival; DFS, disease-free survival; f/u, follow-up; perc, percutaneous; RFS, recurrence-free survival.
[a] Biopsy not routinely performed.

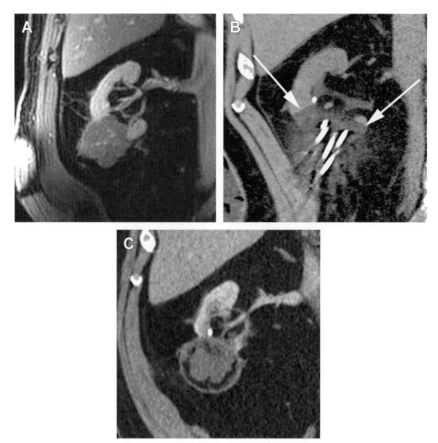

Fig. 5. Long-term follow-up after cryoablation of a 6.0-cm papillary RCC in the right kidney. (*A*) Coronal MR imaging with intravenous contrast shows a 6.0-cm mass in the lower part of the right kidney. (*B*) Coronal reconstructed CT image shows a total of 5 cryoprobes in the mass with the iceball extending beyond the tumor margin (*arrows*). (*C*) Coronal reconstructed CT with intravenous contrast 6 years after ablation shows fat necrosis at the ablation site and no recurrent tumor.

and colleagues[61] found that size was not associated with treatment failure. Unfortunately, the ablation of such large tumors is frequently associated with an increased risk of complications.[57]

Microwave Ablation

The expanding use of MWA in the management of renal masses has become evident with a growing body of literature to support its role in treatment. Initial results of intraoperative MWA have been quite favorable.[85] More recent larger series detailing the percutaneous experience have shown success similar to RFA. Yu and colleagues[54] achieved 98% technical success and 3-year recurrence-free survival of 92% in the MWA of 49 RCCs; there were no technical or technique failures in those with tumors smaller than 4 cm. The University of Wisconsin group recently showed 100% technical and short-term (mean 8 month) technique effectiveness in the treatment of 55 clinical T1a RCCs using MWA.[65]

Surgical Comparison Studies

Meta-analyses comparing surgery with ablative techniques have been published, but these frequently include series with heterogeneous

---

Box 1
Potential complications of percutaneous renal ablation

Perirenal hemorrhage

Hematuria

Nerve injury

Urothelial injury

Bowel injury

Infection

Pneumothorax

Thromboembolism

Medical event

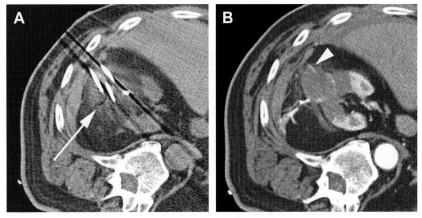

Fig. 6. Clinically unimportant bleeding immediately after cryoablation. (*A*) CT without intravenous contrast during the ablation of a 3.9-cm mass in the upper part of the right kidney shows a subtle crack in the iceball evident by a hypoattenuating irregular line extending obliquely from the probes (*arrow*). (*B*) CT with intravenous contrast immediately after ablation shows active extravasation at the site of the iceball crack. A small amount of extravasation is also present at the cryoprobe tract (*arrowhead*). The patient's postprocedure course was unremarkable, without clinical evidence of bleeding.

techniques (specifically, surgical and percutaneous approaches) and lack stratification based on recognized limitations of device. An oft-cited review showing the inferiority of RFA to cryoablation and surgery failed to recognize the marked strength of RFA in treating small (<3 cm) renal masses.[15] It is important to appreciate and take advantage of the strengths of each ablation method in treating renal tumors.

Using a combined prospectively maintained renal tumor registry including over 1800 patients, Thompson and colleagues[86] published a comparison of PN, RFA, and cryoablation in the treatment T1 renal masses at a single institution. The 3-year recurrence-free survival for T1a tumors was 98% for all 3 populations. Perhaps more impressive was the similar rate of 3-year recurrence-free survival in patients treated for T1b tumors, in whom there was no significant difference between PN and cryoablation.

A comparison of MWA and open RN in the management of T1a RCC showed similar rates of estimated 5-year RCC-related survival at 97.1% and 97.8%, respectively.[87] Of the 65 tumors treated with MWA, there was a single case of local tumor progression.

Complications

Complications following renal ablation are infrequent (**Box 1**). In a review of complications related to ablation and surgery, the AUA consensus panel found that major urologic complications occurred following 4.9% and 6.0% of cryoablation and RFA procedures, respectively.[6] This rate compares

with 6.3% following open PN and 9.0% following laparoscopic PN.

In detailing the complications following 573 renal ablation procedures, Atwell and colleagues[57] found both overall (13.2%) and major (8.4%) complication rates to be higher following cryoablation compared with RFA (9.8% and 4.7%, respectively), although tumors treated with cryoablation were larger and more often centrally located.

Bleeding is the most common complication related to cryoablation and may be associated with tumor size, central location, and number of cryoprobes. Cracking of the iceball can occur and may be associated with bleeding (**Fig. 6**).[88]

The most common complications following RFA are nerve and urothelial injury. Nerve injuries with secondary sensory or motor neuropathy usually resolve within 6 months but may occasionally last longer. Ureteral strictures can be devastating and are difficult to definitively manage without surgery.

REFERENCES

1. Motzer RJ, Agarwal N, Beard C, et al. Kidney cancer. J Natl Compr Canc Netw 2011;9(9):960–77.
2. American Cancer Society. Available at: http://www.cancer.org/cancer/kidneycancer/detailedguide/kidney-cancer-adult-key-statistics. Accessed December 19, 2014.
3. Ridge CA, Pua BB, Madoff DC. Epidemiology and staging of renal cell carcinoma. Semin Intervent Radiol 2014;31(1):3–8.
4. Ljungberg B, Bensalah K, Bex S, et al. EAU guidelines on renal cell carcinoma: 2014 update. Eur Urol 2015;67(5):913–24.

5. Edge SB, American Joint Committee on Cancer, American Cancer Society. AJCC cancer staging handbook : from the AJCC cancer staging manual. 7th edition. New York: Springer; 2010. p. xix, 718.

6. Campbell SC, Novick AC, Belldegrun A, et al. Guideline for management of the clinical T1 renal mass. J Urol 2009;182(4):1271–9.

7. Hafez KS, Fergany AF, Novick AC. Nephron sparing surgery for localized renal cell carcinoma: impact of tumor size on patient survival, tumor recurrence and TNM staging. J Urol 1999;162(6):1930–3.

8. Krabbe LM, Bagrodia A, Margulis V, et al. Surgical management of renal cell carcinoma. Semin Intervent Radiol 2014;31(1):27–32.

9. Lee CT, Katz J, Shi W, et al. Surgical management of renal tumors 4 cm. or less in a contemporary cohort. J Urol 2000;163(3):730–6.

10. Crepel M, Jeldres C, Sun M, et al. A population-based comparison of cancer-control rates between radical and partial nephrectomy for T1A renal cell carcinoma. Urology 2010;76(4):883–8.

11. Huang WC, Elkin EB, Levey AS, et al. Partial nephrectomy versus radical nephrectomy in patients with small renal tumors–is there a difference in mortality and cardiovascular outcomes? J Urol 2009; 181(1):55–61 [discussion: 61–2].

12. Leibovich BC, Blute M, Cheville JC, et al. Nephron sparing surgery for appropriately selected renal cell carcinoma between 4 and 7 cm results in outcome similar to radical nephrectomy. J Urol 2004;171(3):1066–70.

13. Patard JJ, Shvarts O, Lam JS, et al. Safety and efficacy of partial nephrectomy for all T1 tumors based on an international multicenter experience. J Urol 2004;171(6 Pt 1):2181–5 [quiz: 2435].

14. Hollingsworth JM, Miller DC, Daignault S, et al. Rising incidence of small renal masses: a need to reassess treatment effect. J Natl Cancer Inst 2006; 98(18):1331–4.

15. Kunkle DA, Egleston BL, Uzzo RG. Excise, ablate or observe: the small renal mass dilemma–a meta-analysis and review. J Urol 2008;179(4):1227–33 [discussion: 1233–4].

16. Chawla SN, Crispen PL, Hanlon AL, et al. The natural history of observed enhancing renal masses: meta-analysis and review of the world literature. J Urol 2006;175(2):425–31.

17. Kunkle DA, Crispen PL, Chen DY, et al. Enhancing renal masses with zero net growth during active surveillance. J Urol 2007;177(3):849–53 [discussion: 853–4].

18. Patel N, Cranston D, Akhtar MZ, et al. Active surveillance of small renal masses offers short-term oncological efficacy equivalent to radical and partial nephrectomy. BJU Int 2012;110(9):1270–5.

19. Smaldone MC, Kutikov A, Egleston BL, et al. Small renal masses progressing to metastases under active surveillance: a systematic review and pooled analysis. Cancer 2012;118(4):997–1006.

20. Donat SM, Diaz M, Bishoff JT, et al. Follow-up for clinically localized renal neoplasms: AUA guideline. J Urol 2013;190(2):407–16.

21. Li D, Pua BB, Madoff DC. Role of embolization in the treatment of renal masses. Semin Intervent Radiol 2014;31(1):70–81.

22. Schwartz MJ, Smith EB, Trost DW, et al. Renal artery embolization: clinical indications and experience from over 100 cases. BJU Int 2007;99(4):881–6.

23. May M, Brookman-Amissah S, Pflanz S, et al. Preoperative renal arterial embolisation does not provide survival benefit in patients with radical nephrectomy for renal cell carcinoma. Br J Radiol 2009;82(981):724–31.

24. Zielinski H, Szmigielski S, Petrovich Z. Comparison of preoperative embolization followed by radical nephrectomy with radical nephrectomy alone for renal cell carcinoma. Am J Clin Oncol 2000;23(1):6–12.

25. Subramanian VS, Stephenson AJ, Goldfarb DA, et al. Utility of preoperative renal artery embolization for management of renal tumors with inferior vena caval thrombi. Urology 2009;74(1):154–9.

26. Maxwell NJ, Saleem Amer N, Rogers E, et al. Renal artery embolisation in the palliative treatment of renal carcinoma. Br J Radiol 2007;80(950):96–102.

27. Mukund A, Gamanagatti S. Ethanol ablation of renal cell carcinoma for palliation of symptoms in advanced disease. J Palliat Med 2010;13(2):117–20.

28. Munro NP, Woodhams S, Nawrocki JD, et al. The role of transarterial embolization in the treatment of renal cell carcinoma. BJU Int 2003;92(3):240–4.

29. Onishi T, Oishi Y, Suzuki Y, et al. Prognostic evaluation of transcatheter arterial embolization for unresectable renal cell carcinoma with distant metastasis. BJU Int 2001;87(4):312–5.

30. Arima K, Yamakado K, Kinbara H, et al. Percutaneous radiofrequency ablation with transarterial embolization is useful for treatment of stage 1 renal cell carcinoma with surgical risk: results at 2-year mean follow up. Int J Urol 2007;14(7):585–90 [discussion: 590].

31. Mondshine RT, Owens S, Mondschein JI, et al. Combination embolization and radiofrequency ablation therapy for renal cell carcinoma in the setting of co-existing arterial disease. J Vasc Interv Radiol 2008; 19(4):616–20.

32. Nakasone Y, Kawanaka K, Ikeda O, et al. Sequential combination treatment (arterial embolization and percutaneous radiofrequency ablation) of inoperable renal cell carcinoma: single-center pilot study. Acta Radiol 2012;53(4):410–4.

33. Woodrum DA, Atwell TD, Farrell MA, et al. Role of intraarterial embolization before cryoablation of large renal tumors: a pilot study. J Vasc Interv Radiol 2010;21(6):930–6.

34. Yamakado K, Nakatsuka A, Kobayashi S, et al. Radiofrequency ablation combined with renal arterial embolization for the treatment of unresectable renal cell carcinoma larger than 3.5 cm: initial experience. Cardiovasc Intervent Radiol 2006;29(3):389–94.

35. Winokur RS, Pua BB, Madoff DC. Role of combined embolization and ablation in management of renal masses. Semin Intervent Radiol 2014;31(1):82–5.

36. Goldberg SN, Gazelle GS, Mueller PR. Thermal ablation therapy for focal malignancy: a unified approach to underlying principles, techniques, and diagnostic imaging guidance. AJR Am J Roentgenol 2000;174(2):323–31.

37. Dupuy DE, Goldberg SN. Image-guided radiofrequency tumor ablation: challenges and opportunities–part II. J Vasc Interv Radiol 2001;12(10): 1135–48.

38. Gervais DA, McGovern FJ, Arellano RS, et al. Radiofrequency ablation of renal cell carcinoma: part 1, Indications, results, and role in patient management over a 6-year period and ablation of 100 tumors. AJR Am J Roentgenol 2005;185(1):64–71.

39. Huffman SD, Huffman NP, Lewandowski RJ, et al. Radiofrequency ablation complicated by skin burn. Semin Intervent Radiol 2011;28(2):179–82.

40. Simon CJ, Dupuy DE, Mayo-Smith WW. Microwave ablation: principles and applications. Radiographics 2005;25(Suppl 1):S69–83.

41. Clark PE, Woodruff RD, Zagoria RJ, et al. Microwave ablation of renal parenchymal tumors before nephrectomy: phase I study. AJR Am J Roentgenol 2007;188(5):1212–4.

42. Skinner MG, Iizuka MN, Kolios MC, et al. A theoretical comparison of energy sources–microwave, ultrasound and laser–for interstitial thermal therapy. Phys Med Biol 1998;43(12):3535–47.

43. Theodorescu D. Cancer cryotherapy: evolution and biology. Rev Urol 2004;6(Suppl 4):S9–19.

44. Chosy SG, Nakada SY, Lee FT Jr, et al. Monitoring renal cryosurgery: predictors of tissue necrosis in swine. J Urol 1998;159(4):1370–4.

45. Levy D, Avallone A, Jones JS. Current state of urological cryosurgery: prostate and kidney. BJU Int 2010;105(5):590–600.

46. Saliken JC, McKinnon JG, Gray R. CT for monitoring cryotherapy. AJR Am J Roentgenol 1996;166(4): 853–5.

47. Campbell SC, Krishnamurthi V, Chow G, et al. Renal cryosurgery: experimental evaluation of treatment parameters. Urology 1998;52(1):29–33 [discussion: 33–4].

48. Gehl J. Electroporation: theory and methods, perspectives for drug delivery, gene therapy and research. Acta Physiol Scand 2003;177(4):437–47.

49. Dupuy DE. Radiofrequency ablation: an outpatient percutaneous treatment. Med Health R I 1999; 82(6):213–6.

50. Uppot RN, Silverman SG, Zagoria RJ, et al. Imaging-guided percutaneous ablation of renal cell carcinoma: a primer of how we do it. AJR Am J Roentgenol 2009;192(6):1558–70.

51. Zagoria RJ. Imaging of small renal masses: a medical success story. AJR Am J Roentgenol 2000; 175(4):945–55.

52. Clark TW, Millward SF, Gervais DA, et al. Reporting standards for percutaneous thermal ablation of renal cell carcinoma. J Vasc Interv Radiol 2009;20(7 Suppl):S409–16.

53. Psutka SP, Feldman AS, McDougal WS, et al. Long-term oncologic outcomes after radiofrequency ablation for T1 renal cell carcinoma. Eur Urol 2013;63(3): 486–92.

54. Yu J, Liang P, Yu XL, et al. US-guided percutaneous microwave ablation of renal cell carcinoma: intermediate-term results. Radiology 2012;263(3):900–8.

55. Zagoria RJ, Pettus JA, Rogers M, et al. Long-term outcomes after percutaneous radiofrequency ablation for renal cell carcinoma. Urology 2011;77(6): 1393–7.

56. Varkarakis IM, Allaf ME, Inagaki T, et al. Percutaneous radio frequency ablation of renal masses: results at a 2-year mean followup. J Urol 2005;174(2): 456–60 [discussion: 460].

57. Atwell TD, Carter RE, Schmit GD, et al. Complications following 573 percutaneous renal radiofrequency and cryoablation procedures. J Vasc Interv Radiol 2012;23(1):48–54.

58. Atwell TD, Farrell MA, Callstrom MR, et al. Percutaneous cryoablation of large renal masses: technical feasibility and short-term outcome. AJR Am J Roentgenol 2007;188(5):1195–200.

59. Atwell TD, Schmit GD, Boorjian SA, et al. Percutaneous ablation of renal masses measuring 3.0 cm and smaller: comparative local control and complications after radiofrequency ablation and cryoablation. AJR Am J Roentgenol 2013;200(2):461–6.

60. Rosenberg MD, Kim CY, Tsivian M, et al. Percutaneous cryoablation of renal lesions with radiographic ice ball involvement of the renal sinus: analysis of hemorrhagic and collecting system complications. AJR Am J Roentgenol 2011;196(4):935–9.

61. Blute ML Jr, Okhunov Z, Moreira DM, et al. Image-guided percutaneous renal cryoablation: preoperative risk factors for recurrence and complications. BJU Int 2013;111(4 Pt B):E181–5.

62. Cantwell CP, Wah TM, Gervais DA, et al. Protecting the ureter during radiofrequency ablation of renal cell cancer: a pilot study of retrograde pyeloperfusion with cooled dextrose 5% in water. J Vasc Interv Radiol 2008;19(7):1034–40.

63. Bodily KD, Atwell TD, Mandrekar JN, et al. Hydrodisplacement in the percutaneous cryoablation of 50 renal tumors. AJR Am J Roentgenol 2010;194(3): 779–83.

64. Farrell MA, Charboneau JW, Callstrom MR, et al. Par-anephric water instillation: a technique to prevent bowel injury during percutaneous renal radiofre-quency ablation. AJR Am J Roentgenol 2003; 181(5):1315–7.

65. Moreland AJ, Ziemlewicz TJ, Best SL, et al. High-powered microwave ablation of t1a renal cell carci-noma: safety and initial clinical evaluation. J Endourol 2014;28(9):1046–52.

66. Onik G, Onik C, Medary I, et al. Life-threatening hy-pertensive crises in two patients undergoing hepatic radiofrequency ablation. AJR Am J Roentgenol 2003;181(2):495–7.

67. Balageas P, Cornelis F, Le Bras Y, et al. Ten-year experience of percutaneous image-guided radiofre-quency ablation of malignant renal tumours in high-risk patients. Eur Radiol 2013;23(7):1925–32.

68. Wah TM, Irving HC, Gregory W, et al. Radiofre-quency ablation (RFA) of renal cell carcinoma (RCC): experience in 200 tumours. BJU Int 2014; 113(3):416–28.

69. Breen DJ, Rutherford EE, Stedman B, et al. Manage-ment of renal tumors by image-guided radiofre-quency ablation: experience in 105 tumors. Cardiovasc Intervent Radiol 2007;30(5):936–42.

70. Best SL, Park SK, Youssef RF, et al. Long-term out-comes of renal tumor radio frequency ablation strat-ified by tumor diameter: size matters. J Urol 2012; 187(4):1183–9.

71. Ferakis N, Bouropoulos C, Granitsas T, et al. Long-term results after computed-tomography-guided percutaneous radiofrequency ablation for small renal tumors. J Endourol 2010;24(12):1909–13.

72. Veltri A, Gazzera C, Busso M, et al. T1a as the sole selection criterion for RFA of renal masses: random-ized controlled trials versus surgery should not be postponed. Cardiovasc Intervent Radiol 2014; 37(5):1292–8.

73. Laeseke PF, Sampson LA, Haemmerich D, et al. Multiple-electrode radiofrequency ablation creates confluent areas of necrosis: in vivo porcine liver re-sults. Radiology 2006;241(1):116–24.

74. Dodd GD 3rd, Frank MS, Aribandi M, et al. Radio-frequency thermal ablation: computer analysis of the size of the thermal injury created by overlap-ping ablations. AJR Am J Roentgenol 2001; 177(4):777–82.

75. Uchida M, Imaide Y, Sugimoto K, et al. Percuta-neous cryosurgery for renal tumours. Br J Urol 1995;75(2):132–6 [discussion: 136–7].

76. Atwell TD, Farrell MA, Callstrom MR, et al. Percuta-neous cryoablation of 40 solid renal tumors with US guidance and CT monitoring: initial experience. Radiology 2007;243(1):276–83.

77. Littrup PJ, Ahmed A, Aoun HD, et al. CT-guided percutaneous cryotherapy of renal masses. J Vasc Interv Radiol 2007;18(3):383–92.

78. Permpongkosol S, Link RE, Kavoussi LR, et al. Percutaneous computerized tomography guided cryoablation for localized renal cell carcinoma: factors influencing success. J Urol 2006;176(5): 1963–8 [discussion: 1968].

79. Shingleton WB, Sewell PE Jr. Percutaneous renal tu-mor cryoablation with magnetic resonance imaging guidance. J Urol 2001;165(3):773–6.

80. Silverman SG, Tuncali K, vanSonnenberg E, et al. Renal tumors: MR imaging-guided percutaneous cryotherapy–initial experience in 23 patients. Radi-ology 2005;236(2):716–24.

81. Gupta A, Allaf ME, Kavoussi LR, et al. Computerized tomography guided percutaneous renal cryoabla-tion with the patient under conscious sedation: initial clinical experience. J Urol 2006;175(2):447–52 [dis-cussion: 452–3].

82. Schmit GD, Thompson RH, Kurup AN, et al. Percutaneous cryoablation of solitary sporadic renal cell carcinomas. BJU Int 2012;110(11 Pt B): E526–31.

83. Georgiades CS, Rodriguez R. Efficacy and safety of percutaneous cryoablation for stage 1A/B renal cell carcinoma: results of a prospective, single-arm, 5-year study. Cardiovasc Intervent Radiol 2014;37(6):1494–9.

84. Schmit GD, Atwell TD, Callstrom MR, et al. Percuta-neous cryoablation of renal masses >or=3 cm: effi-cacy and safety in treatment of 108 patients. J Endourol 2010;24(8):1255–62.

85. Guan W, Bai J, Liu J, et al. Microwave ablation versus partial nephrectomy for small renal tumors: intermediate-term results. J Surg Oncol 2012; 106(3):316–21.

86. Thompson RH, Atwell T, Schmit G, et al. Comparison of partial nephrectomy and percutaneous ablation for cT1 renal masses. Euro Urol 2015;67:252–9.

87. Yu J, Liang P, Yu XL, et al. US-guided percuta-neous microwave ablation versus open radical nephrectomy for small renal cell carcinoma: intermediate-term results. Radiology 2014;270(3): 880–7.

88. Schmit GD, Atwell TD, Callstrom MR, et al. Ice ball fractures during percutaneous renal cryoablation: risk factors and potential implications. J Vasc Interv Radiol 2010;21(8):1309–12.

89. del Cura JL, Zabala R, Iriarte JI, et al. Treatment of renal tumors by percutaneous ultrasound-guided ra-diofrequency ablation using a multitined electrode: effectiveness and complications. Eur Urol 2010; 57(3):459–65.

90. Karam JA, Ahrar K, Vikram R, et al. Radiofrequency ablation of renal tumours with clinical, radiographi-cal and pathological results. BJU Int 2013;111(6): 997–1005.

91. Lorber G, Glamore M, Doshi M, et al. Long-term onco-logic outcomes following radiofrequency ablation

with real-time temperature monitoring for T1a renal cell cancer. Urol Oncol 2014;32(7):1017–23.

92. Takaki H, Soga N, Kanda H, et al. Radiofrequency ablation versus radical nephrectomy: clinical outcomes for stage T1b renal cell carcinoma. Radiology 2014;270(1):292–9.

93. McClure TD, Chow DS, Tan N, et al. Intermediate outcomes and predictors of efficacy in the radiofrequency ablation of 100 pathologically proven renal cell carcinomas. J Vasc Interv Radiol 2014;25(11): 1682–8 [quiz: 1689].

94. Breen DJ, Bryant TJ, Abbas A, et al. Percutaneous cryoablation of renal tumours: outcomes from 171 tumours in 147 patients. BJU Int 2013;112(6):758–65.

95. Buy X, Lang H, Garnon J, et al. Percutaneous renal cryoablation: prospective experience treating 120 consecutive tumors. AJR Am J Roentgenol 2013; 201(6):1353–61.

96. Kim EH, Tanagho YS, Bhayani SB, et al. Percutaneous cryoablation of renal masses: Washington University experience of treating 129 tumours. BJU Int 2013;111(6):872–9.

Adrenal Imaging and Intervention

Brian C. Allen, MD[a],*, Isaac R. Francis, MBBS[b]

KEYWORDS

- Adrenal adenoma • Adrenocortical carcinoma • Pheochromocytoma
- Absolute percentage washout • Relative percentage washout • Cushing syndrome
- Conn syndrome

KEY POINTS

- Incidental adrenal masses are common and most are benign.
- Imaging appearances suspicious for malignancy include large size (>4 cm), growth, heterogeneity, irregular margins, and necrosis.
- Adrenal masses may be biochemically active and produce excess glucocorticoids, aldosterone, androgens, and/or catecholamines.
- Computed tomography can differentiate most adenomas and nonadenomas using absolute or relative percentage washout, because adenomas tend to enhance earlier and stronger, and deenhance earlier and to a greater degree than do most nonadenomas.

INTRODUCTION

The adrenal glands are complex endocrine organs composed of 2 distinct regions: the adrenal cortex and the adrenal medulla. The cortex is composed of 3 zones: the outer zona glomerulosa, which is the site of aldosterone production; the middle zona fasciculata, which is the site of cortisol and sex steroid production; and the inner zona reticularis, which secretes cortisol, androgens, and estrogens, and is the source of cholesterols for steroidogenesis. The adrenal medulla is the central aspect of the gland and primarily secretes catecholamines.[1]

The adrenal glands are a common site for benign and malignant primary tumors as well as metastatic disease. Cross-sectional imaging allows both the detection and characterization of many adrenal masses, making percutaneous biopsy unnecessary in many cases.

This article reviews imaging protocols for adrenal imaging, including computed tomography (CT), MR imaging, and fluorine-18 fluorodeoxyglucose (FDG) PET/CT. Diagnostic algorithms are described for the imaging evaluation of incidentally detected adrenal masses, the noninvasive detection of adrenal tumors in patients with known biochemical abnormalities, and staging of patients with known primary malignancies. In addition, imaging-guided interventions for the diagnosis and therapy for various adrenal tumors are discussed.

NORMAL ANATOMY

The normal adrenal glands are inverted Y-shaped or V-shaped organs in the suprarenal space, enclosed by the Gerota fascia. The adrenal glands have straight or concave margins with bodies measuring less than 10 to 12 mm in length and

Disclosure: The authors have nothing to disclose.
[a] Abdominal Imaging, Department of Radiology, Duke University Medical Center, 2301 Erwin Road, Box 3808, Durham, NC 27710, USA; [b] Abdominal Imaging, Department of Radiology, University of Michigan Hospitals, 1500 East Medical Center Drive, Room BID540, Ann Arbor, MI 48109-5030, USA
* Corresponding author.
E-mail address: brian.allen@duke.edu

Radiol Clin N Am 53 (2015) 1021–1035
http://dx.doi.org/10.1016/j.rcl.2015.05.004
0033-8389/15/$ – see front matter © 2015 Elsevier Inc. All rights reserved.

limbs measuring less than 5 to 6 mm in thickness.[2] There are usually 3 adrenal arteries, arising most commonly from the inferior phrenic artery, the aorta, and the renal artery. There are usually single adrenal veins. The right adrenal vein drains directly into the inferior vena cava and the left adrenal vein drains into the inferior phrenic vein and then the renal vein. Vascular anatomy is difficult to identify on routine cross-sectional imaging, and is occasionally identified during CT angiography, but is extremely important for intravascular catheter-based diagnostic and interventional techniques.

On CT, the normal adrenal glands are symmetric and of homogeneous soft tissue density. On MR imaging, the adrenal glands are of intermediate signal intensity on T1-weighted (T1w) imaging, and are isointense to slightly hypointense to liver on T2-weighted (T2w) imaging.[3] There is a wide range of normal uptake in the adrenal glands on FDG-PET, from no uptake to moderate uptake.[4] In general, the uptake within the adrenal glands on FDG-PET is similar to or less than background liver.

IMAGING PROTOCOLS

The imaging evaluation of known or suspected adrenal abnormalities typically consists of CT, MR imaging, or PET/CT. Metaiodobenzyl-guanidine (MIBG; preferred) and, less commonly, octreotide scintigraphy may be used to identify pheochromocytomas, but these targeted nuclear medicine studies should be used selectively in patients with a high pretest probability of disease (eg, patients with a family history, patients with an associated hereditary disorder, patients with biochemical evidence of excess sympathetic hormones).[5]

CT imaging of the adrenal glands typically consists of a multiphase study including an unenhanced scan, a 1-minute delayed-enhanced scan, and a 15-minute delayed-enhanced scan (**Box 1**). The unenhanced scan is used to identify lipid-rich adenomas, which can be diagnosed when an adrenal nodule is homogeneous and measures less than 10 Hounsfield units (HU). If a mass can be characterized as a lipid-rich adenoma on the unenhanced scan, intravenous contrast is not required. For adrenal masses that are homogeneous and measure greater than 10 HU in a patient with suspected metastasis, intravenous contrast administration and washout calculations are necessary. The unenhanced, 1-minute, and 15-minute scans are used to calculate absolute percentage washout (APW) and/or relative percentage washout (RPW) in order to differentiate lipid-poor adenomas from metastases. Details of how to perform these calculations and the formulae used are described later.

MR imaging of the adrenal glands is generally performed with a phased-array body coil with the patient supine (see **Box 1**). A typical adrenal protocol begins with a coronal localizer using a fast sequence such as single-shot turbo spin echo/single-shot fast spin echo (ssFSE), which provides an anatomic overview of the abdomen. Gradient dual-echo T1w (in-phase and opposed-phase) imaging with the longer echo time assigned to the in-phase echo is fundamental in adrenal nodule evaluation. In-phase and opposed-phase imaging allow detection of intravoxel lipid within adrenal masses, manifesting as nonlinear signal loss on the opposed-phase images. The presence of macroscopic fat within an adrenal mass can be seen on opposed-phase images by the characteristic India ink artifact at fat-water interfaces. Axial

---

Box 1
Simplified imaging protocols

CT imaging protocol

Unenhanced CT to identify lipid-rich adenomas (<10 Hounsfield units [HU])

One-minute and 15-minute delayed-enhanced CT to differentiate lipid-poor adenomas from metastases using absolute percentage washout (APW) or relative percentage washout (RPW)

MR imaging protocol

Coronal and axial T2w single-shot fast spin echo localizer

Axial and coronal T1w dual-echo gradient echo to assess for lipid in lipid-rich adenomas and India ink artifact in myelolipomas

Fat-suppressed T2w fast spin echo to assess for pseudocysts, cysts, and the occasional light–bulb-bright pheochromocytoma

(Optional) Fat-suppressed T1w gradient echo before and dynamically after intravenous contrast material to assess for venous thrombus in patients with suspected adrenocortical carcinoma

fat-suppressed T2w images are useful to evaluate for the typical marked hyperintensity of cysts and pseudocysts, and the so-called lightbulb-bright sign of some pheochromocytomas. Multiphase contrast-enhanced imaging is sometimes performed using a three-dimensional (3D), fat-suppressed T1w gradient echo sequence; however, the contrast washout–based calculations used with CT are not accepted or widely used for MR imaging because of the non-normalized units of signal intensity. For this reason, many MR adrenal mass protocols forgo the use of contrast-enhanced imaging for adrenal nodule characterization. In patients with dominant adrenal masses suspicious for adrenocortical carcinoma, contrast-enhanced imaging is helpful to determine whether there is vascular invasion.

FDG-PET/CT typically is used as a staging examination in patients with certain known primary malignancies. Qualitative visual assessment of radiotracer uptake compared with background liver activity and quantitative analysis using standardized uptake values (SUV) are the methods used to determine whether a lesion is suspicious for a malignancy.[6] Adrenal nodules with uptake greater than background liver are likely malignant, adrenal nodules with uptake less than background liver are likely benign, and adrenal nodules with uptake similar to background liver are equivocal. FDG-PET/CT can also be used for the detection of distant metastatic disease in patients with probable malignancy.

IMAGING FINDINGS/PATHOLOGY
Incidental Adrenal Masses

Incidental adrenal masses (ie, adrenal masses measuring >1 cm that are discovered on an imaging study performed for an indication other than for the adrenal gland) are common, occurring in up to 7% of adults, and are often referred to as incidentalomas.[7] Most incidentally discovered adrenal masses are benign, and the most commonly discovered incidental adrenal mass is a nonhyperfunctioning adenoma.[8] The purpose of diagnostic imaging is to differentiate benign masses from those that may require treatment. Benign, so-called leave-alone, masses include nonhyperfunctioning adenomas, myelolipomas, cysts, pseudocysts, and unclassified lesions with long-term stability (**Box 2**).

Benign lesions with specific imaging findings
Myelolipoma Myelolipomas are benign adrenal masses composed of variable amounts of fat, myeloid cells, and erythroid cells. Their imaging appearance is characteristic, with the

---

Box 2
Simplified differential diagnosis

Benign
  Adenoma
  Pseudocyst
  Hemorrhage
  Myelolipoma
  Cyst
  Pheochromocytoma
  Granulomatous disease
Malignant
  Metastasis
  Adrenocortical carcinoma
  Pheochromocytoma

---

identification of macroscopic fat within an adrenal mass (**Box 3**). On CT imaging, macroscopic fat, similar in attenuation to the adjacent retroperitoneal fat, is seen on both unenhanced and intravenous contrast-enhanced examinations (**Fig. 1**). In general, unenhanced CT is more sensitive for the diagnosis of macroscopic fat than is contrast-enhanced CT because of pseudoenhancement effects. On MR imaging, the fat component of a myelolipoma is hyperintense on T1w images without fat suppression and becomes hypointense on T1w images with fat suppression. A similar change in signal is seen on T2w imaging (hyperintense on T2w imaging without fat suppression,

---

Box 3
Diagnostic criteria for adrenal masses

Less than 10 HU and homogeneous on unenhanced CT is diagnostic of a lipid-rich adenoma

APW greater than 60% and RPW greater than 40% are suggestive of lipid-poor adenoma

Nonlinear signal loss within an adrenal nodule on opposed-phase imaging is suggestive of a lipid-rich adenoma

Large quantities of macroscopic fat (India ink artifact) within an adrenal mass are diagnostic of myelolipoma

Adrenal cysts (rare) and adrenal pseudocysts (uncommon) are of fluid density or signal intensity and do not enhance

Malignant adrenal masses tend to be large (>4 cm) and heterogeneous with central necrosis and irregular margins

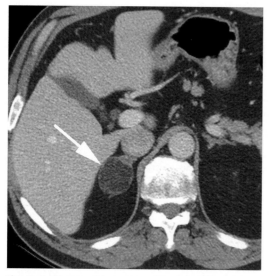

Fig. 1. A 61-year-old woman with right adrenal mye-lolipoma. Axial contrast-enhanced CT shows a 3-cm right adrenal mass (*arrow*), composed primarily of macroscopic lipid.

hypointense on T2w imaging with fat suppression). On T1w opposed-phase images, a characteristic India ink artifact is seen at the fat-water interfaces of the mass. This artifact is diagnostic of the presence of macroscopic fat and characteristic of myelolipoma (**Fig. 2**). Myelolipomas are occasionally complicated by calcifications and hemorrhage, but necrosis is rare.[2] Some adrenocortical cancers can contain small quantities of macroscopic fat (generally <10% of the total volume).

Cyst True cysts of the adrenal gland are rare, benign, homogeneous, and do not enhance

following intravenous contrast administration (**Fig. 3**). On CT, they measure water density (<20 HU); on MR imaging, they are fluid signal intensity. Occasionally, an internal septation or peripheral calcification is seen. Complicated cysts may have areas of apparent wall thickening or irregularity that generally do not enhance. The presence of nodular or thick septal enhancement within a cystic adrenal mass is an indication for resection.

Other adrenal lesions

Adrenal hemorrhage and pseudocysts Adrenal hemorrhage is often asymptomatic, but patients may present with flank pain. Bilateral adrenal hemorrhage may present as a life-threatening condition with high mortality related to the underlying disease and superimposed endocrine dysfunction.[9] Causes of adrenal hemorrhage include anticoagulation (ie, supratherapeutic treatment), septicemia (ie, classically related to meningococcus [Waterhouse-Friderichsen syndrome]), iatrogenic events (eg, adrenal biopsy, ipsilateral partial nephrectomy), trauma, and spontaneous hemorrhage of an underlying adrenal tumor (rare).

On imaging, the appearance of adrenal hemorrhage depends on the time of imaging following the event. On CT, acute and subacute adrenal hemorrhage may appear as a round or oval high-attenuation mass that does not enhance following intravenous contrast administration. Hemorrhage may also present as an infiltrative/amorphous mass, or as adreniform enlargement that should decrease in size over time.[9]

The MR appearance of adrenal hemorrhage depends on the age of the blood products and the

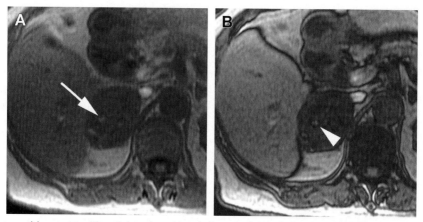

Fig. 2. A 67-year-old woman with a right adrenal myelolipoma. (*A*) Axial T1w in-phase image shows a large, heterogeneous right adrenal mass with hyperintense foci (*arrow*), representing macroscopic lipid. (*B*) Axial T1w opposed-phase image shows a dark-rimmed India ink artifact (*arrowhead*) around the bright foci, which represents signal loss at the interface between the fat-containing and the water-containing components of the myelolipoma.

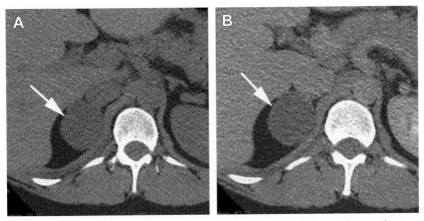

Fig. 3. A 35-year-old man with right adrenal cyst. (*A*) Axial unenhanced CT image shows a homogeneous water attenuation right adrenal mass (*arrow*). (*B*) Axial contrast-enhanced CT image in the nephrographic phase shows no enhancement of this mass (*arrow*).

relative amount of deoxyhemoglobin, methemoglobin, and hemosiderin.[10] Subacute hemorrhage is usually heterogeneously hyperintense on T1w imaging because of methemoglobin.

Chronic hemorrhage usually manifests as either dense calcification or a pseudocyst. Pseudocysts are fluid signal intensity centrally with peripheral calcifications or hemosiderin (hypointense on T2w imaging). Occasionally, a thin peripheral enhancing rim can be seen.

Granulomatous disease In the acute phase, granulomatous disease can manifest as no abnormality (common) or bilateral adrenal nodules (rare). In the chronic phase, granulomatous disease can show no abnormality (common) or bilateral calcifications (common).

Malignant lesions

Imaging appearances suspicious for adrenal malignancy (metastases, adrenocortical carcinoma, malignant pheochromocytoma) include new or enlarging enhancing adrenal masses without history of intercurrent severe atypical infection, large size (>4 cm), heterogeneity, irregular margins, and necrosis (see **Box 3**). Patients with these imaging characteristics require evaluation with biochemical studies, biopsy, and/or resection. Note that suspected adrenocortical cancer should not be biopsied to avoid the risk of tumor spillage.

In patients who have one or more adrenal nodules without suspicious imaging features but who have a suspicious history (eg, personal history of malignancy, concern for metastatic disease), further imaging with adrenal protocol CT, adrenal protocol MR, and/or FDG-PET/CT can help differentiate adenoma from metastasis.

American College of Radiology Incidental Findings Committee: management recommendations

Incidental adrenal masses are adrenal masses measuring greater than 1 cm that are discovered on cross-sectional imaging performed for an indication other than the evaluation of the adrenal glands (**Fig. 4**). The American College of Radiology (ACR) has devised a flow chart for the evaluation of incidentally discovered adrenal masses.[7] If an adrenal mass can be characterized definitively as a benign lesion (eg, cyst, pseudocyst, calcification, myelolipoma) then no further work-up is required. If a homogeneous adrenal mass measures 1 to 4 cm and shows a density of less than 10 HU on unenhanced CT or nonlinear generalized signal loss on opposed-phase MR imaging, a lipid-rich adenoma may be diagnosed in most situations. Exceptions on MR imaging include patients with known clear cell renal cell carcinoma or hepatocellular carcinoma because such metastases can appear identical. Some adrenocortical cancers can contain lipid, but are not homogeneous. If an adrenal mass is unchanged for longer than 1 year, it is likely to be benign but may or may not be functional (eg, hyperfunctioning adenoma, benign pheochromocytoma).

In patients with an indeterminate adrenal mass, a personal history of cancer, and no prior imaging that can be used to assess stability of the adrenal mass, further evaluation should be considered with CT, MR imaging, or FDG-PET/CT. If a mass cannot be characterized as an adenoma; if it is enlarging; or if it has other suspicious features of malignancy, such as heterogeneity, margin irregularity, or internal necrosis, percutaneous biopsy may be indicated; particularly if the adrenal gland is the only site of potential metastasis.

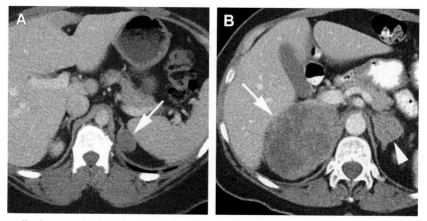

Fig. 4. Incidentally discovered adrenal masses in 2 different patients. (*A*) A 37-year-old woman with a homogeneous, low-attenuation, smoothly marginated left adrenal mass measuring less than 3 cm (*arrow*) on this contrast-enhanced CT image. These imaging features suggest a benign mass, which was confirmed by stability on follow-up imaging. (*B*) A 53-year-old man with a large, heterogeneous right adrenal mass (*arrow*) with irregular margins. These imaging features suggest a malignant mass, subsequently proved to represent metastatic melanoma. A small left adrenal metastasis is also present (*arrowhead*).

In general, the primary role of adrenal protocol CT and adrenal protocol MR is for the differentiation of adenoma from metastasis in at-risk patients. It should not be performed in all patients with an incidental adrenal nodule; it is not capable of predicting adrenal mass hyperfunction; and it is not helpful in further characterizing heterogeneous, necrotic, large (>4 cm), or otherwise complicated adrenal masses.

BIOCHEMICALLY ACTIVE ADRENAL MASSES

Biochemically active adrenal masses may arise from the adrenal cortex or adrenal medulla. Cortical tumors produce excess glucocorticoids, aldosterone, or androgens, and medullary tumors produce excess catecholamines.

Cushing Syndrome

Excess production of cortisol leads to the characteristic signs and symptoms of Cushing syndrome, including obesity, insulin resistance, depression, and hypertension. Hypercortisolism may be subclinical in about 5% of cases.[11] Most cases of Cushing syndrome are caused by stimulation of the adrenal by a pituitary adenoma that secretes excess adrenocorticotropic hormone (ACTH). Primary adrenal tumors (eg, adenoma, adrenocortical carcinoma) are the cause in about 20% of cases and ectopic ACTH production (ie, extrapituitary) is seen in approximately 1% of cases. The evaluation of patients with Cushing syndrome begins with biochemical testing and pituitary MR imaging. If a pituitary adenoma is not detected, adrenal CT or MR imaging is performed next. If

both pituitary and adrenal causes are excluded, then a CT of the chest, abdomen, and pelvis is performed to identify an ectopic source. Biochemical tests include 24-hour urine free cortisol, late-night salivary cortisol test, and overnight dexamethasone suppression test.[11]

Conn Syndrome

Conn syndrome results from increased aldosterone level, which leads to sodium retention, hypertension, and potassium wasting. Clinically, the diagnosis is suspected in patients with hypertension and hypokalemia, and is then confirmed by measuring serum aldosterone to renin levels.[11] Conn syndrome may result from an adrenal cortical tumor or adrenal hyperplasia. Thin-section CT (slice thickness 2–3 mm) is the first imaging test used in patients with primary hyperaldosteronism. Its purpose is to help subtype the disease and to exclude the possibility of a hyperfunctioning adrenocortical cancer. Multiphasic imaging with 15-minute delays is usually not necessary because the clinical suspicion is typically unrelated to metastatic disease, and washout calculations are not designed to discriminate between primary adrenal masses.

Because of the high prevalence of incidental nonhyperfunctioning adrenal nodules and the insensitivity of CT to small (<1 cm) adrenal nodules,[12] the usefulness of CT for localizing the source of hyperfunction is limited, particularly in patients more than 40 years of age, who are more likely to have an unrelated adrenal nodule. Therefore, in patients greater than or equal to 40 years old with primary hyperaldosteronism who desire a surgical cure, adrenal venous sampling by an experienced radiologist is required to localize the sites of aldosterone production. If the source is unilateral, then ipsilateral adrenalectomy is usually curative. If the source is bilateral (eg, adrenal hyperplasia), then the management is usually medical (eg, spironolactone).

Pheochromocytoma

Pheochromocytomas are neuroendocrine tumors that arise from the chromaffin cells of the adrenal medulla and lead to excess catecholamine production. The excess catecholamines may cause headache, hypertension, diaphoresis, tachycardia, and anxiety. Pheochromocytomas are associated with multiple syndromes, including multiple endocrine neoplasia 2A and 2B, von Hippel-Lindau, neurofibromatosis 1, and the Carney triad.[13] Mutations in the succinate dehydrogenase gene complex also predispose patients to the development of hereditary pheochromocytomas.[14]

The biochemical work-up for suspected pheochromocytoma consists of plasma metanephrines and urinary metanephrines, which have a combined sensitivity of 97% to 99%.[15]

Most (90%) pheochromocytomas arise from the adrenal gland and most (90%) are benign. Approximately 10% are extra-adrenal (ie, paraganglioma) and approximately 10% are malignant. On CT imaging, pheochromocytomas have a variable appearance but tend to be hypervascular, with avid arterial-phase enhancement.[16] Rarely (<1%), pheochromocytomas mimic lipid-rich adenomas by measuring less than 10 HU on unenhanced CT (Box 4).[17] In addition, although most (~75%) pheochromocytomas show slow washout of less than 60% APW and less than 40% RPW, a substantial minority (~25%) mimic the washout patterns of lipid-poor adenomas.[18]

On MR imaging, most pheochromocytomas are hyperintense on T2w imaging, but a substantial minority are not (Fig. 5).[19] Classically, pheochromocytoma has been described as light-bulb bright on T2w imaging, but this is not always the case. Pheochromocytomas tend to be heterogeneous and may show flow voids on T2w imaging, giving them a salt-and-pepper appearance. Following contrast administration, pheochromocytomas avidly enhance.[13]

MIBG scintigraphy is a nuclear medicine examination that has been used to localize pheochromocytomas and has both high sensitivity (95%–100%) and high specificity (100%).[20] MIBG scintigraphy should be used in certain patient populations, such as those with relevant family history or hereditary disorders, and in those patients with positive biochemical markers but negative CT or MR imaging.[5] It has also been used in the detection of distant metastatic disease in patients with malignant pheochromocytomas. Although most

---

Box 4
Pearls and pitfalls

Pearls:

A homogeneous adrenal nodule that is less than 10 HU on unenhanced CT is diagnostic of a lipid-rich adenoma.

If an adrenal mass measures greater than 30 HU on unenhanced CT, adrenal CT with washout may be a better option than MR imaging with chemical shift imaging.

Pheochromocytoma may mimic adrenal adenoma. Biopsy of pheochromocytoma can be avoided by obtaining preprocedural biochemical studies.

Malignant adrenal tumors and metastases tend to be large (>4 cm) and heterogeneous with central necrosis and irregular margins.

Pitfalls:

Some (~25%) pheochromocytomas show APW greater than 60% and could be confused with adenoma.

Adrenocortical carcinoma, pheochromocytoma, clear cell renal cell carcinoma, and hepatocellular carcinoma metastases may contain intravoxel lipid and may show heterogeneous signal loss on opposed-phase imaging.

Collision tumors (ie, metastatic disease to the adrenal gland with a coexisting benign lesion) are rare, but when present, 2 distinct regions of varying signal intensity within the same adrenal mass are generally seen.

Biopsy of a suspected adrenocortical carcinoma is contraindicated because of the risk of tumor spillage and needle-track seeding. Such masses should move directly to open resection.

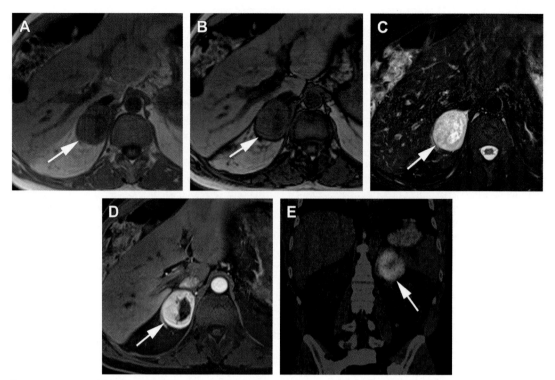

Fig. 5. A 57-year-old man with right adrenal pheochromocytoma. (*A*) Axial T1w in-phase image shows a hetero-geneous right adrenal mass (*arrow*). (*B*) Axial T1w opposed-phase image does not show any signal drop within the mass (*arrow*). (*C*) Axial T2w fat-suppressed image shows a hyperintense, heterogeneous mass (*arrow*). (*D*) Axial contrast-enhanced T1w fat-suppressed image in the arterial phase shows that this mass (*arrow*) is hypervas-cular with a necrotic portion. (*E*) I-123 MIBG single-photon emission CT image in the coronal plane in another patient shows an MIBG-avid left adrenal mass, proved subsequently by surgical resection to be a pheochromocy-toma (*arrow*). ([*E*] *Courtesy of* Keyanoosh Hosseinzadeh, MD, Wake Forest University School of Medicine, Winston-Salem, NC.)

pheochromocytomas are avid on PET/CT, MIBG scintigraphy is superior for the detection of pheo-chromocytomas, particularly those that are benign.[20] In cases in which there is biochemical evidence of pheochromocytoma but negative MIBG imaging, octreotide scanning can be used as an alternative, but it is not a first-line test.

Operative resection is the primary treatment of pheochromocytoma. Recently, transarterial embo-lization and percutaneous thermal ablation have been used to treat pheochromocytoma, particu-larly in poor operative candidates.[21,22] In patients undergoing local therapy or local tissue sampling (rare) of a suspected pheochromocytoma, alpha blockade is recommended in advance to avoid an adrenergic crisis. Iodine-131 MIBG therapy may be used for systemic treatment of select patients with metastatic pheochromocytoma.[23]

Adrenocortical Carcinoma

Adrenocortical carcinoma is a rare malignancy with an incidence of 1 to 2 per million people per

year. Most cases are sporadic, but there is an as-sociation with Li-Fraumeni cancer syndrome, Carney complex, Beckwith-Wiedemann syn-drome, familial adenomatous polyposis coli and multiple endocrine neoplasia type 1.[24] There is a slight female predilection and a bimodal age distri-bution, with tumors seen in infants and children less than 5 years old, and in older patients in the fourth to fifth decades of life. Adrenocortical carci-noma is a functional (hormone-producing) tumor in 60% of cases, although this is less common in adults. The tumors may secrete androgens, cortisol, estrogens, or aldosterone, which can lead to Cushing syndrome, virilization, or feminiza-tion.[24] In adults, adrenocortical carcinoma often presents as a large mass that is sometimes palpable, and with abdominal or flank pain. Thirty percent of patients present with metastatic dis-ease to regional and para-aortic lymph nodes, lung, liver, and bones.[24]

On CT, adrenocortical carcinomas tend to be large, usually measuring greater than 4 cm. In addition, tumor margins tend to be irregular, and central necrosis and hemorrhage are common, particularly when the tumor is larger than 6 cm.[25] Calcification may be seen in up to 30% of these tumors.[25] Some adrenocortical cancers contain lipid and small quantities of fat. Adrenocortical carcinoma generally enhances heterogeneously following the intravenous administration of contrast. There may be local invasion of adjacent structures, and venous extension is common. Hussain and colleagues[26] found size greater than 4 cm and heterogeneous enhancement to be the most important imaging factors for the characterization of adrenocortical carcinoma. Adrenocortical carcinoma generally has APW and RPW values of less than 60% and 40%, respectively, compatible with nonadenomas.[27]

On MR imaging, adrenocortical carcinoma is heterogeneously isointense to slightly hypointense to liver on T1w imaging, but is hyperintense if hemorrhage is present. These masses are heterogeneous and hyperintense on T2w imaging (**Fig. 6**). On opposed-phase imaging, regions of heterogeneous signal loss representing intravoxel lipid or small regions (<10% total volume) of India ink artifact representing macroscopic fat may be seen (see **Box 4**).[28] Adrenocortical carcinoma shows avid, heterogeneous enhancement with slow washout.[29] In general, washout calculations are not performed for, or helpful in, the evaluation of adrenocortical carcinoma because of their size and heterogeneity.

FDG-PET/CT has a high sensitivity and high specificity for malignant adrenal masses, including adrenocortical carcinoma, with a sensitivity of up to 100% and a specificity of 88% to 97%. It is also used for the detection of distant metastatic disease.[30,31]

Surgery is the optimal treatment of adrenocortical carcinoma and may be performed even with tumor thrombus extending to the right heart.

Transarterial embolization can be used for oncologic palliation, pain relief, hormone suppression, and to decrease tumor bulk and vascularity before surgical resection.[32] Percutaneous ablation in patients who are poor operative candidates or with unresectable tumors has been shown to be effective for short-term local control, particularly for small tumors, but long-term data are not available.[33] Percutaneous biopsy of a suspected adrenocortical carcinoma in a surgical candidate is not advised because it can result in tumor spillage that renders the patient incurable.

ADRENAL MASSES IN THE SETTING OF KNOWN PRIMARY MALIGNANCY
Computed Tomography

The adrenal glands are a common site for benign adenoma formation (2%–5% of patients) and metastatic disease development. In the setting of known primary malignancy, differentiating adenoma from metastasis is important because the diagnosis of adrenal metastasis can change the clinical stage and treatment plan.

However, up to 70% of adrenal adenomas contain intracellular lipid (cholesterol, fatty acids, and neutral fat), which reduces the unenhanced CT density of adenomas to less than that of other soft tissue nodules like metastases.[34] A meta-analysis has shown that a threshold of 10 HU or less, which is the most widely used threshold, has a sensitivity of 71% and a specificity of 98% for the diagnosis of lipid-rich adenoma (see **Box 3, Fig. 7**).[35]

However, 10% to 40% of adenomas are lipid-poor and measure greater than 10 HU on unenhanced CT.[35] Lipid-poor adenomas may be characterized by adrenal washout calculations using 1-minute delayed-enhanced and 15-minute

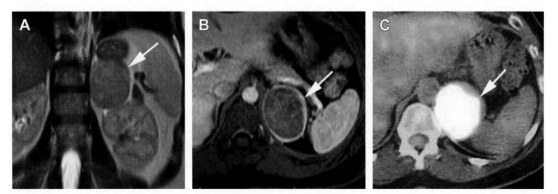

Fig. 6. A 67-year-old woman with adrenocortical carcinoma. (*A*) Coronal ssFSE image shows a heterogeneous left adrenal mass (*arrow*). (*B*) Axial contrast-enhanced T1w fat-suppressed image shows a hypovascular, heterogeneous mass (*arrow*). (*C*) Axial fused PET/CT image shows that the mass is FDG avid (*arrow*).

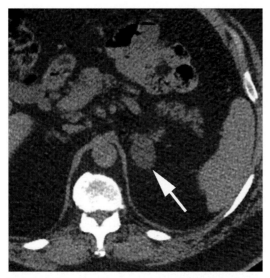

Fig. 7. A 59-year-old man with a left adrenal adenoma. Unenhanced axial CT image shows a small, homogeneous mass that measures −2 HU, which is compatible with a lipid-rich adenoma (*arrow*).

delayed-enhanced CT imaging, because adenomas (both lipid rich and lipid poor) show earlier and more rapid washout than do metastases (**Figs. 8** and **9**).[36] APW and RPW may be used to characterize these lipid-poor adenomas. APW is calculated as (1-minute HU − 15-minute HU)/ (1-minute HU − unenhanced HU) × 100. RPW is rarely used; it is used when the unenhanced imaging is not available and an incidental nodule is detected in real time in an at-risk patient who is still near the CT scanner and can complete delayed imaging. It is calculated as: (1-minute HU − 15-minute HU)/1-minute HU × 100.

An APW greater than or equal to 60% has sensitivity of 88% to 98% and a specificity of 92% to 96% for the diagnosis of adrenal adenoma; an RPW greater than or equal to 40% has a sensitivity of 96% and a specificity of 100% for the diagnosis of adrenal adenoma (see **Box 3**).[36–38] The calculated area under the curve for washout in general is 97% for the differentiation of adrenal adenomas from metastases.[36]

Dual-energy CT has shown some promise for differentiating lipid-rich from lipid-poor lesions.[39] Virtual unenhanced and true unenhanced datasets are similar, but not exact, which could lead to the misclassification of some lesions.[40] CT histogram analysis has been explored as well,[41] but the diagnostic accuracy is not ideal and it does not see routine clinical use.

MR Imaging

Chemical shift MR imaging takes advantage of the lipid content of adenomas, in which intravoxel lipid is seen as nonlinear signal loss within a nodule on opposed-phase imaging (see **Box 3**). It is important for the longer echo time of the dual-echo sequence to be the in-phase echo to ensure that the signal loss is related to lipid and not to T2* effects. Adenomas characteristically show homogeneous signal loss on opposed-phase imaging, but occasionally heterogeneous signal loss is seen instead (**Fig. 10**).[42] Following contrast administration, adenomas generally enhance homogeneously, but the presence of cystic change or hemorrhage within some adenomas may cause heterogeneous enhancement.[43] Signal intensity washout calculations are not commonly used for the characterization of adrenal nodules in the

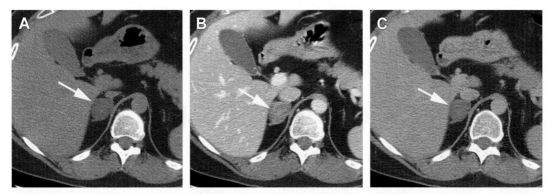

Fig. 8. A 33-year-old woman with right adrenal adenoma. (*A*) Axial unenhanced CT image shows a homogeneous right adrenal mass (*arrow*) that measures 25 HU. Because the mass measured greater than 10 HU, intravenous contrast was administered for further characterization. (*B*) Axial contrast-enhanced CT image in the portal venous phase shows a homogeneously enhancing mass (*arrow*) that measures 90 HU. (*C*) At 15 minutes, the adrenal mass (*arrow*) measures 46 HU. Absolute percentage enhancement washout is calculated at 68%, which is compatible with a lipid-poor adenoma.

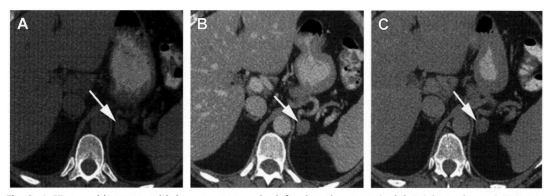

Fig. 9. A 57-year-old woman with breast cancer and a left adrenal metastasis. (*A*) Axial unenhanced CT image shows a homogeneous left adrenal mass (*arrow*) that measures 13 HU. Because the mass measured greater than 10 HU, intravenous contrast was administered for further characterization. (*B*) Axial contrast-enhanced CT image in the portal venous phase shows a homogeneously enhancing mass (*arrow*) that measures 54 HU. (*C*) At 15 minutes, the adrenal mass (*arrow*) measures 37 HU. Absolute percentage enhancement washout is calculated at 41%, making this a nonadenoma. Biopsy was performed, confirming metastasis. (*Courtesy of* Keyanoosh Hosseinzadeh, MD, Wake Forest University School of Medicine, Winston-Salem, NC.)

way APW is used with CT. In general, apparent diffusion coefficient (ADC) values are not useful in differentiating adrenal masses, but, in indeterminate masses, higher ADC values are more likely to be benign.[44]

Both qualitative and quantitative methods may be used to detect signal loss in adrenal adenomas. Visual qualitative analysis of signal loss in an adrenal mass may be compared with splenic signal intensity change; this has been shown to be as effective as quantitative methods.[45] Quantitative methods include the adrenal/spleen ratio and the signal intensity index (SII).[41] SII is calculated as (SI in − SI out)/SI in, and an SII greater than 16.5% is classically characteristic of an adenoma.[46] However, the SII threshold varies by the field strength and pulse sequence selection (eg, two dimensional vs 3D).

Overall, MR imaging with chemical shift imaging has a sensitivity of 87% to 100% and a specificity of 92% to 100% for the diagnosis of adrenal adenoma.[47–49] When comparing CT washout with chemical shift MR imaging for adenoma diagnosis, the CT APW was superior, with a reported sensitivity, specificity, and accuracy of 84%, 79%, and 83%, compared with 67%, 89%, and 74%, respectively, for SII calculations.[50] A potential pitfall is seen in adenomas with low lipid/water ratio, or lipid-poor adenomas, in which there may be no appreciable signal loss on opposed-phase

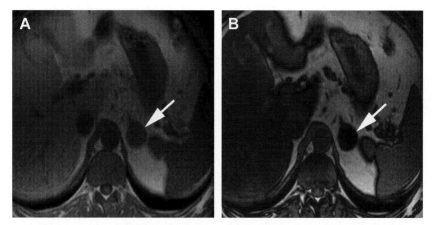

Fig. 10. A 37-year-old man with a left adrenal adenoma. (*A*) Axial T1w in-phase image shows a small, homogeneous left adrenal mass (*arrow*). (*B*) Axial T1w opposed-phase image shows homogeneous signal decrease in the mass (*arrow*), compatible with a lipid-rich adenoma. This patient also had signal decrease in the liver, compatible with hepatic steatosis.

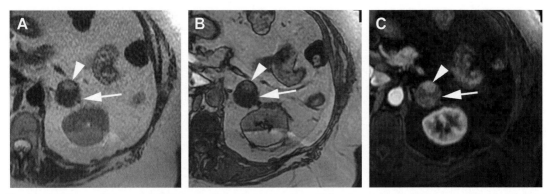

Fig. 11. A 72-year-old woman with renal cell carcinoma and a collision tumor in the left adrenal gland. (*A*) Axial T1w in-phase image shows a left adrenal mass with 2 distinct regions: a hypointense region (*arrow*) and a hyperintense region (*arrowhead*). (*B*) Axial T1w opposed-phase image shows calculated signal decrease in the larger region (*arrow*), compatible with a lipid-rich adenoma. There is no signal decrease in the second region (*arrowhead*). (*C*) Axial T1w fat-suppressed image following intravenous contrast shows that the non-adenoma portion of the left adrenal mass is hypervascular (*arrowhead*) compared to the adenoma portion (*arrow*).

imaging. Studies have evaluated the utility of chemical shift imaging for adenomas that measure greater than 10 HU on unenhanced CT, and have shown that chemical shift imaging may be inferior to APW for adrenal masses that are greater than 20 to 30 HU on unenhanced CT.[51,52]

An important pitfall of chemical shift imaging is that nonadenomas can also show signal loss on opposed-phase imaging. These nonadenomas include adrenocortical carcinoma (rare, generally large and heterogeneous), pheochromocytoma (rare), and certain metastases from primary lipid-containing tumors such as clear cell renal cell carcinoma and hepatocellular carcinoma (see **Box 4**).[53,54] Patients with such metastases generally have a personal history of that tumor type.

Another potential pitfall is the rare collision tumor, in which a metastasis arises adjacent to a benign adrenal mass (**Fig. 11**). When present, 2 distinct regions of varying signal intensity are generally seen.

PET/Computed Tomography/MR Imaging

FDG-PET/CT has been shown to be highly sensitive and specific for the identification of benign and malignant adrenal masses (**Fig. 12**). Quantitative (SUV) and qualitative (signal intensity relative to background liver) methods have been used. For the identification of benign masses, FDG-PET/CT has a reported sensitivity, specificity, positive predictive value, negative predictive value,

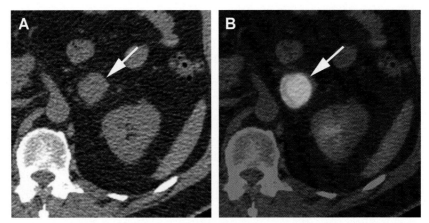

Fig. 12. 64-year-old man with lung cancer and left adrenal metastasis. (*A*) Axial unenhanced CT image from a staging PET/CT shows a left adrenal mass (*arrow*). (*B*) Axial fused PET/CT image shows that this mass is FDG avid, compatible with a metastasis (*arrow*). This patient had other metastases, so the nodule was not biopsied, but resolved with systemic treatment on follow-up imaging.

Box 5
What the referring physician needs to know

Benign leave-alone masses, such as myelolipomas, cysts, pseudocysts, and nonhyperfunctioning adenomas, do not require further characterization or imaging.

Potentially malignant masses, including new or enlarging masses, masses greater than 4 cm, heterogeneous masses, and those with irregular margins or necrosis, require further evaluation with biochemical studies, biopsy, and/or resection. Suspected adrenocortical cancer should not be biopsied before resection.

CT or MR imaging may be used to differentiate adenomas from metastases. CT and MR imaging cannot differentiate functioning from nonfunctioning adenomas, or adenomas from some pheochromocytomas.

and accuracy of 99%, 100%, 100%, 93%, and 99%, respectively.[6] FDG-PET/CT also excels at the detection of distant metastatic disease in patients with adrenocortical carcinoma or adrenal metastasis. False-positive findings on FDG-PET/CT can be seen in some adrenal adenomas, adrenal hyperplasia, and in inflammatory conditions that affect the adrenal glands. False-negative FDG-PET/CT is occasionally seen in the setting of coexistent adrenal hemorrhage or extensive necrosis.

Percutaneous Biopsy

Percutaneous biopsy of the adrenal gland has become much less common since the advent of noninvasive methods of adrenal nodule characterization. However, in the setting of an indeterminate adrenal mass in a patient with a known primary malignancy, percutaneous biopsy may be required. Although ultrasonography-guided adrenal mass biopsy is feasible, CT-guided adrenal mass biopsy is more common. CT-guided adrenal mass biopsy has been shown to be both safe and accurate, with an overall accuracy of 90% and a major complication rate of only 2.8% in a 10-year series of 270 patients.[55]

CT-guided adrenal mass biopsy is often performed with the patient in the ipsilateral decubitus position to compress the ipsilateral lung, minimizing the risk of pneumothorax and decreasing ipsilateral motion. Angling the CT gantry is also commonly used to allow visualization of the entire needle along an angled caudal-to-cephalad approach. This approach also minimizes the risk of pneumothorax. For right adrenal nodules, this is often challenging because of the location of the right kidney, so a transhepatic approach may be used instead.

Pneumothorax and tumor seeding are uncommon risks of most adrenal biopsies, with 1 caveat: a suspected adrenocortical carcinoma should not be biopsied in a surgical candidate because it can render the patient incurable from tumor spillage

(the patient instead should move directly to resection). Before biopsy of an indeterminate adrenal mass, the diagnosis of a pheochromocytoma should be excluded by biochemical analysis to avoid an adrenergic crisis.[56]

SUMMARY

The adrenal glands are a common site for benign and malignant tumors. Incidental adrenal masses are commonly encountered and almost always benign. Management guidelines are based on mass size, mass morphologic characteristics, and patient history. In patients with biochemical evidence of hormonal excess, imaging and image-guided intervention (ie, adrenal vein sampling) plays critical roles in localizing the site of hormone production and in guiding therapy. In patients with a known primary malignancy, CT, MR imaging, and FDG-PET/CT allow the noninvasive differentiation of adenoma from metastasis in most cases. In some situations, percutaneous biopsy or surgical resection may be required for indeterminate or aggressive adrenal masses (**Box 5**).

REFERENCES

1. Greenfield LJ, Mulholland MW. Surgery: scientific principles and practice. 3rd edition. Philadelphia: Lippincott Williams & Wilkins; 2001.
2. Lockhart ME, Smith JK, Kenney PJ. Imaging of adrenal masses. Eur J Radiol 2002;41(2):95–112.
3. Krebs TL, Wagner BJ. The adrenal gland: radiologic-pathologic correlation. Magn Reson Imaging Clin N Am 1997;5(1):127–46.
4. Bagheri B, Maurer AH, Cone L, et al. Characterization of the normal adrenal gland with 18F-FDG PET/CT. J Nucl Med 2004;45(8):1340–3.
5. Greenblatt DY, Shenker Y, Chen H. The utility of metaiodobenzylguanidine (MIBG) scintigraphy in patients with pheochromocytoma. Ann Surg Oncol 2008;15(3):900–5.

6. Boland GW, Blake MA, Holalkere NS, et al. PET/CT for the characterization of adrenal masses in patients with cancer: qualitative versus quantitative accuracy in 150 consecutive patients. AJR Am J Roentgenol 2009;192(4):956–62.

7. Berland LL, Silverman SG, Gore RM, et al. Managing incidental findings on abdominal CT: white paper of the ACR incidental findings committee. J Am Coll Radiol 2010;7(10):754–73.

8. Song JH, Chaudhry FS, Mayo-Smith WW. The incidental indeterminate adrenal mass on CT (>10 H) in patients without cancer: is further imaging necessary? Follow-up of 321 consecutive indeterminate adrenal masses. AJR Am J Roentgenol 2007;189(5):1119–23.

9. Sacerdote MG, Johnson PT, Fishman EK. CT of the adrenal gland: the many faces of adrenal hemorrhage. Emerg Radiol 2012;19(1):53–60.

10. Bradley WG Jr. MR appearance of hemorrhage in the brain. Radiology 1993;189(1):15–26.

11. Zeiger MA, Thompson GB, Duh QY, et al. The American Association of Clinical Endocrinologists and American Association of Endocrine Surgeons medical guidelines for the management of adrenal incidentalomas. Endocr Pract 2009;15(Suppl 1):1–20.

12. Dunnick NR, Leight GS Jr, Roubidoux MA, et al. CT in the diagnosis of primary aldosteronism: sensitivity in 29 patients. AJR Am J Roentgenol 1993;160(2):321–4.

13. Elsayes KM, Narra VR, Leyendecker JR, et al. MRI of adrenal and extraadrenal pheochromocytoma. AJR Am J Roentgenol 2005;184(3):860–7.

14. Lefebvre M, Foulkes WD. Pheochromocytoma and paraganglioma syndromes: genetics and management update. Curr Oncol 2014;21(1):e8–17.

15. Lenders JW, Pacak K, Walther MM, et al. Biochemical diagnosis of pheochromocytoma: which test is best? JAMA 2002;287(11):1427–34.

16. Northcutt BG, Raman SP, Long C, et al. MDCT of adrenal masses: can dual-phase enhancement patterns be used to differentiate adenoma and pheochromocytoma? AJR Am J Roentgenol 2013;201(4):834–9.

17. Blake MA, Krishnamoorthy SK, Boland GW, et al. Low-density pheochromocytoma on CT: a mimicker of adrenal adenoma. AJR Am J Roentgenol 2003;181(6):1663–8.

18. Patel J, Davenport MS, Cohan RH, et al. Can established CT attenuation and washout criteria for adrenal adenoma accurately exclude pheochromocytoma? AJR Am J Roentgenol 2013;201(1):122–7.

19. Miyajima A, Nakashima J, Baba S, et al. Clinical experience with incidentally discovered pheochromocytoma. J Urol 1997;157(5):1566–8.

20. Shulkin BL, Thompson NW, Shapiro B, et al. Pheochromocytomas: imaging with 2-[fluorine-18]fluoro-2-deoxy-D-glucose PET. Radiology 1999;212(1):35–41.

21. Wolf FJ, Dupuy DE, Machan JT, et al. Adrenal neoplasms: effectiveness and safety of CT-guided ablation of 23 tumors in 22 patients. Eur J Radiol 2012;81(8):1717–23.

22. Kumar P, Bryant T, Breen D, et al. Transarterial embolization and doxorubicin eluting beads-transarterial chemoembolization (DEB-TACE) of malignant extra-adrenal pheochromocytoma. Cardiovasc Intervent Radiol 2011;34(6):1325–9.

23. Gonias S, Goldsby R, Matthay KK, et al. Phase II study of high-dose [131I]metaiodobenzylguanidine therapy for patients with metastatic pheochromocytoma and paraganglioma. J Clin Oncol 2009;27(25):4162–8.

24. Bharwani N, Rockall AG, Sahdev A, et al. Adrenocortical carcinoma: the range of appearances on CT and MRI. AJR Am J Roentgenol 2011;196(6):W706–14.

25. Fishman EK, Deutch BM, Hartman DS, et al. Primary adrenocortical carcinoma: CT evaluation with clinical correlation. AJR Am J Roentgenol 1987;148(3):531–5.

26. Hussain S, Belldegrun A, Seltzer SE, et al. Differentiation of malignant from benign adrenal masses: predictive indices on computed tomography. AJR Am J Roentgenol 1985;144(1):61–5.

27. Slattery JM, Blake MA, Kalra MK, et al. Adrenocortical carcinoma: contrast washout characteristics on CT. AJR Am J Roentgenol 2006;187(1):W21–4.

28. Ferrozzi F, Bova D. CT and MR demonstration of fat within an adrenal cortical carcinoma. Abdom Imaging 1995;20(3):272–4.

29. Szolar DH, Korobkin M, Reittner P, et al. Adrenocortical carcinomas and adrenal pheochromocytomas: mass and enhancement loss evaluation at delayed contrast-enhanced CT. Radiology 2005;234(2):479–85.

30. Groussin L, Bonardel G, Silvera S, et al. 18F-Fluorodeoxyglucose positron emission tomography for the diagnosis of adrenocortical tumors: a prospective study in 77 operated patients. J Clin Endocrinol Metab 2009;94(5):1713–22.

31. Becherer A, Vierhapper H, Potzi C, et al. FDG-PET in adrenocortical carcinoma. Cancer Biother Radiopharm 2001;16(4):289–95.

32. Fowler AM, Burda JF, Kim SK. Adrenal artery embolization: anatomy, indications, and technical considerations. AJR Am J Roentgenol 2013;201(1):190–201.

33. Wood BJ, Abraham J, Hvizda JL, et al. Radiofrequency ablation of adrenal tumors and adrenocortical carcinoma metastases. Cancer 2003;97(3):554–60.

34. Korobkin M, Giordano TJ, Brodeur FJ, et al. Adrenal adenomas: relationship between histologic lipid and CT and MR findings. Radiology 1996;200(3):743–7.

35. Boland GW, Lee MJ, Gazelle GS, et al. Characterization of adrenal masses using unenhanced CT: an

analysis of the CT literature. AJR Am J Roentgenol 1998;171(1):201–4.

36. Korobkin M, Brodeur FJ, Francis IR, et al. CT time-attenuation washout curves of adrenal adenomas and nonadenomas. AJR Am J Roentgenol 1998; 170(3):747–52.

37. Caoili EM, Korobkin M, Francis IR, et al. Delayed enhanced CT of lipid-poor adrenal adenomas. AJR Am J Roentgenol 2000;175(5):1411–5.

38. Caoili EM, Korobkin M, Francis IR, et al. Adrenal masses: characterization with combined unenhanced and delayed enhanced CT. Radiology 2002;222(3):629–33.

39. Morgan DE, Weber AC, Lockhart ME, et al. Differentiation of high lipid content from low lipid content adrenal lesions using single-source rapid kilovolt (peak)-switching dual-energy multidetector CT. J Comput Assist Tomogr 2013;37(6):937–43.

40. Ho LM, Marin D, Neville AM, et al. Characterization of adrenal nodules with dual-energy CT: can virtual unenhanced attenuation values replace true unenhanced attenuation values? AJR Am J Roentgenol 2012;198(4):840–5.

41. Jhaveri KS, Wong F, Ghai S, et al. Comparison of CT histogram analysis and chemical shift MRI in the characterization of indeterminate adrenal nodules. AJR Am J Roentgenol 2006;187(5):1303–8.

42. Gabriel H, Pizzitola V, McComb EN, et al. Adrenal lesions with heterogeneous suppression on chemical shift imaging: clinical implications. J Magn Reson Imaging 2004;19(3):308–16.

43. Semelka RC, Shoenut JP, Lawrence PH, et al. Evaluation of adrenal masses with gadolinium enhancement and fat-suppressed MR imaging. J Magn Reson Imaging 1993;3(2):337–43.

44. Sandrasegaran K, Patel AA, Ramaswamy R, et al. Characterization of adrenal masses with diffusion-weighted imaging. AJR Am J Roentgenol 2011; 197(1):132–8.

45. Mayo-Smith WW, Lee MJ, McNicholas MM, et al. Characterization of adrenal masses (<5 cm) by use of chemical shift MR imaging: observer performance versus quantitative measures. AJR Am J Roentgenol 1995;165(1):91–5.

46. Fujiyoshi F, Nakajo M, Fukukura Y, et al. Characterization of adrenal tumors by chemical shift fast low-angle shot MR imaging: comparison of four methods of quantitative evaluation. AJR Am J Roentgenol 2003;180(6):1649–57.

47. Outwater EK, Siegelman ES, Radecki PD, et al. Distinction between benign and malignant adrenal masses: value of T1-weighted chemical-shift MR imaging. AJR Am J Roentgenol 1995;165(3):579–83.

48. Israel GM, Korobkin M, Wang C, et al. Comparison of unenhanced CT and chemical shift MRI in evaluating lipid-rich adrenal adenomas. AJR Am J Roentgenol 2004;183(1):215–9.

49. Haider MA, Ghai S, Jhaveri K, et al. Chemical shift MR imaging of hyperattenuating (>10 HU) adrenal masses: does it still have a role? Radiology 2004; 231(3):711–6.

50. Koo HJ, Choi HJ, Kim HJ, et al. The value of 15-minute delayed contrast-enhanced CT to differentiate hyperattenuating adrenal masses compared with chemical shift MR imaging. Eur Radiol 2014;24(6): 1410–20.

51. Outwater EK, Siegelman ES, Huang AB, et al. Adrenal masses: correlation between CT attenuation value and chemical shift ratio at MR imaging with in-phase and opposed-phase sequences. Radiology 1996;200(3):749–52.

52. Seo JM, Park BK, Park SY, et al. Characterization of lipid-poor adrenal adenoma: chemical-shift MRI and washout CT. AJR Am J Roentgenol 2014;202(5): 1043–50.

53. Shinozaki K, Yoshimitsu K, Honda H, et al. Metastatic adrenal tumor from clear-cell renal cell carcinoma: a pitfall of chemical shift MR imaging. Abdom Imaging 2001;26(4):439–42.

54. Sydow BD, Rosen MA, Siegelman ES. Intracellular lipid within metastatic hepatocellular carcinoma of the adrenal gland: a potential diagnostic pitfall of chemical shift imaging of the adrenal gland. AJR Am J Roentgenol 2006;187(5):W550–1.

55. Welch TJ, Sheedy PF 2nd, Stephens DH, et al. Percutaneous adrenal biopsy: review of a 10-year experience. Radiology 1994;193(2):341–4.

56. Casola G, Nicolet V, vanSonnenberg E, et al. Unsuspected pheochromocytoma: risk of blood-pressure alterations during percutaneous adrenal biopsy. Radiology 1986;159(3):733–5.

Pancreatic Solid and Cystic Neoplasms
Diagnostic Evaluation and Intervention

Mahmoud M. Al-Hawary, MD[a],*, Isaac R. Francis, MD[b],
Michelle A. Anderson, MD, MSc[c]

KEYWORDS

• Pancreas • Neoplasms • Solid • Cystic • Imaging • Intervention

KEY POINTS

• Typical imaging techniques for the evaluation of pancreatic neoplasms include computed tomography, MR imaging, and, in selected cases, endoscopic ultrasound.
• High-quality dedicated imaging is essential for the diagnosis and assessment of pancreatic tumor extent, both of which are required to determine the best therapy for patients.
• Endoscopic ultrasound facilitates tissue or cyst fluid sampling in solid and cystic pancreatic neoplasms to help establish the diagnosis or narrow the differential diagnosis.
• The mainstay of treatment of pancreatic neoplasms is complete surgical resection when possible.
• Several noninvasive and invasive methods for treating solid and cystic pancreatic neoplasms are being investigated when surgery is not possible or is contraindicated.

INTRODUCTION

Malignant pancreatic neoplasms are usually aggressive tumors with high mortality rates mainly attributed to the high prevalence of advanced disease at presentation and to the lack of significant advancement in medical therapies over the recent decades. The mainstay of curative treatment in most malignant pancreatic neoplasms depends on complete R0 surgical resection of the tumor (ie, no microscopic residual disease following resection) when possible. Focal ablation therapies are increasingly used in locally advanced tumors, unresectable tumors, or in poor surgical candidates and are mainly aimed at pain palliation and potentially improved survival. Common solid pancreatic neoplasms include pancreatic ductal adenocarcinoma (PDA) and pancreatic neuroendocrine tumor (NET). Common premalignant and malignant cystic pancreatic neoplasms include intraductal papillary mucinous neoplasm (IPMN) and mucinous cystic neoplasm (MCN). The incidence and rate of detection of common pancreatic solid and cystic lesions has been increasing in recent years.[1–3] The increase in detection rates is at least in part caused by the improvement in resolution of the imaging modalities, overall increased utilization of imaging for other indications, and an increased awareness of cystic pancreatic neoplasms. Commonly used imaging techniques and protocols, imaging findings, and available

Disclosures: None.
[a] Division of Abdominal Imaging, Department of Radiology, University of Michigan Hospitals, 1500 East Medical Center Drive, Room B1 D502, Ann Arbor, MI 48109, USA; [b] Division of Abdominal Imaging, Department of Radiology, University of Michigan Hospitals, 1500 East Medical Center Drive, Room B1 D540, Ann Arbor, MI 48109, USA; [c] Division of Gastroenterology, Department of Internal Medicine, University of Michigan Hospitals, 1500 East Medical Center Drive, Ann Arbor, MI 48109, USA
* Corresponding author.
E-mail address: alhawary@med.umich.edu

radiologic.theclinics.com

interventions and therapies of common solid and cystic pancreatic neoplasms are discussed in this article.

IMAGING TECHNIQUES AND PROTOCOLS
Computed Tomography

Thin-section multiphasic multidetector computed tomography (MDCT) of the abdomen is the most commonly used imaging tool in the evaluation of known or suspected pancreatic lesions.[4–6] CT utilization is primarily driven by the wider availability of CT scanners (compared with MR imaging) and the familiarity of interpreting radiologists with the imaging findings on CT (Fig. 1). The scan protocol outlined (Table 1) makes optimal use of both oral and intravenous contrast material with acquisition parameters that improve focal pancreatic mass detection, focal pancreatic mass extent, and the identification of metastatic disease. The small slice thickness helps achieve the highest spatial resolution possible to optimize visualization and to allow the identification of fine details, such as small focal lesion detection, pancreatic duct dilatation, pancreatic duct communication, tumor-to-vascular relationships, and alteration in vascular contour (Fig. 2). The use of neutral oral contrast material (such as water or other similar-density oral contrast agents) removes the uncommon artifacts caused by high-density oral contrast material and the masking effect of positive oral contrast that can hinder the volumetric reconstruction of the acquired images. Oral contrast also ensures distension of the adjacent stomach and duodenum, potentially improving the detection of local invasion. Selecting an intravenous low-osmolality iodinated contrast agent with a higher iodine concentration (eg, 370 mg Iodine/mL) helps to distinguish hyperenhancing or hypoenhancing lesions from the surrounding pancreatic parenchyma and improves the delineation of the peripancreatic vascular structures (Fig. 3). The reduced volume of intravenous contrast material in combination with reduced scan kilovolts peak settings (100–120 kVp or less) has been shown to increase the attenuation of iodinated contrast material without degrading the diagnostic imaging quality.[7,8] The dual-phase acquisition in the pancreatic parenchymal and subsequently the portal venous phase ensures optimal enhancement of the pancreatic parenchyma and adjacent arteries on the pancreatic phase and optimal enhancement of the remaining solid abdominal organs—most importantly the liver and peripancreatic veins—during the portal phase. Split bolus single-acquisition MDCT with spectral imaging at different kiloelectron volts has been shown to be at least equal to dual-phase single-energy CT in the assessment of vascular, liver, and pancreatic attenuation and tumor conspicuity, with a reduction in the radiation dose to the patients.[9] Scan coverage can be extended to cover the pelvic region with or without the thorax for complete assessment of metastatic disease or other incidental abnormalities that may influence treatment. Such additional staging scans are usually obtained based on institutional preferences, national guidelines, and scan indications.

CT reconstruction algorithms are essential for optimizing the review of the acquired thin-section MDCT images to facilitate the assessment of the pancreas and the surrounding vascular structures (Table 2). These algorithms depend on the slice thickness used in the acquisition, the availability of dedicated image review stations, and a volumetric image reconstruction client capable of generating high-fidelity multi-planar, maximum-intensity projections and 3-dimensional (3D) volumetric images.

MR Imaging

Contrast-enhanced MR imaging and contrast-enhanced magnetic resonance cholangiopancreatography (MRCP) of the abdomen have been shown to be of equal diagnostic accuracy to contrast-enhanced MDCT for the staging of solid pancreatic neoplasms and can be used interchangeably with MDCT depending on local practice preferences[5,10,11] (Fig. 4). However, MRCP is superior to CT for the evaluation of cystic pancreatic lesions given its improved signal-to-noise ratio

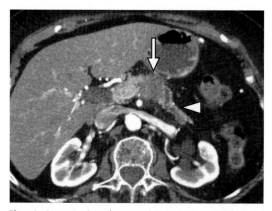

Fig. 1. Pancreatic adenocarcinoma on MDCT. Axial MDCT image through the pancreas demonstrates a focal hypodense lesion in the proximal pancreatic body (arrow) with associated atrophy of the pancreatic parenchyma and concomitant dilatation of the pancreatic duct in the distal body/tail region (arrowhead).

Table 1
MDCT pancreatic protocol

Scan Type	Helical
Slice thickness (detector configuration)	Thinnest possible, preferably submillimeter when available
Gap	None
Oral contrast	Low-density oral contrast or water
Intravenous contrast[a]	Low-osmolality iodinated contrast material with a high iodine concentration ($\geq$300 mg Iodine/mL) and a high injection rate $\geq$4 mL/s
Phase acquisition	Pancreatic parenchymal phase at 40–50 s after commencement of contrast material injection followed by portal venous phase at 65–70 s

[a] Lower iodine concentration and/or volume can be used if lower kilovolts peak setting or spectral CT imaging is used.

and the ability to obtain high-resolution images of the pancreatic and biliary ducts using the natural endogenous contrast provided by fluid-containing structures.[12] This ability is particularly valuable in detecting internal enhancement or solid mural nodules within cystic lesions, focal main pancreatic and biliary duct strictures, cyst-duct communication, and main duct enhancement. These features help in narrowing of the differential diagnosis and for assessing the malignant potential of cystic lesions.[13]

The contrast-enhanced MR imaging with MRCP imaging protocol includes a combination of sequences, each optimized for the evaluation of the pancreatic parenchyma, focal solid or cystic pancreatic lesions, and the pancreatobiliary tree (**Table 3**). Image subtraction technique

between the pre–T1-weighted gradient echo images and post–T1-weighted gradient echo images following intravenous contrast administration are particularly useful in assessing for underlying mural nodular enhancement in cystic lesions, which may be difficult to assess with CT examinations.[14] Diffusion-weighted imaging has also been shown to improve specificity for predicting the invasive malignant IPMN, which demonstrates lower apparent diffusion coefficient values as compared with the IPMN with no invasive tumors.[15,16] In addition to establishing the diagnosis and staging of focal pancreatic solid or cystic neoplasms, contrast-enhanced MR imaging is often used as a problem-solving tool, for example, the characterization of suspected small and iso-attenuating solid pancreatic tumors

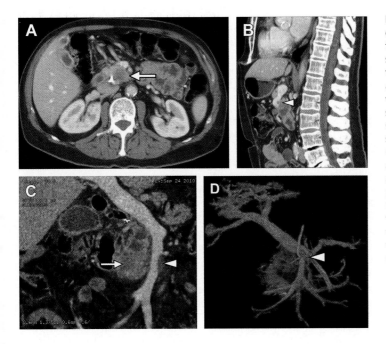

Fig. 2. Pancreatic adenocarcinoma on MDCT with multi-planar and reformatted display. Axial (*A*) and sagittal (*B*) MDCT images through the pancreas demonstrate pancreatic head adenocarcinoma (*arrow*) with evidence of direct tumor invasion into the SMV (*arrowhead*). Curved planar (*C*) and 3D surface-shaded volume-rendered display (*D*) images through the portal vein and superior mesenteric vein in another patient demonstrate pancreatic head adenocarcinoma (*arrow*) with evidence of tumor contact with the superior mesenteric vein and focal narrowing of the vessel caliber at the same level (*arrowhead*).

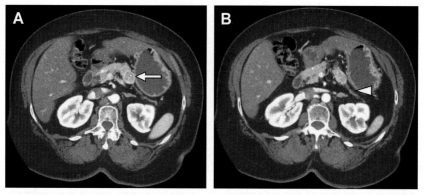

Fig. 3. Pancreatic NET. (*A, B*) Axial MDCT images through the pancreas demonstrate a focal hyperenhancing lesion in the pancreatic body (*arrow*) with associated upstream parenchymal atrophy (*arrowhead*).

on MDCT and the definitive characterization of indeterminate liver lesions noted on initial CT examinations to exclude metastatic disease. Contrast-enhanced MR is also the preferred modality to image the pancreas if contrast-enhanced CT cannot be obtained (eg, severe allergy to iodinated contrast material).

Endoscopic-Guided Ultrasound

High-resolution endoscopic-guided ultrasound (EUS) has become more widely available, and its use has gained broad acceptance in recent years for the diagnosis and management of pancreatic disorders.[17,18] This expanding utilization is caused by the relatively low complication rates and the ability to obtain high-resolution images of the pancreas through placement of the endoscopic ultrasound transducer in direct proximity to the pancreas. Moreover, the ability to introduce a fine-needle apparatus through the endoscope facilitates guidance for either aspiration from or injection into focal pancreatic lesions and has added further value to the now established role

of EUS in the diagnosis and intervention of pancreatic diseases[19] (**Fig. 5**).

In solid pancreatic mass evaluation, EUS in conjunction with MDCT has been shown to be the most useful imaging combination in the staging of pancreatic cancer.[20] Large-bore biopsy needles have been introduced that could require fewer samples and provide better samples for histologic analysis, but their use is technically challenging.[21] Similar to routine transcutaneous ultrasound, EUS is operator dependent and requires specialized expertise; therefore, it is best used in centers that have high clinical volume to ensure its optimal use.

SOLID PANCREATIC NEOPLASMS

The most common solid pancreatic neoplasms include PDA and NET. PDA incidence is increasing, with a reported annual percentage change (APC) of 1.2% between the years 1999 and 2010 compared with a negative APC in the preceding years.[1] Survival rates of no more than 5% to 10% at 5 years highlight the aggressiveness

Table 2
Image review of MDCT acquisition

Image Reconstruction	Comment
Axial 2–3 mm thickness	A thin (2–3 mm) reconstruction slice thickness is important to permit adequate spatial resolution, but overly thin slices (<2 mm) can result in unacceptably low signal-to-noise ratio.
MPR in the sagittal and coronal plane at 2–3 mm thickness	MPR improve assessment of the pancreas and surrounding vasculature. Axial images alone do not easily evaluate structures that curve through the axial plane.
MIP and 3D volumetric images	MIP and 3D reconstructions are useful for depicting the peripancreatic vasculature, including an assessment of vascular caliber change, anatomic variants, and the presence and extent of collateral vessels.

Abbreviations: 3D, 3 dimensional; MIP, maximum-intensity projections; MPR, multi-planar reformats.

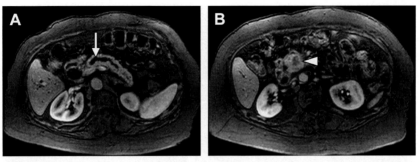

Fig. 4. Pancreatic adenocarcinoma on MR imaging. Axial T1-weighted postcontrast gradient-echo images through the pancreas. (A) Image through the pancreatic body demonstrates main pancreatic duct dilatation (arrow) extending down to the pancreatic head. (B) Image through the pancreatic head demonstrates a focal hypointense lesion (arrowhead) most consistent with adenocarcinoma.

of this tumor.[22] Similarly, high-grade NETs, which are classified based on the presence of high mitotic rate and Ki67 antibody labeling index (immunochemistry stain for tumor cells), can be locally aggressive and produce metastases.[23,24]

The decision regarding resectability status should be made by consensus at multidisciplinary meetings following the acquisition of dedicated pancreatic imaging for accurate staging. Use of a radiology staging reporting template is preferred to ensure a complete assessment and reporting of all imaging criteria that are essential for optimal staging. This template would help improve the treatment decision-making process.[25] Solid pancreatic neoplasm staging is based on 3

imaging findings categories that would influence the feasibility of complete resection and the type of surgery performed. These categories include

- Tumor location in the pancreas
- Absence or presence of tumor extension to the adjacent arteries and/or veins and type of tumor-vascular contact
- Invasion of adjacent organs and distant metastasis (including nonregional lymph node involvement)

The most commonly used reference for the staging and treatment of PDA is published by the National Comprehensive Cancer Network.[26,27]

Table 3
MR imaging pancreatic protocol

Sequences	Comment	Plane	Slice Thickness
T2-weighted single-shot fast spin-echo	Localizer	Coronal +/− axial	≤6 mm
T1-weighted dual-echo gradient echo	For evaluation of lipid- and fat-containing lesions	Axial	≤6 mm
T2-weighted fast spin-echo with fat saturation	Highlight solid and cystic lesions	Axial	≤6 mm
Diffusion-weighted imaging	Growing role in the detection and possibly characterization of some solid and cystic lesions	Axial	≤6 mm
Dynamic 3D T1-weighted gradient echo with fat saturation before and after gadolinium-based contrast material administration	Unenhanced, pancreatic, venous, and equilibrium phases Performed to detect and characterize lesions and assess peripancreatic vasculature	Axial	2–3 mm (3D)
Heavily T2-weighted 3D fast-recovery fast spin echo MRCP with 3D reconstructions	Evaluate for ductal strictures, establish cyst-duct communication	Coronal	1–3 mm (3D)

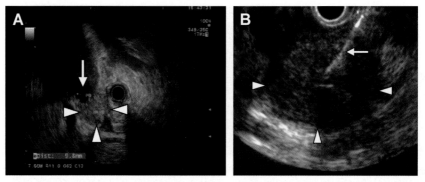

Fig. 5. EUS with fine-needle aspiration. (*A*) Image capture during EUS demonstrates a focal hypoechoic lesion in the pancreatic head (*arrowheads*) consistent with pancreatic adenocarcinoma. Dilated pancreatic duct (*arrow*). (*B*) Image capture during needle aspiration in another patient demonstrates the echogenic needle (*arrow*) passing through the tumor (*arrowheads*).

Nonmetastatic PDAs are categorized into 3 different categories based primarily on the type of vascular contact:

- Resectable: no tumor contact with surrounding vessels
- Borderline resectable: tumor contact with the surrounding vessels that can potentially be downstaged and completely resected following neoadjuvant chemotherapy with or without radiation therapy
- Locally advanced or unresectable: tumor contact or vascular occlusion prohibiting safe complete resection of the tumor with no residual disease

Other modalities of therapy when surgery is not feasible or possible have been described. Percutaneous or intraoperative thermal ablation of locally advanced or unresectable nonmetastatic PDA is emerging as a feasible treatment alternative to systemic therapy. Studies with small numbers of patients show that this may be done with relatively low morbidity and mortality and probable positive impact on patient survival.[28,29] EUS-guided ablation has also been shown to be feasible in treating locally advanced pancreatic cancers with low risk of complications.[30,31] Successful use of ablation has been reported in patients with small pancreatic NETs who are poor surgical candidates.[32] Limitations to ablation therapy include injury to bile ducts, pancreatic ducts, vascular structures, and bowel segments that are in close proximity to the treated tumor. Large prospective studies are needed to determine whether there are survival benefits associated with these techniques.

Reports are emerging about the use of high-intensity focused ultrasound (HIFU) in the treatment of unresectable PDA and NET.[33–37] HIFU is a noninvasive method of solid tumor ablation therapy in which an external ultrasound energy source is used to induce heating or cavitation.[38] Most studies of pancreatic HIFU have included small groups of patients in whom HIFU was used primarily as a palliative measure to reduce pain; few immediate side effects have been reported.[39,40] The effect of HIFU on survival is unclear given the small sample sizes in reported studies, but a modest survival benefit has been suggested.[34]

Based on previous reports of success using percutaneous injection of alcohol for ablation of NETs, EUS-guided ethanol ablation of NETs of the pancreas has been explored as a treatment option for patients who are poor surgical candidates or refuse surgery.[41,42] EUS fine-needle injection is made using the linear echoendoscope in 1 to 2 treatment sessions to deliver an average of 0.8 mL (range 0.12–3.0 mL) 98% ethanol to the tumor.[41] Complications with this technique include pain, pancreatitis, bleeding leading to hematoma formation, and ulceration of the enteral wall.[43] Other antitumor therapies, including photodynamic therapy, brachytherapy, and other novel agents, for pancreatic cancer that can be delivered locally to the site of the tumor using EUS have also been recently introduced but remain investigational at this time.[44,45]

Intraoperative, percutaneous, and more recently EUS-guided gold fiducial placement at the site of localized advanced pancreatic cancer has become more widely accepted; their use for guiding radiation therapy is highly recommended by many experts[46–48] (**Fig. 6**). The visible markers on radiograph and CT help to more accurately guide real-time tracking of localized stereotactic body radiation therapy targeting the site of the tumor, which will allow the delivery of high-dose therapeutic radiation to the tumor with less risk of injury to the surrounding structures[49] (**Fig. 7**).

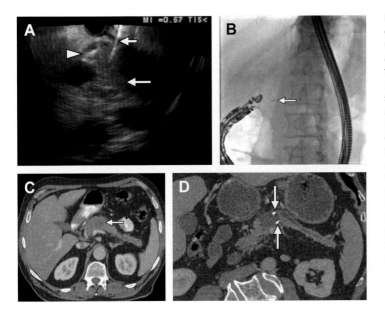

Fig. 6. Tumor localization with EUS-guided placement of gold fiducials using linear echoendoscope in preparation for image-guided radiation therapy. (*A*) EUS image capture during placement of the fiducial clips show a 22-gauge needle (*short arrow*) within the pancreatic mass (*long arrow*). Adjacent placed fiducial clip is seen (*arrowhead*). (*B*) Spot radiograph confirms the placement of the clips (*arrow*). (*C*) Axial MDCT image through the pancreas demonstrates a focal hypodense lesion in the pancreatic body (*arrow*). (*D*) Curved reformatted CT image following the placement of the fiducial clips along the anterior and posterior edge of the mass (*arrows*).

CYSTIC PANCREATIC NEOPLASMS

There has been a significant increase in the detection rate of cystic pancreatic lesions in the last decade mainly caused by the increased utilization of cross-sectional imaging modalities, such as CT and MR imaging.[50] The most common cystic pancreatic neoplasms that have a malignant potential are MCN and IPMN. Both are mucin producing and can exist in a spectrum of forms ranging from premalignant (with low-, moderate-, or high-grade dysplasia) to frankly malignant lesions (invasive carcinoma).[51] The characteristic lining of MCNs is nearly identical to ovarian mucinous tumors exhibiting a papillary architecture. In contrast to MCNs, IPMNs communicate with the pancreatic duct (either the main duct or a branch) and are lined with mucin-secreting, columnar, ductal epithelium, which always displays at least low-grade dysplasia. Various subtypes (gastric, intestinal, pancreaticobiliary, oncocytic) with associated clinical features of significance have been described.[52]

IPMN is typically a tumor present in older men.[53] These tumors can be divided into 3 distinct groups that carry different prognostic significance.[54] These groups include

- Side-branch type: This form is associated with less malignant potential compared with the other types and can be followed by imaging if no concerning features (eg, solid nodule) are present (**Fig. 8**).[54] It is the only cystic lesion among the cystic pancreatic neoplasms that communicates with the main pancreatic duct, and this finding is used as a diagnostic criterion to differentiate IPMN from other cystic tumors.
- Main-duct type: This form primarily involves the main pancreatic duct and can be either focal or diffuse. It carries the highest risk of malignancy relative to the side-branch type.
- Combined or mixed type: This form contains imaging features of both the side-branch–type and main-duct–type IPMNs and is generally considered similar to the main-duct type in regard to the risk of malignancy.

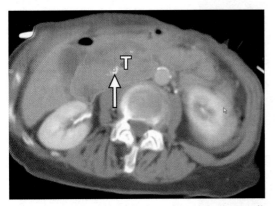

Fig. 7. Image-guided radiation therapy using radiopaque markers. Axial CT image for intensity-modulated radiation therapy, with planning centered at the level of the fiducial marker (*arrow*) to better localize the field of radiation. T, tumor.

The presence of high-risk features, such as severe main pancreatic duct dilation (≥10 mm

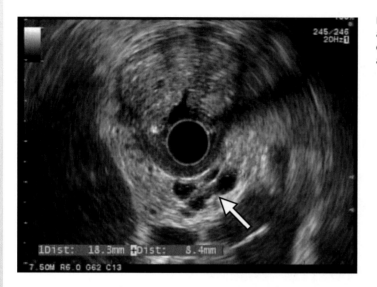

Fig. 8. Side-branch IPMN on EUS. Image capture demonstrates a focal cystic lesion with septa in the pancreatic head (*arrow*).

caliber), and/or an enhancing solid component are an indication of a potentially malignant lesion that warrants surgical removal if not contraindicated[55] (**Figs. 9** and **10**). Intermediate-risk features, such as large cyst size (≥3 cm), nonenhancing mural nodules, a thickened or enhancing cyst wall, septa, or moderate main pancreatic duct dilatation (5–9 mm), are indications for close follow-up to exclude a potentially malignant lesion.

MCNs are rare relative to IPMN and are reported almost exclusively (98%) in middle-aged women in their fifth or sixth decade of life. MCNs exhibit a histologic spectrum that ranges from the benign mucinous cystadenoma to the malignant

cystadenocarcinoma[53] (**Fig. 11**). These tumors are typically composed of an encapsulated round or oval dominant cyst. Additional features include peripheral calcifications (seen in up to 15% of cases), internal septa, and/or nodularity. Presence of septations, wall or septal calcifications, thick surrounding wall, and/or enhancing nodularity is each a worrisome feature for potential malignancy.

The roles for cross-sectional imaging coupled with interventional procedures, such as EUS for morphologic assessment and cyst fluid analysis in the diagnostic evaluation of cystic pancreatic lesions, is continuously evolving. An important function in the evaluation of these lesions is to

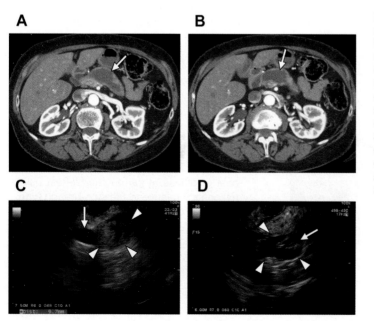

Fig. 9. Main-duct IPMN with high-risk features. (*A, B*) Axial MDCT images through the pancreas demonstrate main pancreatic duct dilatation throughout the gland measuring more than 1 cm in diameter (*arrow*). (*C*) EUS image demonstrates a dilated main pancreatic duct measuring 10 mm (*arrow*) and a nodule/mucin plug within the duct (*arrowheads*). (*D*) EUS image demonstrates a cystic lesion (*arrowheads*) with a large peripheral nodule (*arrow*).

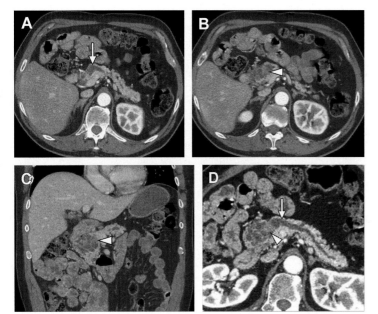

Fig. 10. Main-duct IPMN with concerning high-risk features. (*A, B*) Axial MDCT, (*C*) coronal, and (*D*) curved reformat images through the pancreas demonstrate main-duct dilatation (*arrows*) with focal enlargement in the head region and associated nodular density along the duct (*arrowheads*).

distinguish mucinous (premalignant or malignant IPMN and MCN) from nonmucinous cystic lesions (benign serous tumors or pseudocysts). EUS is an excellent tool that can help guide fine-needle aspiration of pancreatic cyst fluid contents, which can be used to analyze for the presence of mucin, known tumor markers (eg, carcinoembryonic antigen [CEA], carbohydrate-associated antigen [CA] 19-9, CA-125), pancreatic enzymes (eg, amylase), as well as histocytologic analysis. Different combinations of these markers have been shown to differentiate mucinous from nonmucinous lesions but have a limited role in differentiating benign from malignant mucinous cysts.[56,57]

Intracystic fluid with a very low amylase concentration (<250 U/L) virtually excludes a pseudocyst, whereas intracystic fluid with a high amylase level (≥250 U/L) can be seen in both pseudocysts and IPMNs. A low CEA level less than 5 ng/mL and a low CA 19-9 level less than 37 U/mL each suggests a serous tumor or pseudocyst, whereas a high CEA level greater than 800 ng/mL favors a MCN. A CEA of 192 ng/mL or greater has been shown to differentiate mucinous from nonmucinous pancreatic cysts with a sensitivity of 75%, a specificity of 83%, and an overall accuracy of 79%.[56] One report has suggested that the combination of cyst fluid CEA and CA-125 may be helpful to differentiate MCN from IPMN, but thus far no thresholds have proven definitive.[58]

The yield of tumor cells on fine-needle aspiration of cystic lesions of the pancreas is notoriously low; therefore, a negative fine-needle aspiration is not a reliable indicator to exclude malignancy.[59] DNA cyst fluid analysis for *K-ras* mutations may offer improved specificity for

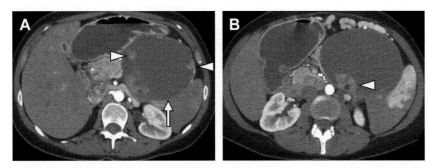

Fig. 11. MCN. (*A, B*) Axial contrast-enhanced MDCT images through the pancreas demonstrate a large unilocular cystic lesion (*arrow*) with soft tissue nodules along the posterior wall (*arrowheads*). Pathology revealed mucinous tumor with invasive carcinoma.

mucinous tumors, in particular when combined with a high CEA level.[60]

EUS pancreatic cyst ablation with ethanol, paclitaxel, or other agents has been used for nonoperative management of some patients who are otherwise not eligible for definitive therapy with resection.[61,62] Histopathologic examination of the cysts in patients who have undergone resection following such therapies have demonstrated variable degrees of ablation of the epithelium lining the cyst cavity ranging from 0% to 100%. Further studies describing the safety of these approaches, the best agents for ablation, and the optimal lesions for therapy are needed. Current applications of these unproven techniques should occur exclusively in a research setting.

SUMMARY

The imaging approach and management of pancreatic neoplasms are continuously evolving. This evolution is mainly caused by the widespread availability and utilization of high-resolution imaging tools, such as MDCT, MR imaging/MRCP, and EUS, which have led to both the increased detection and better characterization of both solid and cystic pancreatic neoplasms. Although there has been no significant change in the basic treatment and mortality rates of pancreatic neoplasms, whereby cure can only be achieved with complete surgical resection, several noninvasive and invasive nonsurgical treatments have become available and are being increasingly used. These treatments range from ethanol injection into pancreatic cysts to alcohol, HIFU, and thermal ablation in solid pancreatic tumors. Although these methods are reported to have low complication rates and may reduce patient symptoms, their effect on patient survival remains unknown. Controlled series are needed to establish their role in the management of these patients.

REFERENCES

1. Howlader N, Noone AM, Krapcho M, et al. SEER cancer statistics review, 1975–2009 (vintage 2009 populations). Bethesda (MD): National Cancer Institute. Available at: http://seer.cancer.gov/statfacts/html/pancreas.html. Accessed December 23, 2014.
2. Laffan TA, Horton KM, Klein AP, et al. Prevalence of unsuspected pancreatic cysts on MDCT. AJR Am J Roentgenol 2008;191(3):802–7.
3. de Jong K, Nio CY, Hermans JJ, et al. High prevalence of pancreatic cysts detected by screening magnetic resonance imaging examinations. Clin Gastroenterol Hepatol 2010;8(9):806–11.
4. Zamboni GA, Kruskal JB, Vollmer CM, et al. Pancreatic adenocarcinoma: value of multidetector CT angiography in preoperative evaluation. Radiology 2007;245(3):770–8.
5. Sahani DV, Shah ZK, Catalano OA, et al. Radiology of pancreatic adenocarcinoma: current status of imaging. J Gastroenterol Hepatol 2008;23(1):23–33.
6. Tamm EP, Balachandran A, Bhosale PR, et al. Imaging of pancreatic adenocarcinoma: update on staging/resectability. Radiol Clin North Am 2012;50(3):407–28.
7. Kalva SP, Sahani DV, Hahn PF, et al. Using the K-edge to improve contrast conspicuity and to lower radiation dose with a 16-MDCT: a phantom and human study. J Comput Assist Tomogr 2006;30(3):391–7.
8. Clark ZE, Bolus DN, Little MD, et al. Abdominal rapid-kVp-switching dual-energy MDCT with reduced IV contrast compared to conventional MDCT with standard weight-based IV contrast: an intra-patient comparison. Abdom Imaging 2014;40:852–8.
9. Brook OR, Gourtsoyianni S, Brook A, et al. Split-bolus spectral multidetector CT of the pancreas: assessment of radiation dose and tumor conspicuity. Radiology 2013;269(1):139–48.
10. Sheridan MB, Ward J, Guthrie JA, et al. Dynamic contrast-enhanced MR imaging and dual-phase helical CT in the preoperative assessment of suspected pancreatic cancer: a comparative study with receiver operating characteristic analysis. AJR Am J Roentgenol 1999;173(3):583–90.
11. Tamm EP, Bhosale PR, Lee JH. Pancreatic ductal adenocarcinoma: ultrasound, computed tomography, and magnetic resonance imaging features. Semin Ultrasound CT MR 2007;28(5):330–8.
12. Kim SH, Lee JM, Lee ES, et al. Intraductal papillary mucinous neoplasms of the pancreas: evaluation of malignant potential and surgical resectability by using MR imaging with MR cholangiography. Radiology 2014;274:723–33.
13. Manfredi R, Graziani R, Motton M, et al. Main pancreatic duct intraductal papillary mucinous neoplasms: accuracy of MR imaging in differentiation between benign and malignant tumors compared with histopathologic analysis. Radiology 2009;253(1):106–15.
14. Do RK, Katz SS, Gollub MJ, et al. Interobserver agreement for detection of malignant features of intraductal papillary mucinous neoplasms of the pancreas on MDCT. AJR Am J Roentgenol 2014;203(5):973–9.
15. Kang KM, Lee JM, Shin CI, et al. Added value of diffusion-weighted imaging to MR cholangiopancreatography with unenhanced MR imaging for predicting malignancy or invasiveness of intraductal

papillary mucinous neoplasm of the pancreas. J Magn Reson Imaging 2013;38(3):555–63.

16. Jang KM, Kim SH, Min JH, et al. Value of diffusion-weighted MRI for differentiating malignant from benign intraductal papillary mucinous neoplasms of the pancreas. AJR Am J Roentgenol 2014; 203(5):992–1000.

17. Agarwal B, Abu-Hamda E, Molke KL, et al. Endoscopic ultrasound-guided fine needle aspiration and multidetector spiral CT in the diagnosis of pancreatic cancer. Am J Gastroenterol 2004;99(5): 844–50.

18. Varadarajulu S, Eloubeidi MA. The role of endoscopic ultrasonography in the evaluation of pancreatico-biliary cancer. Surg Clin North Am 2010;90(2):251–63.

19. Mizuno N, Hara K, Hijioka S, et al. Current concept of endoscopic ultrasound-guided fine needle aspiration for pancreatic cancer. Pancreatology 2011; 11(Suppl 2):40–6.

20. Soriano A, Castells A, Ayuso C, et al. Preoperative staging and tumor resectability assessment of pancreatic cancer: prospective study comparing endoscopic ultrasonography, helical computed tomography, magnetic resonance imaging, and angiography. Am J Gastroenterol 2004;99(3):492–501.

21. Lee YN, Moon JH, Kim HK, et al. Core biopsy needle versus standard aspiration needle for endoscopic ultrasound-guided sampling of solid pancreatic masses: a randomized parallel-group study. Endoscopy 2014;46(12):1056–62.

22. Conlon KC, Klimstra DS, Brennan MF. Long-term survival after curative resection for pancreatic ductal adenocarcinoma. Clinicopathologic analysis of 5-year survivors. Ann Surg 1996;223(3):273–9.

23. Reid MD, Balci S, Saka B, et al. Neuroendocrine tumors of the pancreas: current concepts and controversies. Endocr Pathol 2014;25(1):65–79.

24. Burns WR, Edil BH. Neuroendocrine pancreatic tumors: guidelines for management and update. Curr Treat Options Oncol 2012;13(1):24–34.

25. Al-Hawary MM, Francis IR, Chari ST, et al. Pancreatic ductal adenocarcinoma radiology reporting template: consensus statement of the society of abdominal radiology and the American Pancreatic Association. Gastroenterology 2014;146(1): 291–304.e1.

26. Tempero MA, Arnoletti JP, Behrman SW, et al. Pancreatic adenocarcinoma, version 2.2012: featured updates to the NCCN guidelines. J Natl Compr Canc Netw 2012;10(6):703–13.

27. Tempero MA, Arnoletti JP, Behrman SW, et al. NCCN guidelines version 1.2015. Available at: http://www. nccn.org/professionals/physician_gls/pdf/pancreatic. pdf. Accessed December 23, 2014.

28. Girelli R, Frigerio I, Salvia R, et al. Feasibility and safety of radiofrequency ablation for locally advanced pancreatic cancer. Br J Surg 2010; 97(2):220–5.

29. Fegrachi S, Besselink MG, van Santvoort HC, et al. Radiofrequency ablation for unresectable locally advanced pancreatic cancer: a systematic review. HPB (Oxford) 2014;16(2):119–23.

30. Arcidiacono PG, Carrara S, Reni M, et al. Feasibility and safety of EUS-guided cryothermal ablation in patients with locally advanced pancreatic cancer. Gastrointest Endosc 2012;76(6):1142–51.

31. Yoon WJ, Brugge WR. Endoscopic ultrasonography-guided tumor ablation. Gastrointest Endosc Clin N Am 2012;22(2):359–69, xi.

32. Rossi S, Viera FT, Ghittoni G, et al. Radiofrequency ablation of pancreatic neuroendocrine tumors: a pilot study of feasibility, efficacy, and safety. Pancreas 2014;43(6):938–45.

33. Li PZ, Zhu SH, He W, et al. High-intensity focused ultrasound treatment for patients with unresectable pancreatic cancer. Hepatobiliary Pancreat Dis Int 2012;11(6):655–60.

34. Wu F, Wang ZB, Zhu H, et al. Feasibility of US-guided high-intensity focused ultrasound treatment in patients with advanced pancreatic cancer: initial experience. Radiology 2005;236(3):1034–40.

35. Lee JY, Choi BI, Ryu JK, et al. Concurrent chemotherapy and pulsed high-intensity focused ultrasound therapy for the treatment of unresectable pancreatic cancer: initial experiences. Korean J Radiol 2011;12(2):176–86.

36. Orgera G, Krokidis M, Monfardini L, et al. High intensity focused ultrasound ablation of pancreatic neuroendocrine tumours: report of two cases. Cardiovasc Intervent Radiol 2011;34(2):419–23.

37. Chen Q, Zhu X, Chen Q, et al. Unresectable giant pancreatic neuroendocrine tumor effectively treated by high-intensity focused ultrasound: a case report and review of the literature. Pancreatology 2013; 13(6):634–8.

38. Kennedy JE, Ter Haar GR, Cranston D. High intensity focused ultrasound: surgery of the future? Br J Radiol 2003;76(909):590–9.

39. Orsi F, Zhang L, Arnone P, et al. High-intensity focused ultrasound ablation: effective and safe therapy for solid tumors in difficult locations. AJR Am J Roentgenol 2010;195(3):W245–52.

40. Gao HF, Wang K, Meng ZQ, et al. High intensity focused ultrasound treatment for patients with local advanced pancreatic cancer. Hepatogastroenterology 2013;60(128):1906–10.

41. Levy MJ, Thompson GB, Topazian MD, et al. US-guided ethanol ablation of insulinomas: a new treatment option. Gastrointest Endosc 2012;75(1): 200–6.

42. Lee MJ, Jung CH, Jang JE, et al. Successful endoscopic ultrasound-guided ethanol ablation of multiple insulinomas accompanied with multiple

endocrine neoplasia type 1. Intern Med J 2013; 43(8):948–50.

43. Deprez PH, Claessens A, Borbath I, et al. Successful endoscopic ultrasound-guided ethanol ablation of a sporadic insulinoma. Acta Gastroenterol 2008; 71(3):333–7.

44. Ashida R, Chang KJ. Interventional EUS for the treatment of pancreatic cancer. J Hepatobiliary Pancreat Surg 2009;16(5):592–7.

45. Nakai Y, Chang KJ. Endoscopic ultrasound-guided antitumor agents. Gastrointest Endosc Clin N Am 2012;22(2):315–24, x.

46. Sanders MK, Moser AJ, Khalid A, et al. EUS-guided fiducial placement for stereotactic body radiotherapy in locally advanced and recurrent pancreatic cancer. Gastrointest Endosc 2010; 71(7):1178–84.

47. Trumm CG, Haussler SM, Muacevic A, et al. CT fluoroscopy-guided percutaneous fiducial marker placement for CyberKnife stereotactic radiosurgery: technical results and complications in 222 consecutive procedures. J Vasc Interv Radiol 2014;25(5): 760–8.

48. Abbas H, Chang B, Chen ZJ. Motion management in gastrointestinal cancers. J Gastrointest Oncol 2014; 5(3):223–35.

49. Yang W, Fraass BA, Reznik R, et al. Adequacy of inhale/exhale breathhold CT based ITV margins and image-guided registration for free-breathing pancreas and liver SBRT. Radiat Oncol 2014;9:11.

50. Khalid A, Brugge W. ACG practice guidelines for the diagnosis and management of neoplastic pancreatic cysts. Am J Gastroenterol 2007; 102(10):2339–49.

51. Brugge WR, Lauwers GY, Sahani D, et al. Cystic neoplasms of the pancreas. N Engl J Med 2004; 351(12):1218–26.

52. Mino-Kenudson M, Fernandez-del Castillo C, Baba Y, et al. Prognosis of invasive intraductal papillary mucinous neoplasm depends on histological and precursor epithelial subtypes. Gut 2011; 60(12):1712–20.

53. Dewhurst CE, Mortele KJ. Cystic tumors of the pancreas: imaging and management. Radiol Clin North Am 2012;50(3):467–86.

54. Terris B, Ponsot P, Paye F, et al. Intraductal papillary mucinous tumors of the pancreas confined to secondary ducts show less aggressive pathologic features as compared with those involving the main pancreatic duct. Am J Surg Pathol 2000;24(10):1372–7.

55. Tanaka M, Fernandez-del Castillo C, Adsay V, et al. International consensus guidelines 2012 for the management of IPMN and MCN of the pancreas. Pancreatology 2012;12(3):183–97.

56. Brugge WR, Lewandrowski K, Lee-Lewandrowski E, et al. Diagnosis of pancreatic cystic neoplasms: a report of the cooperative pancreatic cyst study. Gastroenterology 2004;126(5):1330–6.

57. van der Waaij LA, van Dullemen HM, Porte RJ. Cyst fluid analysis in the differential diagnosis of pancreatic cystic lesions: a pooled analysis. Gastrointest Endosc 2005;62(3):383–9.

58. Nagashio Y, Hijioka S, Mizuno N, et al. Combination of cyst fluid CEA and CA 125 is an accurate diagnostic tool for differentiating mucinous cystic neoplasms from intraductal papillary mucinous neoplasms. Pancreatology 2014;14(6):503–9.

59. de Jong K, Poley JW, van Hooft JE, et al. Endoscopic ultrasound-guided fine-needle aspiration of pancreatic cystic lesions provides inadequate material for cytology and laboratory analysis: initial results from a prospective study. Endoscopy 2011;43(7): 585–90.

60. Al-Haddad M, DeWitt J, Sherman S, et al. Performance characteristics of molecular (DNA) analysis for the diagnosis of mucinous pancreatic cysts. Gastrointest Endosc 2014;79(1):79–87.

61. DeWitt J. Endoscopic ultrasound-guided pancreatic cyst ablation. Gastrointest Endosc Clin N Am 2012; 22(2):291–302. ix-x.

62. Oh HC, Seo DW, Kim SH, et al. Systemic effect of endoscopic ultrasonography-guided pancreatic cyst ablation with ethanol and paclitaxel. Dig Dis Sci 2014;59(7):1573–7.

Image-Guided Percutaneous Abdominal Mass Biopsy
Technical and Clinical Considerations

Andrew J. Lipnik, MD*, Daniel B. Brown, MD

KEYWORDS

- Percutaneous • Image-guided • Abdominal • Biopsy • Liver • Kidney • Fine-needle aspiration
- Core needle biopsy

KEY POINTS

- Image-guided percutaneous abdominal biopsy is a safe and effective method of obtaining tissue for diagnosis of a variety of pathologic processes.
- Percutaneous biopsy will play an increasing role in the evaluation of response to directed oncologic therapies.
- Tract seeding remains a concern when biopsy is performed for suspected hepatocellular carcinoma (HCC) and is a disastrous outcome in a liver transplant candidate.
- Tract seeding is relatively rare when biopsy of suspected renal cell carcinoma (RCC) is performed, and biopsy is playing an increasing role in treatment algorithms for RCC.

INTRODUCTION

Image-guided percutaneous biopsy of abdominal masses is one of the most frequently performed procedures in many interventional radiology practices. The success of this minimally invasive procedure rests on its excellent safety profile, rapid recovery time, and high diagnostic yield for a variety of pathologic processes. As imaging techniques have steadily improved, the ability to detect and target smaller lesions has likewise improved, allowing diagnosis and therefore treatment at earlier stages of disease.

PREPROCEDURE
General Indications and Contraindications

Patient preparation begins at the time of scheduling when a valid indication for the procedure should be established. General indications and contraindications for biopsy are listed in **Box 1**.

Contraindications to percutaneous biopsy are few and typically relative. Uncorrectable coagulopathy, inaccessible entry site, and an uncooperative patient are most often cited. However, many bleeding diatheses can be corrected; it is a rare location in the abdomen that cannot be safely reached by a fine needle, and general anesthesia remains an option for uncooperative patients. Ultimately, the risk of the biopsy needs to be weighed against the benefit of the information obtained for that particular patient.

Imaging Review

Relevant imaging should be reviewed to make sure that the requested biopsy can be performed with a high likelihood of success and minimum

Disclosure statement: D.B. Brown is a consultant for Cook Medical, Onyx Pharmaceuticals, Vascular Solutions, and Medtronic. A.J. Lipnik has nothing to disclose.
Department of Radiology and Radiological Sciences, Vanderbilt University Medical Center, 1161 21st Avenue South, MCN - Room CCC-1118, Nashville, TN 37232-2675, USA
* Corresponding author.
E-mail address: andrew.j.lipnik@vanderbilt.edu

Radiol Clin N Am 53 (2015) 1049–1059
http://dx.doi.org/10.1016/j.rcl.2015.05.007

Table 1
Coagulation parameters

Laboratory Test	Normal	Suggested Cutoff
INR	0.9–1.1	$\leq$1.6
aPTT	25–35 s	<1.5× control
Platelets	150,000–450,000	>50,000

Abbreviations: aPTT, activated partial thromboplastin time; INR, international normalized ratio.

Adapted from Patel IJ, Davidson JC, Nikolic B, et al. Addendum of newer anticoagulants to the SIR consensus guideline. J Vasc Interv Radiol 2013;24(5):642; with permission.

risk. This imaging review should include (1) whether or not a definitive diagnosis can be made based on imaging alone, obviating biopsy altogether; (2) if there is a more accessible biopsy target than what was requested; (3) if there is a safe route from the skin to the target; and (4) what the optimal imaging modality for guidance will be.

Anticoagulation Status

Typically, the most feared complication of abdominal biopsy is bleeding. As such, special attention during patient preparation should be paid to the patient's coagulation status. This problem is complex with often-conflicting viewpoints in the literature. Guidelines produced by national societies frequently get translated at the department level to suit local practice needs and the specific clinical circumstances of the patient.

Basic coagulation parameters based on the Society of Interventional Radiology consensus guidelines are suggested in **Table 1**.[1,2] Typically, laboratory results obtained in the previous month are acceptable, but the authors require updated laboratory results when the patient is on therapeutic anticoagulation; has a known bleeding disorder; has recently received chemotherapy, which may alter coagulation status; or has known comorbidities that may affect the bleeding parameters such as cirrhosis, malabsorption/malnutrion, significant hepatic metastatic disease, or renal failure.

The authors correct the international normalized ratio (INR) to less than 1.6 and platelets to greater than 50,000 by transfusing fresh frozen plasma (FFP) and platelets, respectively. Atwell and

colleagues[3] demonstrated low overall rates of significant bleeding (0.5%) using these parameters in over 15,000 core needle biopsies, and notably, aspirin use did not affect the rate of major bleeding. However, it should be recognized that there is a paucity of studies to date that demonstrate a correlation between mild to moderate elevation in coagulation parameters and bleeding risk in image-guided procedures.[4] In addition, in patients with mild coagulopathy, attempts to correct the INR rarely result in normalization.[5] Thus, in certain clinical scenarios, the authors believe that it is acceptable to proceed with a biopsy when coagulation status is outside of these parameters, although the potentially elevated bleeding risk is discussed with both the patient and the referring physician. Given the short half-life of FFP and platelets, the authors prefer to have the last unit of blood products infusing during the procedure. Ultimately, the decision to transfuse FFP or platelets depends on the clinical scenario and consideration of the risks of transfusion, including reactions, volume overload, transmitted infections, and transfusion-related acute lung injury, balanced against the perceived increased risk of hemorrhagic complications.[1,6,7]

Basic management of agents affecting anticoagulation is addressed in **Table 2**. However, withholding anticoagulation and antiplatelet agents should always be discussed with the referring physician, particularly in cases of recent cardiac stent placement, because the risk of adverse events from stopping them may significantly outweigh the bleeding risk of the biopsy. In these cases, the biopsy is deferred until the time when anticoagulants can be safely stopped. If the information to be obtained by the biopsy is of urgency, the biopsy occasionally proceeds at higher risk, which is detailed with the patient during informed consent.

Table 2
Basic anticoagulation and antiplatelet management

Agent	Duration Withheld Before Procedure
Coumadin	5 d
Unfractionated heparin	4–6 h
LMWH	1 dose[a]
NSAIDs	Do not withhold
Aspirin	Do not withhold[b]
Plavix	5 d

Abbreviations: LMWH, low-molecular-weight heparin; NSAID, nonsteroidal antiinflammatory drug.
[a] LMWH is held for 2 doses before renal and spleen biopsies.
[b] Aspirin is held 5 days before renal and spleen biopsies.
Adapted from Patel IJ, Davidson JC, Nikolic B, et al. Addendum of newer anticoagulants to the SIR consensus guideline. J Vasc Interv Radiol 2013;24(5):643.

With the advent of newer-generation anticoagulants, management scenarios are more complicated. Although strong evidence for the periprocedural management of these newer medications is often lacking, withholding for 5 half-lives is generally considered safe because this results in 3% residual drug activity.[2,8]

PERFORMANCE OF PROCEDURE
Imaging Guidance

Although there is no single best imaging modality for biopsy guidance, the selection of the proper modality for an individual patient is important.

Ultrasonography
In general, the authors use ultrasonography (US) whenever possible. This technique has several advantages including (1) real-time imaging, (2) multiplanar imaging, (3) no ionizing radiation, (4) portability, (5) fast, (6) inexpensive, and (7) ability to visualize vascular structures. The ability to visualize needle position in real time is particularly useful in targeting lesions that move with respiratory motion and when the lesion is small or adjacent to a critical structure such as a large blood vessel. The ability to image in any plane allows the user to plot complex oblique pathways from the skin to the target lesion, while avoiding critical structures in nonaxial planes, which can be difficult when using computed tomographic (CT) guidance. The lack of ionizing radiation is most important in children and pregnant patients. Limiting radiation has become increasingly relevant as the awareness, tracking, and regulation of radiation doses in all patients has become more necessary. US guidance also typically results in shorter procedure times and lower cost when compared with CT-guided procedures.[9,10] However, US does have limitations visualizing lesions that are obscured by overlying bone, air-containing structures such as lung or gas-filled bowel, as well as deeper structures in obese patients. In addition, the ability to successfully and safely place a biopsy needle in a lesion is operator dependent with a relatively steep learning curve.

Computed tomography
One of the main advantages of CT guidance is its familiarity to all radiologists and the ease of visualizing the spatial relationship between the needle and the lesion. In addition, CT can be necessary to visualize lesions that are not targetable with US. Nonaxial needle paths can be more difficult when using CT guidance, although this can occasionally be offset by a combination of creative patient positioning and angling of the CT gantry. Decreases in scan acquisition times and improvement in postprocessing software allow rapid multiplanar reformats during biopsy, permitting easier plotting of nonaxial needle paths. Although US can often result in faster procedure times than CT, the use of CT fluoroscopy can improve procedure times compared with the use of CT alone.[9]

MR imaging
MR imaging, like US, is nonionizing, uses multiplanar imaging, and has some real-time ability. The main advantage of MR imaging is its high contrast resolution—some lesions may only be identified on MR imaging. However, there are many significant disadvantages including increased cost and procedure time and the lack of widespread adoption of MR-imaging-compatible biopsy tools. Until these disadvantages are overcome, MR imaging will continue to be a rarely used troubleshooting tool for imaging guidance for abdominal biopsy when the target lesion cannot be visualized by other imaging modalities.

Fluoroscopy
Fluoroscopic-guided abdominal biopsy has been almost entirely supplanted by US and CT guidance. However, fluoroscopy is used in conjunction with transvenous biopsy, typically transjugular liver biopsy. Fluoroscopy is less commonly used during transhepatic biliary biopsy—previously obtained access to the biliary tree can be used to obtain brushings or forceps biopsies of strictures. Alternatively, fluoroscopy can be used to direct percutaneous needle biopsy by targeting a previously placed biliary drain or stent.

Navigation systems

Although not routinely used in most clinical practices, commercially available navigation systems have become available that could potentially change the way biopsies are performed. By coregistering/fusing multiple imaging modalities, coupled with electromagnetic tracking ("Medical GPS"), an operator can guide a biopsy needle to a lesion using one modality that is only detectable with another modality.[11] Thus, a lesion that is only seen on PET or MR imaging can be biopsied using US guidance, without requiring the physical presence of the PET or MR imaging scanner.[12] In addition, the tracking software allows preplotting of an optimized needle trajectory, easing precise needle placement while reducing the number of needle passes necessary and decreasing the procedure time.[13]

Sedation

The authors perform most biopsies under moderate conscious sedation. Although this adds to the length of the procedure and requires additional resources compared with using local anesthesia alone, this approach improves patient comfort and satisfaction. Patients must fast for a minimum of 6 to 8 hours before the procedure. A focused history and physical examination confirming the indication for the biopsy is performed. The American Society of Anesthesiologists (ASA) physical status classification is determined and documented, as is a basic airway evaluation. Patients with an ASA score of III or greater, or with a potentially difficult airway, are at elevated risk of sedation-related complications and may require anesthesiology consult. Alternatively, the biopsy may be performed with local anesthesia alone in cooperative patients.

Biopsy Needles

Needle selection depends on the type of organ and the lesion being biopsied, the presumed relative bleeding risk, and operator preference. Needle types are broadly categorized into smaller gauges (20 gauge to 25 gauge) used for fine-needle aspiration (FNA) and larger gauge (14 gauge to 20 gauge) core needles. Both FNA and core needles are used either with a single-needle technique or with a coaxial needle. FNA needles are ideally suited for aspiration of fluid and obtaining cytology specimens, whereas core needles are used whenever lesion histology is necessary. The diagnostic yield of each type of needle depends on the target organ and lesion, although the combined yield is usually higher.[14]

Although it seems intuitive that larger needle size would result in more bleeding complications, this seems to only loosely hold true, with larger needles (14 and 16 gauge) trending to higher bleeding rates than smaller needles (18-, 20-, and 22-gauge).[15]

Biopsy Technique

Patient positioning

Biopsy success is optimized by correct patient positioning, which depends on the target organ and the lesion location within the organ. For liver, pancreas, and spleen biopsies, the authors typically begin with the patient in the supine position, whereas for renal and adrenal biopsies, a posterior approach necessitates prone positioning. When possible, a subcostal approach is preferred to minimize the risk of intercostal vessel injury and pneumothorax. If an intercostal approach is necessary, placing the patient's ipsilateral arm above the head is helpful to open the intercostal space and allow better US imaging of both the lesion and the needle. However, when using this position during deep sedation or general anesthesia, care should be taken because prolonged abduction can result in brachial plexus injuries.[16,17] To increase tumor visibility or displace intervening structures, imaging in the lateral decubitus or semirecumbent positions can be helpful.

Skin preparation

Once adequate targeting of the target is assured, an appropriate skin entry site is marked. The skin is cleaned with povidone-iodine or chlorhexidine solution, appropriate sterile draping is performed, and the subcutaneous skin and soft tissues are anesthetized with 1% lidocaine. Care is taken to raise a generous skin wheal. Lidocaine is deposited at the level of the peritoneum and just external to the capsule of the target organ, because the rich innervations of these structures can lead to patient discomfort during biopsy needle transgression. In larger patients, a longer needle such as a 22-gauge spinal needle may be required to properly anesthetize the projected biopsy needle pathway.

Needle placement

If multiple samples are required, or if needle placement is expected to be technically difficult, the authors use a coaxial technique to minimize the number of capsular punctures. This technique also allows the option of tract embolization. The outer guiding needle is placed at the edge of the lesion using imaging guidance. The inner stylet is removed, and the lesion is sampled with either an FNA or a core needle (Figs. 1 and 2). This process is repeated until an adequate sample is

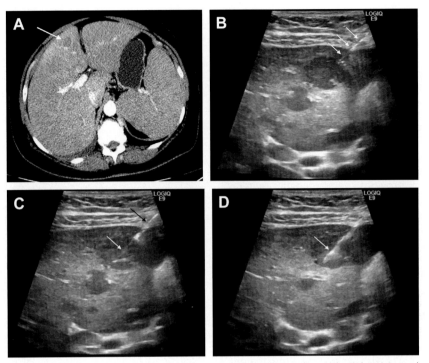

Fig. 1. US-guided liver mass biopsy using coaxial technique. (*A*) Contrast-enhanced axial CT image demonstrating hypoenchancing lesion in segment 4 (*arrow*). (*B*) Subcostal, axial US image demonstrating 17-gauge coaxial guiding needle at the edge of the hypoechoic segment 4 liver mass (*arrows*). Note traversal of normal liver parenchyma before entering the lesion. (*C*) US image with inner stylet of 18-gauge core biopsy needle (*white arrow*) extended to the posterior margin of mass (*black arrow* points to outer 17-gauge guiding needle). (*D*) US image after firing outer cutting cannula (*arrow*).

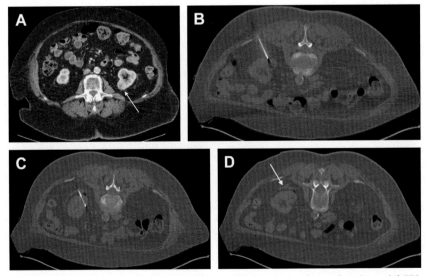

Fig. 2. CT-guided renal mass biopsy using coaxial technique. (*A*) Contrast-enhanced supine axial CT image demonstrating small left lower pole solid renal mass (*arrow*). (*B*) Prone axial CT image with 17-gauge coaxial guiding needle at posterior edge of left renal mass. (*C*) Prone CT image with inner stylet of 18-gauge core biopsy needle extended to posterior margin of mass. (*D*) Prone CT image postbiopsy with small amount of perinephric hemorrhage (*arrow*).

obtained or the procedure is terminated. The ability to obtain a large number of core needle biopsy specimens may be increasingly necessary because the ability to subtype tumors based on molecular markers is used to guide therapy and patient access to research protocols often involves obtaining larger tissue samples.[18]

Sampling technique tips
For larger lesions, the diagnostic yield can be increased by tangentially sampling the outer portion of the lesion, because the inner core is often necrotic and provides nondiagnostic material. When obtaining an FNA sample, a back-and-forth motion is used within the target lesion. Sampling is stopped at the first sign of blood in the hub of the needle. When on-site cytology is used, the FNA sample is obtained without aspirating using a syringe. Capillary action preferentially draws in the sample passively, whereas active aspiration typically introduces more blood into the sample and obscures the diagnostic tissue, making on-site interpretation more difficult. When FNA is used to produce a cell block or for flow cytometry, active aspiration can be used to maximize material acquisition with each pass.

Coaxial versus noncoaxial technique
Theoretic advantages of a coaxial technique include a single puncture of the target organ capsule, ease and speed of obtaining multiple samples, potential for tract embolization, and potentially less risk for tract seeding. Advantages of a noncoaxial technique include smaller needle size and less dwell time of the needle in the patient. This second consideration is potentially advantageous because respiratory motion results in shear stresses transmitted through the needle to the capsule, possibly risking target organ laceration. Ultimately, however, neither technique has proven safer; in a large retrospective study of 1060 hepatic and renal biopsies, coaxial technique (764 biopsies) both with Gelfoam tract embolization (269 biopsies) and without (495 biopsies) was compared with noncoaxial technique (296 biopsies), and no significant difference in either major or minor complications between these techniques was described, or in any subgroup analysis.[19] It is suggested that using a coaxial system may minimize tract seeding, but studies documenting this are limited by short duration of follow-up.[20]

Tract embolization
As mentioned previously, the most feared complication of percutaneous biopsy is bleeding, particularly in patients with ascites or coagulopathy. To this end, multiple strategies have been described to reduce the risk of tract bleeding after biopsy including Gelfoam, coils, fibrin glue, cyanoacrylates, and radiofrequency cautery.[21–26] All the techniques use a coaxial guiding technique, with the earlier iterations using a guiding sheath and later variations performed through a guiding needle. Of these techniques, only radiofrequency cauterization carries the extra advantage of potentially decreased tract seeding as well as hemorrhage. Although studies have demonstrated decreased amounts of bleeding in both heparinized and unheparinized animal models compared with no tract embolization, this has not necessarily translated to clinically significant reductions of postbiopsy hemorrhage in practice.[21,22,27,28] Some studies have suggested that patients with at least moderate coagulopathy can undergo biopsy with relative safety when using a coaxial approach with tract embolization; however, no prospective study comparing high-risk patients with and without tract embolization exists.[29–31] Part of the difficulty in conducting such a study is that the excellent safety profile of percutaneous biopsy would necessitate enrollment of a large number of patients to appropriately power the study.

Specimen handling
Core biopsy samples are placed in 10% formaldehyde solution and sent to surgical pathology for evaluation. Typically, a minimum of 2 to 3 good core samples are obtained, although some research protocols call for considerably more tissue to be obtained. In cases of suspected lymphoma, additional FNA samples are obtained and placed into Roswell Park Memorial Institute (RPMI) solution for flow cytometry. When infectious causes are in the differential diagnosis, the sample is placed in a sterile container for microbiologic evaluation. Occasionally, biopsy samples are sent to outside institutions for molecular studies and have specific handling instructions.

On-site pathologic evaluation
On-site pathologic evaluation is an extremely useful adjunct to the biopsy procedure, allowing rapid initial evaluation of cytologic specimens from FNA samples as well as touch imprint cytology from core needle biopsies. This evaluation improves diagnostic yield while minimizing the risk of multiple needle passes.[32] Real-time assessment can advise whether FNA or core biopsy will improve the diagnostic yield, if sample should be obtained for culture, or if additional material needs to be obtained and placed in a special medium for further evaluation. In general, the nondiagnostic biopsy rate is decreased with on-site evaluation, resulting

in fewer repeat biopsies and improved patient satisfaction.[33]

ORGAN-SPECIFIC CONSIDERATIONS
Liver

Indications and technical considerations
The indication for liver biopsy can be broadly grouped into 2 categories, random liver biopsy for diagnosis of hepatocellular disease and targeted liver biopsy for tissue diagnosis of a liver mass. The indications for liver mass biopsy are listed in **Box 2**. With refinements in abdominal imaging, benign causes can frequently be confidently diagnosed on imaging alone, obviating a biopsy; this is particularly helpful in cases of suspected adenomas and hemangiomas because these highly vascular lesions have higher rates of bleeding after biopsy.

Certain locations in the liver can be more technically difficult in terms of visualizing and accessing the lesion, particularly masses that are closer to the dome and/or more anterior. In these instances, patient cooperation with deep inspiration and/or decubitus or semirecumbent positioning can be essential. When multiple liver lesions with similar diagnostic imaging characteristics are present, the choice of which lesion to biopsy is made based on lesion visibility and location. Every effort is made to choose a lesion and needle trajectory that passes through at least some normal parenchyma before accessing the lesion, preferably at least 3 to 4 cm to minimize the risk of both bleeding and tract seeding.

Box 2
Indications for liver mass biopsy

Benign
    Focal nodular hyperplasia
    Adenoma
    Hemangioma
Malignant
    HCC
    Cholangiocarcinoma
    Lymphoma and PTLD
    Metastatic disease
Infectious
    Abscess

Note: when diagnosis can be made on the basis of imaging alone, biopsy should be avoided.

Abbreviation: PTLD, posttransplant lymphoproliferative disorder.

Results
Diagnostic yield for percutaneous liver biopsy ranges from 83% to 100%.[34,35] However, outcomes vary based on lesion size, pathology, and the use of FNA or core biopsy. Accuracy for diagnosis of HCC has been reported to be greater than 86%, but non-diagnostic biopsies are more frequent in smaller tumors, particularly less than 2 cm.[36,37]

Complications
Although death following percutaneous biopsy is rare, a significant portion of these events occur after liver biopsy. Nevertheless, mortality in large series is under 0.01% and seems to be more frequent in patients with cirrhosis or in those with underlying malignancy.[38] Major hemorrhage requiring transfusion or intervention ranges from 0% to 3.4%.[3,39,40]

In addition to bleeding, tract seeding is a feared complication of liver mass biopsy most frequently associated with HCC. Various retrospective studies have found rates of tract seeding ranging from 0% to 5.1%.[20,41] Two large meta-analyses of 1340 and 2242 patients demonstrated an incidence of 2.7% and median risk of 2.29%, respectively.[42,43] High rates of tract seeding have also been suggested after liver biopsy for colorectal metastases, although it can be difficult to distinguish postbiopsy peritoneal implants from metastatic peritoneal implants in a patient with preexisting metastatic disease.[44] These rates should be compared with those from large surveys of percutaneous biopsy from all sites and malignancy types with an overall rate of 0.005% to 0.009%.[45]

Hepatocellular carcinoma
The utility of biopsy in the diagnosis of HCC remains controversial, with most of the discussion centered on the potential for tract seeding.[46] This complication in a patient listed for transplant is a catastrophic outcome, making the only potential curative intervention for patients with cirrhosis with liver cancer no longer available.

Given the above-mentioned concerns, HCC is unusual compared with most other neoplasms in that imaging diagnosis is acceptable for treatment. Per the National Comprehensive Cancer Network guidelines, the diagnosis of HCC in a lesion greater than 1 cm can be made by documenting arterial enhancement with venous washout on CT or MR imaging.[47] This finding is most important in the setting of transplant eligibility. According to the Organ Procurement and Transplantation Network/United Network for Organ Sharing policy for liver transplant allocation, no biopsy is necessary when a lesion meets the above-mentioned diagnostic criteria and falls within the Milan criteria (a single lesion$\geq$2 cm but<5 cm, or 3 lesions each$\geq$1 cm but<3 cm). These patients are not only eligible for liver transplant but also receive Model for End-Stage Liver Disease exception points such that their starting score is 22.[48]

Given the above-mentioned factors, the authors typically do not biopsy lesions in patients with cirrhosis except in troubleshooting situations when the lesion does not fulfill imaging criteria for HCC or there is a concerning history of additional malignancy that would alter the treatment algorithm.

Ascites

Certain special considerations apply to liver mass biopsies. While the presence of ascites can be negated during random liver biopsy by the use of the transjugular biopsy technique, lesion targeting almost always requires a percutaneous approach. Historically, ascites has been considered a contraindication to liver biopsy. However, studies suggesting higher complication rates are often compromised by lack of imaging guidance and confounding clinical variables such as bleeding diatheses that are often present in the same patient population. In a retrospective study of 476 patients (173 with ascites and 303 without ascites) who underwent percutaneous imaged-guided (18 or 20 gauge) liver biopsy (69% targeted lesion and 31% random parenchyma), the presence of ascites did not result in a significant difference in the major complication rate.[40]

Some have advocated for prebiopsy ascites drainage. The theoretic advantage of this approach is to restore the tamponade effect of the abdominal wall on the site of liver entry. In addition, leaving a drain in place during the immediate postbiopsy period may aid in early diagnosis and treatment of a hemorrhagic complication by identifying sanguineous drainage. Arguments against draining ascites include the additive risk of the drainage procedure and the loss of possible tamponade effect of the ascites fluid itself. Unfortunately, the utility of draining ascites before biopsy has not been addressed in a meaningful way in the literature. The authors prefer to drain ascites before biopsy only in the setting of massive ascites when it improves the technical ability to target the lesion, with early removal of the drain after the postbiopsy period of observation has elapsed without evidence of complication.

Kidney

Indications and technical considerations

Historically, renal mass biopsy has played a limited role in the diagnosis of renal masses, often being reserved for cases of suspected lymphoma or focal infection or in cases of known extrarenal malignancy. The indications for renal mass biopsy are listed in **Box 3**. The historically high failure rate of renal mass biopsy to reliably make a diagnosis of malignancy, with up to a 25% false-negative rate, has limited the role of this technique.[46,49,50] Failure of renal mass biopsy is related to both the heterogeneity of the renal masses and associated sampling error and difficulty in distinguishing masses on histology alone, with surgical explant pathologic evaluation considered the gold standard.[49] With increasing use of cross-sectional imaging, renal masses are more frequently incidentally detected with downward stage migration (typically masses$\leq$4 cm). There is a relatively high rate of benign disease (20% to 50%) in small renal masses, and many small malignant masses have an indolent course.[49,51] As a result, the role of active surveillance and ablation has increased, particularly in suboptimal candidates for extirpation.[49,51] This group of patients, coupled with improved techniques resulting in better diagnostic yields, has expanded the role for renal mass biopsy.

The patient is placed in a prone position, and a subcostal approach is preferred for ease of targeting, to limit the risk of bleeding from intercostal vessels and minimize the risk of pneumothorax. When an intercostal approach is unavoidable, placing a pillow underneath the patient's abdomen to reduce the natural lumbar lordosis can widen the intercostal space and improve visualization. Hypertension, both chronic and acute at the time of biopsy, is a known risk factor for hemorrhagic complications after native kidney biopsy.[52] Thus, management of blood pressure is a critical component of patient management during the

---

Box 3
Indications for renal mass biopsy

Classic indications

Known extrarenal malignancy

Suspected lymphoma

Suspected infection

Tissue diagnosis for unresectable renal mass

Emerging indications

Grading of tumor

Diagnosis before ablation

Recurrence after ablation

Aid management of small renal masses

biopsy and periprocedural period, and a blood pressure threshold of 140/90 has been suggested.[52,53] The authors prefer US guidance for its real-time visualization of the needle, which is particularly helpful given the respiratory motion of the kidney. However, when the kidney cannot be targeted because of obesity, or interposed bowel or lung, and when altering patient position is unsuccessful, CT guidance may be needed to confidently perform the biopsy. In contrast to liver biopsies, no effort is made to cross normal renal parenchyma before entering the lesion.

Results

In a meta-analysis of 2474 patients biopsied before 2001, a reevaluation of the biopsy results suggested that the historical rate of false-negative results was probably inflated because many studies misclassified nondiagnostic and technical failures as false-negatives and found a biopsy failure rate of 8.9%, false-negative rate of 4.4%, false-positive rate of 1.2%, and accuracy of 88.9%.[50] The same analysis looked at 227 biopsies after 2001 and found a biopsy failure rate of 3.5%, false-negative rate of 0.7%, false-positive rate of 0.9%, and accuracy of 88%.[50] Outcomes have continued to improve. A retrospective study in 2007 of 125 renal mass biopsies yielded a similar rate of nondiagnostic biopsies of 4%, with sensitivity and specificity of 97.7% and 100%, respectively.[54] This study suggested that clinical management was affected by at least 60% of the biopsy results, underscoring the increasing relevance of renal mass biopsy.

Complications

Major complication rates of renal mass biopsy are relatively infrequent with a reported rate of bleeding complications requiring transfusion of 1% to 2% despite identification of hemorrhage in 91% of patients on postbiopsy CT.[50,55] In contrast to HCC, tract seeding has been noted to be quite rare, occurring in less than 0.01%.[56] However, the tract seeding rate has been suggested to be higher in transitional cell carcinomas.[56,57] In native renal biopsy, the risk of bleeding complications increases with patient hypertension, elevated creatinine levels, amyloid, and larger needle size.[52,58,59] Other complications are rare: mortality, 0.02%; nephrectomy, 0.01%; macroscopic hematuria, 3.5%; transfusion, 0.9%; and angiographic intervention, 0.6%.[58]

POSTPROCEDURE
Recovery/Observation

Our postprocedural routine varies depending on the site of biopsy. Vital signs are measured every 15 minutes for the first hour, every 30 minutes for the next 2 hours, and hourly thereafter. The authors observe patients undergoing liver biopsy for 4 hours (including transjugular). Previous guidelines recommended a minimum 6-h observation period.[60] However, a retrospective review of 3214 patients demonstrated similar major complication rates despite the staged reduction in recovery period from 6 to 1 hour.[61] The authors observe renal mass biopsies for 6 hours.

Although most bleeding complications are expected to occur during the proscribed recovery time, patients are given written instructions to call for increasing abdominal, shoulder, flank or chest pain; shortness of breath; bleeding from the skin entry site; abdominal swelling; blood in the stool; fevers or chills; or discharge from the skin entry site. In addition, the patient is instructed to spend the first night postbiopsy within 30 minutes of the hospital and in the company of a responsible adult. Finally, patients are called 24 hours after the procedure to assess for delayed complications.

SUMMARY

Percutaneous image-guided biopsy of abdominal masses is a safe and effective method for obtaining diagnostic tissue for a variety of pathologic processes. Attention to patient preparation, including coagulation status, and choice of imaging modalities are key to the safe performance of the procedure.

REFERENCES

1. Patel IJ, Davidson JC, Nikolic B, et al. Consensus guidelines for periprocedural management of coagulation status and hemostasis risk in percutaneous image-guided interventions. J Vasc Interv Radiol 2012;23(6):727–36.
2. Patel IJ, Davidson JC, Nikolic B, et al. Addendum of newer anticoagulants to the SIR consensus guideline. J Vasc Interv Radiol 2013;24(5):641–5.
3. Atwell TD, Smith RL, Hesley GK, et al. Incidence of bleeding after 15,181 percutaneous biopsies and the role of aspirin. AJR Am J Roentgenol 2010; 194(3):784–9.
4. Segal JB, Dzik WH. Paucity of studies to support that abnormal coagulation test results predict bleeding in the setting of invasive procedures: an evidence-based review. Transfusion 2005;45(9): 1413–25.
5. Abdel-Wahab OI, Healy B, Dzik WH. Effect of fresh-frozen plasma transfusion on prothrombin time and bleeding in patients with mild coagulation abnormalities. Transfusion 2006;46(8):1279–85.

6. Kleinman S, Caulfield T, Chan P, et al. Toward an understanding of transfusion-related acute lung injury: statement of a consensus panel. Transfusion 2004; 44(12):1774–89.

7. Khati NJ, Gorodenker J, Hill MC. Ultrasound-guided biopsies of the abdomen. Ultrasound Q 2011;27(4): 255–68.

8. Douketis JD, Berger PB, Dunn AS, et al. The perioperative management of antithrombotic therapy: American College of Chest Physicians Evidence-Based Clinical Practice Guidelines (8th Edition). Chest 2008;133(6 Suppl):299s–339s.

9. Sheafor DH, Paulson EK, Kliewer MA, et al. Comparison of sonographic and CT guidance techniques: does CT fluoroscopy decrease procedure time? AJR Am J Roentgenol 2000;174(4):939–42.

10. Sheafor DH, Paulson EK, Simmons CM, et al. Abdominal percutaneous interventional procedures: comparison of CT and US guidance. Radiology 1998;207(3):705–10.

11. Abi-Jaoudeh N, Kruecker J, Kadoury S, et al. Multimodality image fusion-guided procedures: technique, accuracy, and applications. Cardiovasc Intervent Radiol 2012;35(5):986–98.

12. Krucker J, Xu S, Venkatesan A, et al. Clinical utility of real-time fusion guidance for biopsy and ablation. J Vasc Interv Radiol 2011;22(4):515–24.

13. Appelbaum L, Sosna J, Nissenbaum Y, et al. Electromagnetic navigation system for CT-guided biopsy of small lesions. AJR Am J Roentgenol 2011;196(5): 1194–200.

14. Stewart CJ, Coldewey J, Stewart IS. Comparison of fine needle aspiration cytology and needle core biopsy in the diagnosis of radiologically detected abdominal lesions. J Clin Pathol 2002;55(2):93–7.

15. Gazelle GS, Haaga JR, Rowland DY. Effect of needle gauge, level of anticoagulation, and target organ on bleeding associated with aspiration biopsy. Work in progress. Radiology 1992;183(2):509–13.

16. Desai KR, Nemcek AA Jr. Iatrogenic brachial plexopathy due to improper positioning during radiofrequency ablation. Semin Intervent Radiol 2011; 28(2):167–70.

17. Shankar S, Vansonnenberg E, Silverman SG, et al. Brachial plexus injury from CT-guided RF ablation under general anesthesia. Cardiovasc Intervent Radiol 2005;28(5):646–8.

18. Marshall D, Laberge JM, Firetag B, et al. The changing face of percutaneous image-guided biopsy: molecular profiling and genomic analysis in current practice. J Vasc Interv Radiol 2013;24(8):1094–103.

19. Hatfield MK, Beres RA, Sane SS, et al. Percutaneous imaging-guided solid organ core needle biopsy: coaxial versus noncoaxial method. AJR Am J Roentgenol 2008;190(2):413–7.

20. Maturen KE, Nghiem HV, Marrero JA, et al. Lack of tumor seeding of hepatocellular carcinoma after percutaneous needle biopsy using coaxial cutting needle technique. AJR Am J Roentgenol 2006; 187(5):1184–7.

21. Falstrom JK, Moore MM, Caldwell SH, et al. Use of fibrin sealant to reduce bleeding after needle liver biopsy in an anticoagulated canine model: work in progress. J Vasc Interv Radiol 1999; 10(4):457–62.

22. Kim EH, Kopecky KK, Cummings OW, et al. Electrocautery of the tract after needle biopsy of the liver to reduce blood loss. Experience in the canine model. Invest Radiol 1993;28(3):228–30.

23. Allison DJ, Adam A. Percutaneous liver biopsy and track embolization with steel coils. Radiology 1988; 169(1):261–3.

24. Chuang VP, Alspaugh JP. Sheath needle for liver biopsy in high-risk patients. Radiology 1988;166(1 Pt 1):261–2.

25. Probst P, Rysavy JA, Amplatz K. Improved safety of splenoportography by plugging of the needle tract. AJR Am J Roentgenol 1978;131(3):445–9.

26. Smith TP, McDermott VG, Ayoub DM, et al. Percutaneous transhepatic liver biopsy with tract embolization. Radiology 1996;198(3):769–74.

27. Pritchard WF, Wray-Cahen D, Karanian JW, et al. Radiofrequency Cauterization with Biopsy Introducer Needle. J Vasc Interv Radiol 2004;15(2):183–7.

28. Choi SH, Lee JM, Lee KH, et al. Postbiopsy splenic bleeding in a dog model: comparison of cauterization, embolization, and plugging of the needle tract. AJR Am J Roentgenol 2005;185(4):878–84.

29. Tsang WK, Luk WH, Lo A. Ultrasound-guided plugged percutaneous biopsy of solid organs in patients with bleeding tendencies. Hong Kong Med J 2014;20(2):107–12.

30. Riley SA, Ellis WR, Irving HC, et al. Percutaneous liver biopsy with plugging of needle track: a safe method for use in patients with impaired coagulation. Lancet 1984;2(8400):436.

31. Zins M, Vilgrain V, Gayno S, et al. US-guided percutaneous liver biopsy with plugging of the needle track: a prospective study in 72 high-risk patients. Radiology 1992;184(3):841–3.

32. Moghadamfalahi M, Podoll M, Frey AB, et al. Impact of immediate evaluation of touch imprint cytology from computed tomography guided core needle biopsies of mass lesions: single institution experience. Cytojournal 2014;11:15.

33. Iglesias-Garcia J, Dominguez-Munoz JE, Abdulkader I, et al. Influence of on-site cytopathology evaluation on the diagnostic accuracy of endoscopic ultrasound-guided fine needle aspiration (EUS-FNA) of solid pancreatic masses. Am J Gastroenterol 2011;106(9):1705–10.

34. Welch TJ, Sheedy PF 2nd, Johnson CD, et al. CT-guided biopsy: prospective analysis of 1,000 procedures. Radiology 1989;171(2):493–6.

35. Gazelle GS, Haaga JR. Guided percutaneous biopsy of intraabdominal lesions. AJR Am J Roentgenol 1989;153(5):929–35.

36. Caturelli E, Solmi L, Anti M, et al. Ultrasound guided fine needle biopsy of early hepatocellular carcinoma complicating liver cirrhosis: a multicentre study. Gut 2004;53(9):1356–62.

37. Huang GT, Sheu JC, Yang PM, et al. Ultrasound-guided cutting biopsy for the diagnosis of hepatocellular carcinoma–a study based on 420 patients. J Hepatol 1996;25(3):334–8.

38. Piccinino F, Sagnelli E, Pasquale G, et al. Complications following percutaneous liver biopsy. A multicentre retrospective study on 68,276 biopsies. J Hepatol 1986;2(2):165–73.

39. Giorgio A, Tarantino L, de Stefano G, et al. Complications after interventional sonography of focal liver lesions: a 22-year single-center experience. J Ultrasound Med 2003;22(2):193–205.

40. Little AF, Ferris JV, Dodd GD 3rd, et al. Image-guided percutaneous hepatic biopsy: effect of ascites on the complication rate. Radiology 1996;199(1): 79–83.

41. Takamori R, Wong LL, Dang C, et al. Needle-tract implantation from hepatocellular cancer: is needle biopsy of the liver always necessary? Liver Transpl 2000;6(1):67–72.

42. Silva MA, Hegab B, Hyde C, et al. Needle track seeding following biopsy of liver lesions in the diagnosis of hepatocellular cancer: a systematic review and meta-analysis. Gut 2008;57(11):1592–6.

43. Stigliano R, Marelli L, Yu D, et al. Seeding following percutaneous diagnostic and therapeutic approaches for hepatocellular carcinoma. What is the risk and the outcome? Seeding risk for percutaneous approach of HCC. Cancer Treat Rev 2007; 33(5):437–47.

44. Jones OM, Rees M, John TG, et al. Biopsy of resectable colorectal liver metastases causes tumour dissemination and adversely affects survival after liver resection. Br J Surg 2005;92(9):1165–8.

45. Smith EH. Complications of percutaneous abdominal fine-needle biopsy. Review. Radiology 1991; 178(1):253–8.

46. Brown DB, Gonsalves CF. Percutaneous biopsy before interventional oncologic therapy: current status. J Vasc Interv Radiol 2008;19(7):973–9.

47. Benson AB 3rd, Abrams TA, Ben-Josef E, et al. NCCN clinical practice guidelines in oncology: hepatobiliary cancers. J Natl Compr Canc Netw 2009; 7(4):350–91.

48. Wald C, Russo MW, Heimbach JK, et al. New OPTN/UNOS policy for liver transplant allocation: standardization of liver imaging, diagnosis, classification, and reporting of hepatocellular carcinoma. Radiology 2013;266(2):376–82.

49. Lim A, O'Neil B, Heilbrun ME, et al. The contemporary role of renal mass biopsy in the management of small renal tumors. Front Oncol 2012;2:106.

50. Lane BR, Samplaski MK, Herts BR, et al. Renal mass biopsy–a renaissance? J Urol 2008;179(1):20–7.

51. Frank I, Blute ML, Cheville JC, et al. Solid renal tumors: an analysis of pathological features related to tumor size. J Urol 2003;170(6 Pt 1):2217–20.

52. Eiro M, Katoh T, Watanabe T. Risk factors for bleeding complications in percutaneous renal biopsy. Clin Exp Nephrol 2005;9(1):40–5.

53. Shidham GB, Siddiqi N, Beres JA, et al. Clinical risk factors associated with bleeding after native kidney biopsy. Nephrology (Carlton) 2005;10(3):305–10.

54. Maturen KE, Nghiem HV, Caoili EM, et al. Renal mass core biopsy: accuracy and impact on clinical management. AJR Am J Roentgenol 2007;188(2): 563–70.

55. Ralls PW, Barakos JA, Kaptein EM, et al. Renal biopsy-related hemorrhage: frequency and comparison of CT and sonography. J Comput Assist Tomogr 1987;11(6):1031–4.

56. Silverman SG, Gan YU, Mortele KJ, et al. Renal masses in the adult patient: the role of percutaneous biopsy. Radiology 2006;240(1):6–22.

57. Slywotzky C, Maya M. Needle tract seeding of transitional cell carcinoma following fine-needle aspiration of a renal mass. Abdom Imaging 1994;19(2): 174–6.

58. Corapi KM, Chen JL, Balk EM, et al. Bleeding complications of native kidney biopsy: a systematic review and meta-analysis. Am J Kidney Dis 2012; 60(1):62–73.

59. Nicholson ML, Wheatley TJ, Doughman TM, et al. A prospective randomized trial of three different sizes of core-cutting needle for renal transplant biopsy. Kidney Int 2000;58(1):390–5.

60. Jacobs WH, Goldberg SB. Statement on outpatient percutaneous liver biopsy. Dig Dis Sci 1989;34(3): 322–3.

61. Firpi RJ, Soldevila-Pico C, Abdelmalek MF, et al. Short recovery time after percutaneous liver biopsy: should we change our current practices? Clin Gastroenterol Hepatol 2005;3(9):926–9.

Imaging of the Liver Following Interventional Therapy for Hepatic Neoplasms

Sharon Z. Adam, MD, Frank H. Miller, MD*

KEYWORDS

- Intra-arterial embolotherapies • Ablation • HCC • Hepatic metastases • MR imaging • CT
- Response • Complications

KEY POINTS

- Locoregional interventional procedures are being performed more frequently for both primary hepatic tumors and metastases and have imaging findings and complications that differ from findings after systemic therapies.
- Multiphasic computed tomography (CT) or MR imaging can be used as routine follow-up modalities. Follow-up imaging to evaluate response is usually performed at 1 month and 4 months after treatment and then every 3 to 6 months. After conventional transarterial chemoembolization (TACE), an immediate postprocedural unenhanced CT is performed to assess adequate uptake in the treated lesion, and after ablation earlier imaging is obtained, within the first 1 to 2 weeks (often immediately after the procedure) to ensure complete ablation.
- Response assessment after intra-arterial and ablative procedures is complex. It requires not only measurement of size but also evaluation of necrosis and enhancement patterns and preferably should include functional parameters such as diffusion-weighted imaging (DWI).

INTRODUCTION

The liver is a common site of malignancy. Most malignant liver lesions are metastatic. Primary malignancies such as hepatocellular carcinoma (HCC) are also commonly seen, especially in cirrhotic patients, and are the third leading cause of cancer death in the world.[1] Treatment of hepatic malignancies has evolved tremendously over the past few decades. Curative surgical resection or liver transplantation (for primary malignancies) is still considered optimal when feasible, whereas systemic chemotherapy and external beam irradiation are no longer the only alternatives, and locoregional interventional techniques have been developed to improve survival in patients who are not surgical candidates. These techniques are used not only for palliation when other treatments fail but also as curative treatment when surgery is not feasible or as an adjunct to other types of definitive interventions or treatments, for instance, downstaging patients for curative resection or liver transplantation.[2]

Interpretation of imaging of patients after locoregional therapy can be difficult and distinctly different from imaging after systemic therapy. This article discusses the use of a variety of imaging modalities and imaging findings before and after interventional treatment and describes potential complications of these therapies and their imaging. Guidelines for patient selection for the different

The authors have nothing to disclose.
Department of Radiology, Northwestern University Feinberg School of Medicine, Northwestern Memorial Hospital, 676 North Saint Clair Street, Suite 800, Chicago, IL 60611, USA
* Corresponding author.
E-mail address: fmiller@northwestern.edu

Radiol Clin N Am 53 (2015) 1061–1076
http://dx.doi.org/10.1016/j.rcl.2015.05.009
0033-8389/15/$ – see front matter © 2015 Elsevier Inc. All rights reserved.

locoregional therapies and principles of assessing treatment response using international guidelines are discussed in other articles of this issue (see the article by Molvar and Lewandowski and article by Minocha and Lewandowski, respectively).

OVERVIEW OF TECHNIQUES
Intra-arterial Therapy

Catheter-based therapies administered intra-arterially include bland embolization, TACE, and radioembolization. The type of therapy used is often based on institutional preference and expertise. The rationale behind intra-arterial therapies is the difference between the normal liver's dual blood supply (both arterial and portal venous) and the almost purely arterial blood supply to tumors; this is seen not only in hypervascular tumors, such as HCC, but also in hypovascular tumors, only to a lesser extent. This arterial blood supply is the result of growth factor–mediated neoangiogenesis.[3] Tumors can therefore be treated by targeting the hepatic artery branches that supply them.

Depending on the chosen technique, embolic material alone (in bland embolization), a combination of embolic material with chemotherapeutic drugs (in TACE), or radiation-emitting particles (in radioembolization) are injected. Bland embolization uses embolic material to occlude the arterial blood supply to the tumor, resulting in ischemia and tumor necrosis. TACE can be performed either in the conventional method, in which the cytotoxic drug in emulsified with a radio-opaque ethiodized oil (Lipiodol/Ethiodol) that is injected selectively into the desired artery and then followed by bland embolization, or using drug-eluting beads (DEBs) made of polyvinyl alcohol microspheres loaded with chemotherapeutic agents. DEB-TACE beads are radiolucent and therefore require contrast media to be injected as well during the procedure. Radioembolization, also known as selective internal radiation therapy, combines the low embolic effect of micron-sized spheres with localized high-dose radiotherapy in the form of beta-emitting yttrium 90 (^{90}Y). This method allows much higher doses of radiation to be administered without the risk of radiation-induced hepatic injury. The basis of the imaging findings depends on the different mechanisms that these therapies use.

Ablative Techniques

Ablation of hepatic tumors can be achieved using multiple techniques. Most techniques are thermal or chemical.[4] Newer techniques, such as irreversible electroporation that uses electric current to induce cell death, have been introduced, but they are mostly investigational. Chemical ablation uses ethanol (or much less frequently acetic acid) to induce cellular damage. Thermal ablation is the mainstay of ablation, mostly using radiofrequency (RF) or microwave (MW). Other less frequent forms of thermal ablation include cryoablation, high-intensity focused ultrasound (HIFU), and laser interstitial thermotherapy.

All forms of ablation cause coagulative necrosis of the targeted tumor.[5] Unlike intra-arterial therapies, these techniques do not have any selectivity to tumoral tissue, and their effect depends on location. The effect of thermal ablation relies on reaching an adequate temperature that causes tissue damage, and chemical ablation requires equal distribution of the ablatant in the tumor to allow for adequate exposure.[4]

TIMING OF POSTPROCEDURAL IMAGING
Intra-arterial Therapy

Follow-up imaging at the authors' institution is performed at 1 month after the procedure, 3 months after the first postprocedural scan, and then every 3 to 6 months. Other schedules have been proposed, some advocating more frequent follow-up in the first year or tailoring follow-up according to individually assessed risk.[6] After conventional TACE, an early postprocedural unenhanced CT is performed immediately after the procedure, to ensure adequate delivery of the ethiodized oil to the desired region (Figs. 1 and 2). The desired finding is complete retention of ethiodized oil in the treated lesion, as it has been shown to correlate with complete necrosis of the tumor (whereas incomplete retention may indicate residual viable tumor). When no retention is seen, aberrant vascular supply should be suspected and the procedure should be repeated as soon as possible, after identifying the anatomic variant (see Fig. 2). An early scan can be attempted for the same purpose after DEB-TACE; however, because the beads are not radio-opaque and contrast is injected only for the purpose of visualizing the injection, contrast retention is transient and inconsistent. Retention has been shown to occur in only 76%, more commonly in larger lesions, and it is usually visible only during the first 6 to 12 hours.[7,8] Therefore, it cannot be used reliably to assess distribution and determine the need for further procedures before follow-up imaging and is generally not performed in practice.

Ablative Techniques

Early or immediate imaging is sometimes performed to ensure complete lesion ablation and to

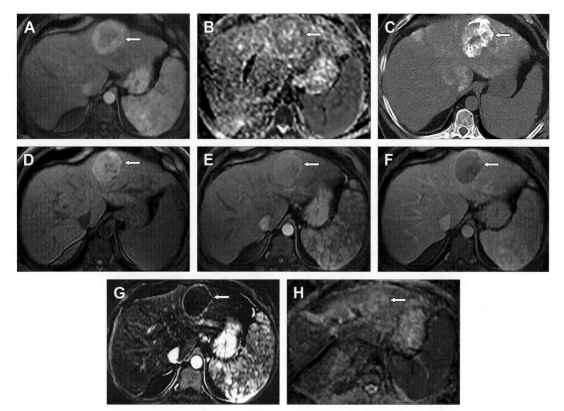

Fig. 1. A 64-year-old man, HCC treated by conventional TACE as a bridge to transplantation. Axial arterial phase T1-weighted image (T1WI) (*A*) and ADC map (*B*) show a large hypervascular tumor in segment 2 with restricted diffusion mostly in the periphery of the tumor (*arrows*). Axial unenhanced CT performed immediately after the procedure (*C*) shows excellent uptake of ethiodized oil in the lesion (*arrow*). MR imaging performed after 1 month demonstrated a mild reduction in size. Axial unenhanced (*D*), arterial phase (*E*), and portal venous phase (*F*) T1WI demonstrate the difficulty in assessing enhancement when there is intrinsic T1 hyperintensity due to hemorrhage (*arrows*). The subtraction image (*G*) shows that only thin rim enhancement is present (*arrow*), without tumoral enhancement, consistent with good response. The post-TACE ADC map (*H*) shows increased ADC values (*arrow*), indicating good response as well. The patient subsequently underwent successful transplantation with no tumor seen on explant.

monitor for potential complications. Timing of this scan differs between institutions. Some institutions perform either triphasic CT or multiphasic MR imaging within 24 hours of ablation,[9] some recommend performing CT immediately after the procedure,[10] and others suggest within 1 to 2 weeks.[11] Ultrasonography (preferably contrast enhanced, where available) can be performed as

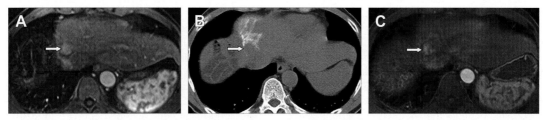

Fig. 2. A 66-year-old man, HCC, prior partial hepatectomy, radioembolization, TACE, and RF ablation of multiple lesions, undergoing conventional TACE for a segment IV lesion. An arterially enhancing tumor is seen on T1-weighted (*A*) baseline MR imaging (*arrow*). On unenhanced CT performed immediately after TACE (*B*), ethiodized oil uptake is seen in segment IV parenchyma. However, there is a focal round filling defect in the midst of the uptake (*arrow*), corresponding to the tumor. Follow-up MR imaging performed after 1 month (*C*) confirms the treatment failure, showing the tumor's unchanged arterial enhancement likely from different blood supply to the tumor (*arrow*).

the immediate postprocedural imaging; however, it is less accurate than CT or MR imaging. In addition, the echogenic focus created by the ablation (which is due to formation of microbubbles in the heated tissue[11]) can cause overestimation or underestimation of the treated volume on ultrasonography and last for 15 minutes to 6 hours therefore limiting its use.[9] If the early scan is performed immediately after the procedure, and untreated regions are detected, additional ablation can be performed immediately.

Further follow-up imaging, CT or MR imaging, at the authors' institution is usually performed using a similar time line as for intra-arterial therapies, at 1 month and then every 3 months.[7,9]

MODALITIES FOR LONG-TERM IMAGING FOLLOW-UP

The modality used for follow-up differs between different institutions based on preference. Both CT and MR imaging can assess the size of the treated lesion. CT is readily available and is excellent for evaluation of the distribution of the ethiodized oil immediately after treatment. Triphasic CT can be used to assess necrosis and enhancement changes after treatment; however, after conventional TACE it may be difficult to assess enhancement because of the presence of hyperdense ethiodized oil.

At the authors' institution, multiphasic MR imaging is preferred for long-term follow-up of HCC and cholangiocarcinomas because it has better contrast resolution and sensitivity to contrast injection, better lesion characterization with multiple sequences, and the ability to add functional sequences such as DWI and perfusion-weighted imaging. These attributes allow for better assessment of residual or recurrent viable tissue and better characterization of additional lesions that may be encountered and may affect treatment decision. The use of DWI is especially important when contrast injection is contraindicated because of renal insufficiency, rendering CT and routine MR imaging sequences suboptimal for assessing response. For metastatic tumors, CT is often preferred because it can be used to simultaneously evaluate the chest, abdomen, and pelvis to evaluate for additional metastases.

PET with fludeoxyglucose (FDG-PET) can be a useful problem-solving tool for assessing response when the known malignancy is FDG-avid and standard imaging features are not definitive or conflicting. It is especially helpful for assessing response in patients with hypovascular tumors, such as colorectal metastases, when assessing response based on enhancement can be difficult. After radioembolization for colorectal metastases, PET has a better response detection rate than CT.[12,13] Compared with size measurements or combined size and necrosis evaluation on CT, reduction of FDG uptake on PET is significantly better at detecting response (6% and 24% vs 63%, respectively).[12] Subsequent CT can detect response in an additional 12%, a finding attributed to the hypovascular nature of colorectal metastases and the resultant difficulties to assess their response on CT, demonstrating that PET can show response earlier than CT. After radioembolization, non-FDG-PET may have an additional role, as recent studies suggest, assessing adequate microsphere distribution in the treated lesion. Understanding the distribution of the microspheres may allow not only early assessment of possible treatment failure but also improvement of dose calculations in the future.[14]

Patients with HCC, especially with underlying cirrhosis, are at risk of developing not only recurrence but also new lesions elsewhere in the liver.[15] Similarly, the nature of the metastatic disease dictates potential multiple new lesions in the liver and elsewhere, and often, patients have occult lesions undetected before treatment.[16] Therefore, follow-up allows for early detection not only of local recurrence or residual tumor but also of new lesions, which is essential for patient management, allowing additional treatment sessions as necessary.

IMAGING APPEARANCE AFTER INTRA-ARTERIAL THERAPIES
Size

As a sole criterion, size is not always sufficient for assessing response. Traditional guidelines for assessment of response to treatment, which are based on size measurements, were originally devised for systemic cytotoxic therapy. After systemic treatment, lesions are expected to reduce significantly in size and optimally disappear. Locoregional therapies induce tumor necrosis, creating a nonviable cavity that reduces in size when the liver remodels itself around it. This remodeling process is slow, and months may be needed for sufficient size changes to become visible, depending on the type of treatment; hence, earlier imaging biomarkers of response are often needed (such as necrosis, diffusion changes, or FDG uptake). Sometimes lesions undergoing locoregional treatment do not decrease in size or never disappear completely.[17,18] However, many lesions treated intra-arterially do show size reduction. Therefore, size evaluation should be a major part of the assessment of follow-up studies and should always be interpreted in context with other imaging markers of response.

Reduction in size after radioembolization may take time to be seen on imaging studies. Radioembolization has a less prominent embolic effect compared with other intra-arterial therapies, and necrosis is mainly caused by the cytotoxic effects of radiation, which are often not immediate. Despite these differences, when time to response based on size criteria alone was compared between radioembolization and TACE, no statistically significant differences were found.[19]

Necrosis, Tumoral and Nodular Enhancement

Necrosis is an important criterion following intra-arterial therapies that is able to detect response earlier than size. Studies have shown that when necrosis is used to assess response (either alone or in combination with size), response can be detected

much earlier (a median time of 29–34 days compared with 68–130 days for size alone,[12,17] which is in accordance with the timing of the first follow-up imaging performed at 1 month). The signal of the necrotic region on T1- and T2-weighted sequences is variable (see **Fig. 1**; **Fig. 3**) and often depends on the baseline appearance of the tumor. Liquefaction of the necrotic lesion, evident as hypodensity of the lesion on CT and typical T2 hypointensity on MR imaging (although intensity may vary),[20,21] is often not seen. Therefore, necrosis is better evaluated as a lack of enhancing tissue, as recommended by the European Association for the Study of the Liver (EASL)[22,23] than by assessing density or intensity on unenhanced CT or MR imaging. The same concept, of assessing response by evaluating the enhancing component of tumors, was used in the

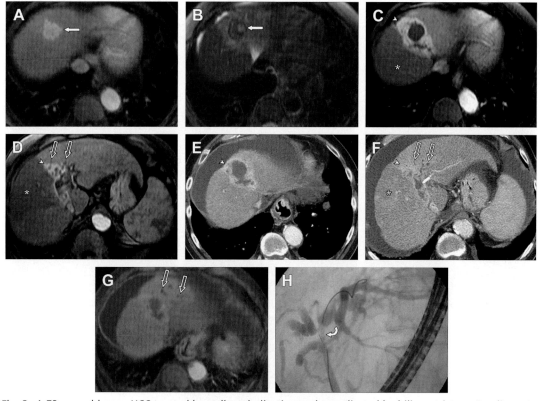

Fig. 3. A 73-year-old man, HCC treated by radioembolization and complicated by biliary stricture. Baseline arterial phase axial T1-weighted image (T1WI) (*A*) shows the hypervascular HCC (*arrow*). MR imaging performed at 1 month posttreatment shows a heterogeneous signal in the treated lesion (*arrow*) on the T2-weighted image (T2WI) (*B*), with surrounding T2 hyperintensity consistent with edema. Axial arterial phase T1WI (*C, D*) show the lesion is now hypointense, without internal enhancing tissue consistent with complete necrosis. The treated vascular territory is arterially hyperenhancing, mostly surrounding the lesion (*arrowhead*), consistent with typical perfusional changes seen after radioembolization. A hypoperfused wedge-shaped region is seen adjacent to the hyperenhancing region (*asterisk*). Mild biliary dilatation peripheral to the lesion (*open arrows*) is present. The same findings are visible on contrast-enhanced CT performed 1 month later (*E, F*). Biliary dilatation gradually worsened as can be seen on the 4-month follow-up contrast-enhanced MR image (*G*) and the stricture (*curved arrow*) required endoscopic dilatation (*H*).

modified Response Evaluation Criteria in Solid Tumors (mRECIST) guidelines.[24] Studies have shown that using lack of enhancement is a good predictor of lesion nonviability and necrosis, and even when lesions remain large, lack of enhancement correlates with complete necrosis on pathology.[25] Both EASL and mRECIST, however, have limitations for assessing locoregional therapies, as discussed in a separate article elsewhere in this issue (see the article by Minocha and Lewandowski). Evaluating enhancement changes is easier when the tumor is hypervascular (HCC or hypervascular metastases), compared with hypovascular malignancies, because the arterial phase shows the lack of arterial enhancement that was previously present (see Fig. 3). Using enhancement as a criterion for hypovascular tumors, such as colorectal metastases, is less reliable, as it is less easily identified on imaging studies. As response guidelines refer to arterial enhancement as the determinant of response, modifications have been suggested to allow for their use in late enhancing tumors such as cholangiocarcinomas.[26]

On CT and MR imaging, enhancement can be assessed by comparing density or signal intensity measurements on the unenhanced and enhanced scans. Subtraction images whereby the unenhanced image is subtracted from the enhanced image can be created (see Fig. 1; Fig. 4) and have been shown to improve readers' confidence when evaluating response on MR imaging.[27] On MR imaging, they are especially helpful when the lesion has intrinsic T1 hyperintensity due to hemorrhage that may make the visual evaluation of enhancement difficult (see Fig. 1).

Radioembolization differs from other embolotherapies in the postprocedural assessment of enhancement. After TACE or bland embolization, which have a strong embolic effect, tumoral enhancement is expected to resolve shortly after treatment. Any tumoral enhancement on follow-up imaging after TACE or bland embolization is suspicious of residual viable tumor (see Figs. 2 and 4) and should be managed as such. Radioembolization, however, has a less prominent embolic effect, and necrosis is caused by radiation, a process that

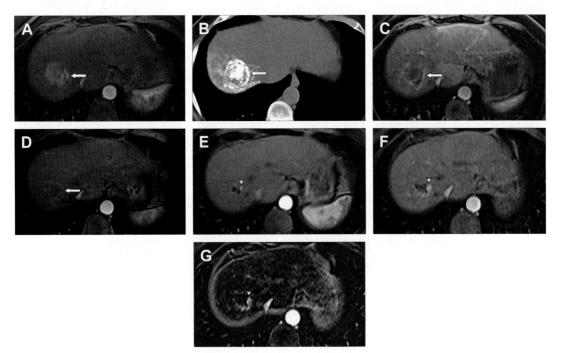

Fig. 4. A 71-year-old woman, HCC treated by conventional TACE. A markedly hypervascular lesion (arrow) is seen on axial arterial phase T1-weighted image (T1WI) (A). Immediately after TACE, axial unenhanced CT demonstrates excellent ethiodized-oil uptake in the lesion (arrow) and surrounding vascular territory (B). Subsequent arterial phase T1WI at 1 month (C), 6 months (D), and 10 months (E) demonstrate necrosis and gradual size reduction with typical rim enhancement (arrows), until 10 months after treatment, when nodular arterial enhancement appears at the periphery of the lesion (arrowhead). Untreated, at 25 months after TACE (F) the lesion has increased in size and the nodular arterial enhancement clearly increased (arrowheads), as evident in the subtraction image (G). This nodular arterial enhancement denotes viable tumor, recurring in the periphery of the treated lesion, and further therapy is planned.

can be lengthy. After radioembolization, tumoral enhancement diminishes over several months, and changes may not be visible on the early follow-up imaging. Peripheral nodular arterial enhancement may be seen after radioembolization and may persist for months after radioembolization and does not necessarily indicate residual viable tumor, as it does after other embolotherapies. Enhancing nodules, seen more often in larger tumors, can even increase in size during the first few months after treatment and have been shown to regress spontaneously after several months (mean duration of 144 days).[17] Complete histologic necrosis has been found even in the presence of nodular enhancement.[28] However, when these findings persist beyond the 6-months follow-up, viable tumor should be suspected.

Rim Enhancement

A thin rim of enhancement, less than 5 mm in width, can be seen surrounding the treated lesion after intra-arterial therapies[7,17,28] (see **Figs. 1** and **4**; **Fig. 5**). After radioembolization, it has been shown to occur in approximately a third of cases, and it was noted to appear as early as the first month and as late as 6 months (mean of 52 days) and persist for several months (mean of 4 months).[17] Most lesions exhibiting rim enhancement after treatment responded well to treatment. This type of enhancement does not usually indicate residual viable tumor and is considered a benign postprocedural finding, most likely caused by an inflammatory response.

Diffusion Restriction

DWI can be used as an additional imaging parameter to assist in the evaluation of response[29–31] and may detect response earlier than conventional

size criteria.[29,32,33] Many hepatic tumors demonstrate restriction of water diffusion on MR imaging, seen as hyperintense signal on DWI and hypointense signal on apparent diffusion coefficient (ADC) maps. This restriction may improve after successful treatment, with a concomitant increase in ADC values (see **Fig. 1**; **Fig. 6**),[21,34,35] which correlates with histologic necrosis.[36] Although this is not always seen, it may help determine treatment response in equivocal cases or when contrast administration is contraindicated and is especially helpful in assessing hypovascular tumors.[20] Newer volumetric ADC techniques that are potentially more accurate for assessing diffusion changes are being studied.[31,37–39] However, on its own, just like other imaging parameters, diffusion is not a perfect tool, and even when diffusion restriction is still present, there may be complete histologic necrosis of lesion.[38]

Perfusion Imaging

New evolving techniques attempt to assess tumor perfusion using different methods. Some perform CT perfusion scans (multiple scans of the target region after contrast administration).[40,41] Others use data from dynamic contrast-enhanced MR imaging quantitatively as an estimator of tumor perfusion. These MR imaging methods can calculate the arterial enhancement fraction that signifies the contribution of the arterial phase to the maximal tumoral enhancement, create perfusion maps[42] or enhancement/perfusion curves (time-signal curves), and calculate curve slopes, time-to-peak, and other parameters.[43] These methods show a difference in tumor perfusion before and after therapy and a correlation with survival and tumor response. Although these are promising techniques, they are time consuming, require dedicated software (with often noticeable

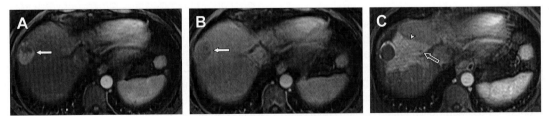

Fig. 5. A 54-year-old woman, multifocal HCC, treated by radioembolization. Before radioembolization, the tumor (*arrow*) exhibited typical arterial enhancement and subsequent washout with capsular enhancement, as seen on axial arterial (*A*) and portal venous (*B*) phase T1-weighted image (T1WI). The tumor responded well to the treatment, with complete necrosis and gradual size reduction seen starting with the 1-month follow-up study. The 4-month follow-up arterial phase T1WI (*C*) still demonstrates peripheral rim enhancement and wedge-shaped hyperenhancing perfusional changes (*arrowhead*). Note a second focus of nonenhancement (*open arrow*) located medially in the treated hyperenhancing wedge-shaped region, which corresponds to a successfully treated small HCC that was unidentifiable in the pretreatment MR imaging. Also note the reduction in segmental hepatic volume after treatment, causing the lesion to appear more exophytic.

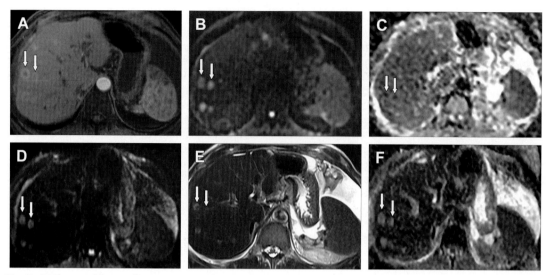

Fig. 6. A 77-year-old man, liver metastases from carcinoid of the small bowel treated by radioembolization. Multiple hepatic hypervascular lesions (*arrows*) are seen before treatment on axial arterial phase T1-weighted image (*A*). On DWI (b value = 500 s/mm^2) the lesions had a high signal (*B*), and on the ADC map they showed a low signal (*C*), confirming restricted diffusion. One month after treatment, the lesions were still hyperintense on DWI (b value = 500 s/mm^2) (*D*) because of their intrinsically high intensity on T2-weighted image (T2 shine through) (*E*) but no longer manifested restricted diffusion, as shown by the increased signal on the ADC map (*F*).

inconsistencies between different software), and are not used routinely in clinical practice.[44]

Ancillary Imaging Findings

Geographic perfusional changes can be seen in the treated vascular territory on contrast-enhanced CT and MR imaging after all types of intra-arterial therapies. These changes appear as ill-defined, usually wedge-shaped, heterogeneous enhancement and are usually hyperenhancing (see **Figs. 3** and **5; Fig. 7**). These changes are transient and usually resolve by the 6-month follow-up imaging.[20,45] Peritumoral edema and hemorrhage can be seen after radioembolization as a result of the radiation effect. Although chemotherapeutic agents have a high selectivity to neoplastic cells, radiation is less selective, because of the high radiosensitivity of the healthy hepatic parenchyma.[46] The short maximal tissue penetration of the beta radiation emitted from ^{90}Y (11 mm) limits the extent of healthy parenchyma affected. Parenchymal edema in a perivascular distribution can be seen after radioembolization. These hypodense regions on CT and T1-hypointense and T2-hyperintense regions on MR imaging may persist for 3 to 6 months.[22,45] These changes must not be confused with treatment failure and tumor infiltration.

Gas bubbles may be seen within the treated necrotic tumor[47] after bland embolization and TACE, can sometimes persist for weeks after

treatment, and should only raise suspicion of infection in an appropriate clinical setting.

Fibrosis and architectural changes may occur after treatment. Intra-arterial therapies often cause volume reduction in the treated segment or lobe (see **Fig. 5**) and also may cause fibrosis, capsular retraction (see **Fig. 7**), and signs of portal hypertension, although usually without clinical sequelae. These changes are a long-term sequelae of treatment and usually appear months after treatment. Hypertrophy of the contralateral lobe may occur, most prominently during the first 6 months after treatment,[48] and can be used to benefit patients for whom hepatic resection after intra-arterial therapy has been planned. When extreme volume reduction and contralateral hypertrophy are seen after radioembolization, they are referred to as radiation lobectomy.[20]

Complications

The most common abdominal complication that can be seen on imaging is nontarget embolization, which can occur in all types of intra-arterial therapies. It is potentially of bigger concern after DEB-TACE and radioembolization because of the higher potency of the therapeutic agent and can be mitigated by pretreatment prophylactic embolization.[3] This complication can occur because of anatomic variants and technical issues during the procedures, collateral flow that was not treated before the procedure, or reflux of the therapeutic particles

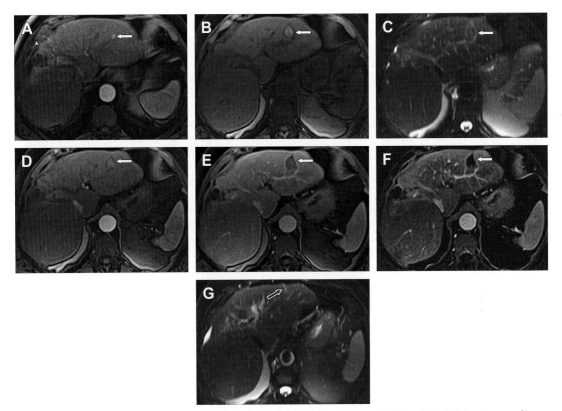

Fig. 7. A 69-year-old man undergoing radiofrequency ablation for recurrent HCC in the left lobe, 1 year after radioembolization of an unresectable right lobe HCC. On axial arterial phase T1-weighted image (T1WI) (*A*), a small hypervascular lesion (*arrow*) is seen in the left lobe. Also seen are chronic postradioembolization changes in the anterior right lobe (*arrowhead*), with architectural distortion and capsular retraction. Note that perfusional changes are still present 1 year after radioembolization. Typical postablation findings are present on MR imaging performed 1 month after treatment. On unenhanced T1WI (*B*), the treated lesion is hyperintense with central hypointensity and is surrounded by an edematous hypointense rim, which is hyperintense on T2-weighted imaging (T2WI) (*C*). Mild rim enhancement, without residual internal tumoral enhancement, is seen on both arterial phase (*D*) and portal phase (*E*) T1WI, and substantiated using subtraction (*F*), consistent with successful ablation. T2WI (*G*) at the level of the needle tract shows a linear hyperintensity (*open arrow*).

into undesired vessels.[7,49,50] This complication most commonly affects the cystic artery, causing ischemic, chemical, or radiation-induced injury to the gallbladder, with a range of imaging findings such as wall thickening, wall enhancement, pericholecystic fluid and even visible discontinuity of the gallbladder wall, sloughed mucosa, and intramural gas in the rare cases of wall gangrene.[51] Gallbladder distension is infrequently seen, as opposed to calculous cholecystitis. Mild hyperenhancement is often seen and considered a benign finding that does not require therapy in the absence of significant symptoms.[52] Even when imaging findings are more pronounced, most cases are asymptomatic and self-limiting.[53] Nontarget embolization is a bigger concern when it involves the stomach or duodenum via the gastroduodenal, right gastric, or accessory left gastric arteries and may lead to gastritis or duodenitis with possible

ulceration.[54] Pancreatitis can also occur,[55] as well as periumbilical dermatitis or skin necrosis, when a patent falciform artery is involved.[56] The imaging features of nontarget embolization are similar to those seen when these are the result of other causes. In cases of nontarget embolization, when conventional TACE is the procedure performed, hyperdense ethiodized oil may be seen on CT in the vessels or organs involved.

Biliary complications can occur because of the exclusive hepatic arterial blood supply to the biliary system, rendering it more susceptible to ischemia after arterial intervention. Mild intrahepatic biliary dilatation seen upstream from the treated lesion is considered an almost normal posttreatment finding and not a complication. Biliary ischemia can lead to strictures (see **Fig. 3**), best visualized on MR cholangiopancreatography (MRCP), and possible bilomas.[7] Biliary complications are more common in patients with baseline biliary obstruction and prior stenting or bilioenteric anastomosis, after DEB-TACE compared with conventional TACE,[7] and in metastatic disease than in HCC,[45,57] because cirrhosis has a protective effect conferred by a hypertrophic peribiliary plexus.[49] Cholangitis has also been reported following intra-arterial therapy.[54]

Hepatic abscesses can also complicate any type of intra-arterial therapy, either as a complication of a biloma or due to bacterial seeding of a necrotic tumor.[50] This condition is more prevalent in patients with prior biliary intervention or surgery.[58]

A rare hepatic complication seen only after radioembolization is radioembolization-induced liver disease, formerly termed radiation hepatitis. This condition is a dose-related clinical diagnosis, based on ascites, elevated bilirubin and alkaline phosphatase levels, and occasionally mild jaundice. It usually occurs 4 to 8 weeks after exposure[59] but can appear as early as 1 week and as late as 7 months.[60] The pathologic process is of sinusoidal obstructive syndrome, also known as veno-occlusive disease, which is manifested by sinusoidal congestion around fibrotically occluded central veins.[61] On imaging, it is seen in the treated vascular territory as hepatic congestion and edema during the early stages. Edema is seen on CT as patchy hypodense areas on unenhanced and enhanced images[62,63] and on MR imaging as T1 hypointensity and T2 hyperintensity.[64] In more severe disease, enhancement abnormalities are seen on multiphasic CT and MR imaging. The affected regions may appear hyperenhancing in the portal venous or delayed phases, probably due to venous drainage abnormalities and delayed clearance of contrast from the parenchyma. In the liver, veins are more susceptible to radiation than arteries,[64] causing decreased portal flow and a compensatory increase in arterial flow. This flow may cause arterial hyperenhancement, which is often patchy because of coexisting edema.[62,65] Unlike viable tumoral tissue, these arterially enhancing regions do not exhibit washout and can therefore be distinguished from viable tumor. These findings may resolve or progress to fibrosis and resulting loss of volume.[62]

Hepatic artery injury, such as spasm, dissection, or thrombosis, is more common when the artery is tortuous.[50] Stenosis may develop as a late complication, usually after repeated manipulation.

IMAGING APPEARANCE AFTER ABLATION THERAPY
Size and Shape of Treated Lesions

Similar to intra-arterial therapies, size is not sufficient for assessing response treatment after ablation therapy, and further imaging parameters, such as lesion appearance and enhancement patterns, should be evaluated. However, after ablation, size plays an important role in evaluating adequacy of treatment. The nonselective nature of ablation techniques requires treating an additional 0.5 to 1 cm margin surrounding the tumor to reach acceptable oncologic control, similar to the principles guiding surgical resection margins (see **Fig. 7**).[10] This margin is particularly important when treating metastases, because they have a less clear lesion-to-liver interface and often have microscopic involvement of the parenchyma surrounding the lesions seen on imaging.[66] Therefore, immediately after the procedure, the ablation zone should be larger than the treated tumor.[11] After successful thermal ablation of tumors in cirrhotic livers, mostly HCCs, the ablation zone may not be larger than the tumor itself, because the higher impedance of cirrhotic tissue renders it less susceptible to thermal insult[66]; this reduces heat dissipation and creates a thermal insulation effect that allows the treated lesion to sustain high temperatures for a longer duration. In accordance with this phenomenon, and despite the narrower ablation margins, outcome after thermal ablation of HCCs (most of which arise in cirrhotic livers) is better than outcome seen in metastases.[7] Fibrotic scar tissue gradually forms around the treated lesion, causing involution of the lesion over 6 to 12 months.[67] The lesions are usually smaller than the pretreatment size by the 1-month follow-up examination.[68] Involution continues over time, but the tumor rarely disappears completely.[4] Reported size is 79% at 1 month, 50% at 4 months, 27% at 10 months, and 11% at 16 months, compared with the immediate postprocedural size.[9] Capsular retraction may occur in peripheral lesions because of this remodeling process around the treated lesion.[7,68]

The shape of the ablation zone is variable, determined by the number and type of probes used, and can be round, oval, or elongated. An irregular shape can be seen when the tumor borders blood vessels, due to the heat dissipating attribute of flowing blood, known as the heat-sink effect.[67] This effect may result in a higher failure rate near large blood vessels because of incomplete ablation of the tumor.[66]

Appearance of Treated Lesions

Lesions that respond to ablation undergo coagulative necrosis and have a variable appearance during the first 4 weeks. On CT they may appear heterogeneous, hypodense, or hyperdense because of the presence of blood as part of coagulative necrosis. On MR imaging (see **Fig. 7**), lesions exhibit heterogeneous T1 hyerintensity and possibly central T1 hypointensity. On T2-weighted images, they are hypointense because of the combination of tissue necrosis and dehydration produced by the intense heating but may be heterogeneous (because of hyperintense foci of blood products or fibrin).[16] Over time the lesions become more homogeneous,[7] and the T1 hyperintensity increases.[9] Liquefactive necrosis may develop, seen as marked T2-weighted hyperintensity[67,69] and requires differentiation from biloma. These variable T1-weighted and T2-weighted appearances limit the use of unenhanced MR imaging, especially in the early postprocedural period. However, localized T1 hypointensity and T2 hyperintensity should raise suspicion for residual or recurrent tumor and should be further evaluated.[66] Dystrophic calcifications may form in the surrounding fibrous tissue, appearing as peripheral calcifications, but they are rare and insignificant.[9,67,68]

The appearance on unenhanced imaging is often not sufficient for evaluating response, and contrast-enhanced imaging is generally necessary for accurate characterization of the treated lesions. Tumoral enhancement is expected to disappear after successful ablation and is used as a marker of successful necrosis, similar to TACE therapies. Any tumoral or peripheral nodular enhancement after ablation represents viable tumor, either residual or recurrent.[7] Subtraction imaging can assist in the evaluation of enhancement, as was explained for intra-arterial therapies (see **Fig. 7**). Assessing viable tumor based on enhancement can be difficult in hypovascular tumors, and a focal area of irregularity in the smooth interface of the ablation zone and adjacent parenchyma should raise suspicion of viable tumor.[68] Multiplanar evaluation of the tumor margins improves assessment of viable tumor, and the coronal and sagittal planes are helpful as tumor is often seen in the periphery of the ablation zone.[70] DWI may help in evaluating viable tumor when the tumor shows baseline restricted diffusion and the size and necrosis criteria are inconclusive or conflicting. After RF ablation, both metastases and HCC exhibit an increase in ADC values during the first 6 months, and after 6 months, ADC values tend to decrease, probably due to fibrosis.[71] Presumably, the same changes in ADC are expected after MW ablation; this may complicate the use of DWI for assessing recurrence in the late follow-up period. It has been shown for HIFU that ADC values remain low when viable tumor remains after treatment and that this can be seen even when enhancement cannot differentiate between the expected periablational enhancement and tumoral enhancement on early posttreatment scans.[72]

A visible linear ablation tract may be seen in the parenchyma and treated lesion on early posttreatment imaging and on follow-up imaging. It is usually hypodense on unenhanced CT and mildly T2 hyperintense on MR imaging (see **Fig. 7**). If the needle tract was ablated (to prevent bleeding or seeding[10]) or bled, it may appear hyperdense on unenhanced CT and exhibit surrounding hyperemia on contrast-enhanced imaging.[7]

Gas bubbles created by coagulative necrosis are a normal finding within the lesion (**Fig. 8A**). These are small bubbles and usually resolve within 1 month.[68] Gas can sometimes be seen in the portal veins as well and usually disappears within 20 minutes, although it may persist for 24 hours.[7,67]

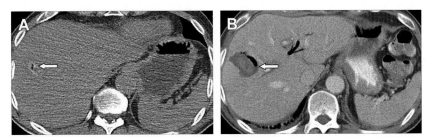

Fig. 8. A 68-year-old man, metastatic pancreatic adenocarcinoma, after Whipple procedure, who developed a hepatic abscess after radiofrequency ablation of a single liver metastasis. Axial unenhanced CT image (*A*) performed immediately after ablation of the right lobe lesion demonstrated a small amount of gas bubbles in the treated lesion, which is an expected postablation finding (*arrow*). Hyperdensity is seen in the lesion, consistent with hemorrhage caused by coagulative necrosis. Axial contrast-enhanced CT (*B*) performed 10 days later because of septic shock, showed a fluid collection with heterogeneous content in the treated lesion, and an increase in the amount of gas seen in the lesion compared with the immediate postprocedural CT. Pneumobilia is also seen in the left lobe. These findings are consistent with abscess formation in a patient with prior bilioenteric anastomosis predisposing to abscess.

Persistence beyond 24 hours implies tissue infarction.[67] A large amount of gas may be seen when 2 ablation techniques are performed concurrently (eg, ethanol ablation and RF ablation), because of a synergistic effect.[67]

Periablational Changes

Perilesional rim enhancement is often normally seen as a result of an inflammatory response and granulation tissue causing reactive hyperemia (see Fig. 7). The rim enhancement is typically thin, although variable degrees of thickness may be seen. It should, however, be completely circumferential.[66] The enhancement is typically visible in the arterial phase but may be seen in addition, or only, in the portal venous phase.[66] On CT, this usually disappears during the first month; however, it may persist for several months on MR imaging.[11]

Perilesional edema can be seen as a sharply marginated hypodense rim on unenhanced CT and T2-hyperintense rim on MR imaging (see Fig. 7). This finding usually persists for 4 to 9 months[7] and should not be mistaken for infiltrating tumor.

Perfusional Changes

Wedge-shaped hyperenhancing regions may be seen in the periphery, adjacent to the treated lesion, especially on the arterial phase. On occasion, this region is T2 hyperintense. Traumatic or thermal injury may cause reduction of portal blood flow with arterial compensation or formation of arterioportal shunts, explaining this phenomenon, which usually resolves in 4 to 6 months.[67]

Complications

The overall complication rate after ablation is low, with large variations reported by different studies, ranging from 0% to 27%.[4,73,74] Most complications are minor. A meta-analysis of 34 studies found very low mortality rates, 0.16% overall (ranging from 0% to 0.88%).[75]

Liver abscess formation, intralesional, perilesional, or perihepatic, is rare, occurring in approximately 0.3%. Abscesses should be suspected only in an appropriate clinical setting, when periprocedural fever persists longer than 10 to 14 days or reappears after resolution, when the procedural gas is not absorbed or even increases in amount (see Fig. 8), when the necrotic ablation zone does not involute or even increases in size, or when the peripheral rim of enhancement is unusually thick.[68,76] Abscesses usually develop over several weeks, in the necrotic lesion or as superinfection of a biloma. However, in diabetic patients they tend to develop earlier and more frequently.[77] The major risk factor is previous bilioenteric anastomosis.[78] Prior biliary interventions (such as stenting) and retention of ethiodized oil after TACE may also increase the risk.[76]

Biliary complications, ranging from mild dilatation to more severe strictures and bilomas, can occur. Transient mild biliary dilatation due to stasis is common (18%[7]), insignificant, and resolves spontaneously when the tumor involutes and inflammation recedes.[67] Persistent dilatation accompanied by lesion involution is assumed to be an irreversible result of thermal damage, which may occur in bile ducts within a 1- to 2-cm radius of the treated lesion.[4] This dilatation is usually seen in the periphery, because proximity to central bile ducts usually precludes thermal ablation and because large vessels exert a relative protective heat-dissipating effect.[68] True strictures occur in only 0.4%.[77] Bilomas may develop adjacent to the treated lesion or the ablation tract[7] in less than 0.3%[79] as a result of biliary damage and leakage and usually resolve spontaneously within 4 months.[68] They should be suspected when the ablation zone does not reduce in size or expands. Bilomas are usually crescent-shaped, but a rounder appearance is possible, and sometimes the communication to the involved duct can be detected, especially on MR imaging.[76] Biliary leakage may also rarely cause fistulization between the biliary system and adjacent organs, most commonly biliocutaneous fistulas.[79] Thickening of the gallbladder wall is reported in 3%, is usually asymptomatic and resolves within 1 week.[77] Significant damage to the gallbladder resulting in cholecystitis is rare, occurring in less than 0.05%, and perforation is even rarer.[80] Cholangitis may also complicate ablation and, as other forms of infection, is more prevalent after bilioenteric anastomosis.[78]

Injury to adjacent viscera, such as colon, stomach, diaphragm, and less commonly small bowel and rib periosteum, can occur with thermal ablation.[4,7] This complication is rare, reported in 0.05% to 0.2%,[75,77] and the colon is most at risk.

Vascular complications are also uncommon. Minor hemorrhage, parenchymal, perihepatic, or intraperitoneal, may occur during and after ablation, but major hemorrhage requiring intervention is rare, occurring in only 0.1%.[77] Arterial pseudoaneurysms, seen as arterially enhancing outpouchings from the hepatic artery, may develop but are usually small and spontaneously thrombose.[7] Small, asymptomatic arterioportal shunts are often seen on the immediate postprocedural imaging or the 1-month follow-up examination, but they usually resolve spontaneously and are clinically insignificant. They are seen as early opacification of the portal vein on the arterial dominant phase. Significant or persistent shunts may exacerbate portal hypertension and should be embolized.[76] Hepatic artery occlusion may also be seen.[76] Bilioportal fistulas and hemobilia have also been reported.[73] In the gallbladder, blood is visible on CT as hyperdense layering content in the acute phase, and on MR imaging as variable-intensity content dependent on the age of hemorrhage.[67] Bilioportal fistulas may also be diagnosed when blood is detected in the bile ducts on contrast-enhanced imaging as contrast fills the ducts and may require transcatheter coil embolization for therapy.[76] Venous thrombosis, mostly of portal veins and less frequently of hepatic veins, has also been reported and should be carefully evaluated to exclude tumor thrombus.[79,81,82] Hepatic infarction is a rare complication, because the liver has a dual blood supply. It is seen as a wedge-shaped unenhancing region in the periphery of the ablation zone, hypodense on CT and T1 hypointense and T2 hyperintense on MR imaging, which sometimes contains tubular gas-filled structures.[9]

Tumor seeding along the needle tract is a late complication reported in 0.1% to 0.5%.[77,79,83] To prevent seeding, the needle tract is usually ablated on withdrawal of the probe.[10] Seeding should be suspected when nodules of irregular tissue that resemble the ablated tumor are detected along the ablation tract and should not be confused with the smooth, transient enhancing hyperemia that can be seen around the tract.[76]

SUMMARY

Many different techniques for locoregional treatment of hepatic tumors exist. Tumors treated by these techniques have specific imaging features and complications that differ from those seen after systemic therapy. Assessing tumor response after these therapies is more complex compared with systemic therapy and may be challenging for radiologists who are unfamiliar with the imaging features. Besides assessing size changes, careful assessment of necrosis and enhancement should be performed, and in equivocal cases, additional imaging modalities and techniques, such as DWI and PET-CT, should be used. Radiologists should be aware of the different findings encountered after these interventions to correctly diagnose response and potential complications.

REFERENCES

1. Bosetti C, Turati F, La Vecchia C. Hepatocellular carcinoma epidemiology. Best Pract Res Clin Gastroenterol 2014;28(5):753–70.

2. Mahnken AH, Pereira PL, de Baere T. Interventional oncologic approaches to liver metastases. Radiology 2013;266(2):407–30.

3. Kritzinger J, Klass D, Ho S, et al. Hepatic embolotherapy in interventional oncology: technology, techniques, and applications. Clin Radiol 2013;68(1):1–15.

4. Hansen PD, Cassera MA, Wolf RF. Ablative technologies for hepatocellular, cholangiocarcinoma, and metastatic colorectal cancer of the liver. Surg Oncol Clin N Am 2015;24(1):97–119.

5. Kulik LM, Chokechanachaisakul A. Evaluation and management of hepatocellular carcinoma. Clin Liver Dis 2015;19(1):23–43.

6. Boas FE, Do B, Louie JD, et al. Optimal imaging surveillance schedules after liver-directed therapy for hepatocellular carcinoma. J Vasc Interv Radiol 2015;26(1):69–73.

7. Brennan IM, Ahmed M. Imaging features following transarterial chemoembolization and radiofrequency ablation of hepatocellular carcinoma. Semin Ultrasound CT MR 2013;34(4):336–51.

8. Golowa YS, Cynamon J, Reinus JF, et al. Value of noncontrast CT immediately after transarterial chemoembolization of hepatocellular carcinoma with drug-eluting beads. J Vasc Interv Radiol 2012; 23(8):1031–5.

9. Kim YS, Rhim H, Lim HK. Imaging after radiofrequency ablation of hepatic tumors. Semin Ultrasound CT MR 2009;30(2):49–66.

10. Sofocleous CT, Sideras P, Petre EN. "How we do it" - a practical approach to hepatic metastases ablation techniques. Tech Vasc Interv Radiol 2013;16(4): 219–29.

11. Rhim H, Goldberg SN, Dodd GD 3rd, et al. Essential techniques for successful radio-frequency thermal ablation of malignant hepatic tumors. Radiographics 2001;21(Spec No):S17–35 [discussion: S36–9].

12. Miller FH, Keppke AL, Reddy D, et al. Response of liver metastases after treatment with yttrium-90 microspheres: role of size, necrosis, and PET. AJR Am J Roentgenol 2007;188(3):776–83.

13. Lewandowski RJ, Thurston KG, Goin JE, et al. 90Y microsphere (TheraSphere) treatment for unresectable colorectal cancer metastases of the liver: response to treatment at targeted doses of 135–150 Gy as measured by [18F]fluorodeoxyglucose positron emission tomography and computed tomographic imaging. J Vasc Interv Radiol 2005;16(12): 1641–51.

14. Gates VL, Salem R, Lewandowski RJ. Positron emission tomography/CT after yttrium-90 radioembolization: current and future applications. J Vasc Interv Radiol 2013;24(8):1153–5.

15. Ko S, Kanehiro H, Hisanaga M, et al. Liver fibrosis increases the risk of intrahepatic recurrence after hepatectomy for hepatocellular carcinoma. Br J Surg 2002;89(1):57–62.

16. Vossen JA, Buijs M, Kamel IR. Assessment of tumor response on MR imaging after locoregional therapy. Tech Vasc Interv Radiol 2006;9(3):125–32.

17. Keppke AL, Salem R, Reddy D, et al. Imaging of hepatocellular carcinoma after treatment with yttrium-90 microspheres. AJR Am J Roentgenol 2007; 188(3):768–75.

18. Yaghmai V, Miller FH, Rezai P, et al. Response to treatment series: part 2, tumor response assessment – using new and conventional criteria. AJR Am J Roentgenol 2011;197(1):18–27.

19. Salem R, Lewandowski RJ, Kulik L, et al. Radioembolization results in longer time-to-progression and reduced toxicity compared with chemoembolization in patients with hepatocellular carcinoma. Gastroenterology 2011;140(2):497–507.e2.

20. Singh P, Anil G. Yttrium-90 radioembolization of liver tumors: what do the images tell us? Cancer Imaging 2013;13(4):645–57.

21. Corona-Villalobos CP, Zhang Y, Zhang WD, et al. Magnetic resonance imaging of the liver after locoregional and systemic therapy. Magn Reson Imaging Clin N Am 2014;22(3):353–72.

22. Atassi B, Bangash AK, Bahrani A, et al. Multimodality imaging following 90Y radioembolization: a comprehensive review and pictorial essay. Radiographics 2008;28(1):81–99.

23. Bruix J, Sherman M, Llovet JM, et al. Clinical management of hepatocellular carcinoma. Conclusions of the Barcelona-2000 EASL conference. European Association for the Study of the Liver. J Hepatol 2001;35(3):421–30.

24. Lencioni R, Llovet JM. Modified RECIST (mRECIST) assessment for hepatocellular carcinoma. Semin Liver Dis 2010;30(1):52–60.

25. Riaz A, Memon K, Miller FH, et al. Role of the EASL, RECIST, and WHO response guidelines alone or in combination for hepatocellular carcinoma: radiologic-pathologic correlation. J Hepatol 2011; 54(4):695–704.

26. Camacho JC, Kokabi N, Xing M, et al. Modified response evaluation criteria in solid tumors and European Association for The Study of the Liver criteria using delayed-phase imaging at an early time point predict survival in patients with unresectable intrahepatic cholangiocarcinoma following yttrium-90 radioembolization. J Vasc Interv Radiol 2014;25(2): 256–65.

27. Winters SD, Jackson S, Armstrong GA, et al. Value of subtraction MRI in assessing treatment response following image-guided loco-regional therapies for hepatocellular carcinoma. Clin Radiol 2012;67(7): 649–55.

28. Riaz A, Kulik L, Lewandowski RJ, et al. Radiologic-pathologic correlation of hepatocellular carcinoma treated with internal radiation using yttrium-90 microspheres. Hepatology 2009;49(4):1185–93.

29. Kamel IR, Reyes DK, Liapi E, et al. Functional MR imaging assessment of tumor response after 90Y microsphere treatment in patients with unresectable hepatocellular carcinoma. J Vasc Interv Radiol 2007; 18(1 Pt 1):49–56.

30. Mannelli L, Kim S, Hajdu CH, et al. Serial diffusion-weighted MRI in patients with hepatocellular carcinoma: prediction and assessment of response to transarterial chemoembolization. Preliminary experience. Eur J Radiol 2013;82(4):577–82.

31. Li Z, Bonekamp S, Halappa VG, et al. Islet cell liver metastases: assessment of volumetric early response with functional MR imaging after transarterial chemoembolization. Radiology 2012;264(1):97–109.

32. Kokabi N, Camacho JC, Xing M, et al. Apparent diffusion coefficient quantification as an early imaging biomarker of response and predictor of survival following yttrium-90 radioembolization for unresectable infiltrative hepatocellular carcinoma with portal vein thrombosis. Abdom Imaging 2014;39(5):969–78.

33. Halappa VG, Bonekamp S, Corona-Villalobos CP, et al. Intrahepatic cholangiocarcinoma treated with local-regional therapy: quantitative volumetric apparent diffusion coefficient maps for assessment of tumor response. Radiology 2012;264(1):285–94.

34. Sahin H, Harman M, Cinar C, et al. Evaluation of treatment response of chemoembolization in hepatocellular carcinoma with diffusion-weighted imaging on 3.0-T MR imaging. J Vasc Interv Radiol 2012;23(2):241–7.

35. Guo Y, Yaghmai V, Salem R, et al. Imaging tumor response following liver-directed intra-arterial therapy. Abdom Imaging 2013;38(6):1286–99.

36. Mannelli L, Kim S, Hajdu CH, et al. Assessment of tumor necrosis of hepatocellular carcinoma after chemoembolization: diffusion-weighted and contrast-enhanced MRI with histopathologic correlation of the explanted liver. AJR Am J Roentgenol 2009;193(4):1044–52.

37. Bonekamp S, Halappa VG, Geschwind JF, et al. Unresectable hepatocellular carcinoma: MR imaging after intraarterial therapy. Part II. Response stratification using volumetric functional criteria after intra-arterial therapy. Radiology 2013;268(2):431–9.

38. Vouche M, Salem R, Lewandowski RJ, et al. Can volumetric ADC measurement help predict response to Y90 radioembolization in HCC? Abdom Imaging 2014. [Epub ahead of print].

39. Gowdra Halappa V, Corona-Villalobos CP, Bonekamp S, et al. Neuroendocrine liver metastasis treated by using intra-arterial therapy: volumetric functional imaging biomarkers of early tumor response and survival. Radiology 2013;266(2):502–13.

40. Hayano K, Lee SH, Yoshida H, et al. Fractal analysis of CT perfusion images for evaluation of antiangiogenic treatment and survival in hepatocellular carcinoma. Acad Radiol 2014;21(5):654–60.

41. Chen G, Ma DQ, He W, et al. Computed tomography perfusion in evaluating the therapeutic effect of transarterial chemoembolization for hepatocellular carcinoma. World J Gastroenterol 2008;14(37):5738–43.

42. Bonekamp S, Bonekamp D, Geschwind JF, et al. Response stratification and survival analysis of hepatocellular carcinoma patients treated with intra-arterial therapy using MR imaging-based arterial enhancement fraction. J Magn Reson Imaging 2014;40(5):1103–11.

43. Chen X, Xiao E, Shu D, et al. Evaluating the therapeutic effect of hepatocellular carcinoma treated with transcatheter arterial chemoembolization by magnetic resonance perfusion imaging. Eur J Gastroenterol Hepatol 2014;26(1):109–13.

44. Gonzalez-Guindalini FD, Botelho MP, Harmath CB, et al. Assessment of liver tumor response to therapy: role of quantitative imaging. Radiographics 2013;33(6):1781–800.

45. Ibrahim SM, Nikolaidis P, Miller FH, et al. Radiologic findings following Y90 radioembolization for primary liver malignancies. Abdom Imaging 2009;34(5):566–81.

46. Lewandowski RJ, Geschwind JF, Liapi E, et al. Transcatheter intraarterial therapies: rationale and overview. Radiology 2011;259(3):641–57.

47. Shah PA, Cunningham SC, Morgan TA, et al. Hepatic gas: widening spectrum of causes detected at CT and US in the interventional era. Radiographics 2011;31(5):1403–13.

48. Theysohn JM, Ertle J, Muller S, et al. Hepatic volume changes after lobar selective internal radiation therapy (SIRT) of hepatocellular carcinoma. Clin Radiol 2014;69(2):172–8.

49. Riaz A, Lewandowski RJ, Kulik LM, et al. Complications following radioembolization with yttrium-90 microspheres: a comprehensive literature review. J Vasc Interv Radiol 2009;20(9):1121–30 [quiz: 1131].

50. Clark TW. Complications of hepatic chemoembolization. Semin Intervent Radiol 2006;23(2):119–25.

51. Wagnetz U, Jaskolka J, Yang P, et al. Acute ischemic cholecystitis after transarterial chemoembolization of hepatocellular carcinoma: incidence and clinical outcome. J Comput Assist Tomogr 2010;34(3):348–53.

52. Atassi B, Bangash AK, Lewandowski RJ, et al. Biliary sequelae following radioembolization with yttrium-90 microspheres. J Vasc Interv Radiol 2008;19(5):691–7.

53. Sag AA, Savin MA, Lal NR, et al. Yttrium-90 radioembolization of malignant tumors of the liver: gallbladder effects. AJR Am J Roentgenol 2014;202(5):1130–5.

54. Riaz A, Awais R, Salem R. Side effects of yttrium-90 radioembolization. Front Oncol 2014;4:198.

55. Lopez-Benitez R, Radeleff BA, Barragan-Campos HM, et al. Acute pancreatitis after embolization of liver tumors: frequency and associated risk factors. Pancreatology 2007;7(1):53–62.

56. Schelhorn J, Ertle J, Schlaak JF, et al. Selective internal radiation therapy of hepatic tumors: procedural implications of a patent hepatic falciform artery. Springerplus 2014;3:595.

57. Yu JS, Kim KW, Jeong MG, et al. Predisposing factors of bile duct injury after transcatheter arterial chemoembolization (TACE) for hepatic malignancy. Cardiovasc Intervent Radiol 2002;25(4):270–4.

58. Mortele KJ, Ros PR. Cystic focal liver lesions in the adult: differential CT and MR imaging features. Radiographics 2001;21(4):895–910.

59. Memon K, Lewandowski RJ, Kulik L, et al. Radioembolization for primary and metastatic liver cancer. Semin Radiat Oncol 2011;21(4):294–302.

60. Lawrence TS, Robertson JM, Anscher MS, et al. Hepatic toxicity resulting from cancer treatment. Int J Radiat Oncol Biol Phys 1995;31(5):1237–48.

61. Maor Y, Malnick S. Liver injury induced by anticancer chemotherapy and radiation therapy. Int J Hepatol 2013;2013:815105.

62. Chiou SY, Lee RC, Chi KH, et al. The triple-phase CT image appearance of post-irradiated livers. Acta Radiol 2001;42(5):526–31.

63. Marn CS, Andrews JC, Francis IR, et al. Hepatic parenchymal changes after intra-arterial Y-90 therapy: CT findings. Radiology 1993;187(1):125–8.

64. Maturen KE, Feng MU, Wasnik AP, et al. Imaging effects of radiation therapy in the abdomen and pelvis: evaluating "innocent bystander" tissues. Radiographics 2013;33(2):599–619.

65. Sheng Y, Wang Q, Li Z, et al. Time-dependent changes in CT of radiation-induced liver injury: a preliminary study in gastric cancer patients. J Huazhong Univ Sci Technolog Med Sci 2010;30(5):683–6.

66. Limanond P, Zimmerman P, Raman SS, et al. Interpretation of CT and MRI after radiofrequency ablation of hepatic malignancies. AJR Am J Roentgenol 2003;181(6):1635–40.

67. Sainani NI, Gervais DA, Mueller PR, et al. Imaging after percutaneous radiofrequency ablation of hepatic tumors: Part 1. Normal findings. AJR Am J Roentgenol 2013;200(1):184–93.

68. Park MH, Rhim H, Kim YS, et al. Spectrum of CT findings after radiofrequency ablation of hepatic tumors. Radiographics 2008;28(2):379–90 [discussion: 390–2].

69. Schima W, Ba-Ssalamah A, Kurtaran A, et al. Post-treatment imaging of liver tumours. Cancer Imaging 2007;7(Spec No A):S28–36.

70. Motoyama T, Ogasawara S, Chiba T, et al. Coronal reformatted CT images contribute to the precise evaluation of the radiofrequency ablative margin

for hepatocellular carcinoma. Abdom Imaging 2014; 39(2):262–8.

71. Lu TL, Becce F, Bize P, et al. Assessment of liver tumor response by high-field (3 T) MRI after radiofrequency ablation: short- and mid-term evolution of diffusion parameters within the ablation zone. Eur J Radiol 2012;81(9):e944–50.

72. Zhang Y, Zhao J, Guo D, et al. Evaluation of short-term response of high intensity focused ultrasound ablation for primary hepatic carcinoma: utility of contrast-enhanced MRI and diffusion-weighted imaging. Eur J Radiol 2011;79(3):347–52.

73. Vogl TJ, Farshid P, Naguib NN, et al. Thermal ablation therapies in patients with breast cancer liver metastases: a review. Eur Radiol 2013;23(3): 797–804.

74. Curley SA, Marra P, Beaty K, et al. Early and late complications after radiofrequency ablation of malignant liver tumors in 608 patients. Ann Surg 2004; 239(4):450–8.

75. Bertot LC, Sato M, Tateishi R, et al. Mortality and complication rates of percutaneous ablative techniques for the treatment of liver tumors: a systematic review. Eur Radiol 2011;21(12):2584–96.

76. Sainani NI, Gervais DA, Mueller PR, et al. Imaging after percutaneous radiofrequency ablation of hepatic tumors: Part 2. Abnormal findings. AJR Am J Roentgenol 2013;200(1):194–204.

77. Liang P, Wang Y, Yu X, et al. Malignant liver tumors: treatment with percutaneous microwave ablation – complications among cohort of 1136 patients. Radiology 2009;251(3):933–40.

78. Flanders VL, Gervais DA. Ablation of liver metastases: current status. J Vasc Interv Radiol 2010;21(8 Suppl):S214–22.

79. Livraghi T, Meloni F, Solbiati L, et al. Complications of microwave ablation for liver tumors: results of a multicenter study. Cardiovasc Intervent Radiol 2012;35(4):868–74.

80. Kim SW, Rhim H, Park M, et al. Percutaneous radiofrequency ablation of hepatocellular carcinomas adjacent to the gallbladder with internally cooled electrodes: assessment of safety and therapeutic efficacy. Korean J Radiol 2009;10(4):366–76.

81. Cha DI, Lee MW, Rhim H, et al. Therapeutic efficacy and safety of percutaneous ethanol injection with or without combined radiofrequency ablation for hepatocellular carcinomas in high risk locations. Korean J Radiol 2013;14(2):240–7.

82. Kim AY, Rhim H, Park M, et al. Venous thrombosis after radiofrequency ablation for hepatocellular carcinoma. AJR Am J Roentgenol 2011;197(6):1474–80.

83. Livraghi T, Solbiati L, Meloni MF, et al. Treatment of focal liver tumors with percutaneous radiofrequency ablation: complications encountered in a multicenter study. Radiology 2003;226(2):441–51.

Assessing Imaging Response to Therapy

Jeet Minocha, MD[a,*], Robert J. Lewandowski, MD, FSIR[b]

KEYWORDS

- World Health Organization (WHO) • Response evaluation criteria in solid tumors (RECIST)
- European Association for the Study of the Liver (EASL) • Modified RECIST (mRECIST)
- Response assessment • Computed tomography (CT) • MR imaging

KEY POINTS

- Accurate assessment of response to locoregional therapies (LRTs) is crucial because objective response can be a surrogate of improved survival.
- Tumor size and necrosis guidelines are the gold standard for assessing imaging response to LRTs.
- Newer imaging modalities (eg, functional MR imaging, PET with fluorodeoxyglucose [FDG-PET]) and biomarkers of response (eg, serum tumor markers) show promise as ancillary tools in assessing response to therapy.

INTRODUCTION

LRTs, such as radiofrequency ablation (RFA), transarterial chemoembolization (TACE), and radioembolization, have proved valuable in the treatment of patients with cancer, most commonly in the liver.[1] Accurate assessment of response to these therapies is crucial because objective response can be a surrogate of improved survival.[2] Imaging plays an essential role in the objective evaluation of tumor response to most cancer therapies, including LRTs. Because imaging response following LRTs has been shown to predict patient survival times,[3] one of the goals of LRTs should be to achieve a radiologic response. Assessing imaging response to LRTs, however, can be challenging and is evolving.

There are several radiologic criteria that are commonly used to assess imaging response to treatment after LRTs, including World Health Organization (WHO),[4] Response Evaluation Criteria in Solid Tumors (RECIST),[5] and European Association for the Study of the Liver (EASL)[6] guidelines.

Volumetric techniques and functional imaging (eg, PET) have also been described.[7–10] No universally accepted criteria exist.

This article reviews the different criteria used to assess radiologic response to LRTs, with special attention to imaging assessment following treatment of hepatocellular carcinoma (HCC).

IMAGING TECHNIQUES

Imaging evaluation of patients treated with LRTs is usually performed with cross-sectional imaging, most commonly computed tomography (CT) or MR imaging . Although there has been considerable interest in other imaging modalities, including PET[8,11] and contrast-enhanced ultrasonography (CEUS),[12,13] these are less commonly used. Accurate imaging assessment of response to therapy requires the following:

- Evaluation of tumor size
- Evaluation of tumor margins
- Evaluation of tumor necrosis

[a] Division of Interventional Radiology, Department of Radiology, University of California San Diego, 200 West Arbor Drive, #8756, San Diego, CA 92103-8756, USA; [b] Section of Interventional Radiology, Department of Radiology, Northwestern Memorial Hospital, Robert H. Lurie Comprehensive Cancer Center, 676 North Saint Clair Street, Suite 800, Chicago, IL 60611, USA
* Corresponding author.
E-mail address: jminocha@ucsd.edu

Radiol Clin N Am 53 (2015) 1077–1088
http://dx.doi.org/10.1016/j.rcl.2015.05.010
0033-8389/15/$ – see front matter © 2015 Elsevier Inc. All rights reserved.

- Detection of residual or recurrent tumor
- Detection of new tumor

The evaluation of treatment success is essential for future treatment decisions and prognosis.[14]

Computed Tomography

CT has been the mainstay of cancer imaging for both initial evaluation and response assessment after treatment. Modern multidetector CT scanners allow thin-section images to be obtained in a single breath-hold with greatly improved speed and resolution, resulting in high-resolution multiplanar reformations.[14] In patients with HCC, multiphase scanning is typically used.[15] The United Network for Organ Sharing currently recommends a multiphasic CT protocol for HCC that includes nonenhanced, late arterial phase, portal venous phase, and delayed phase imaging.[16]

Dual-energy CT (DECT) has become available, and its utility in imaging hypervascular liver masses such as HCC is being evaluated.[17] DECT provides additional information about how tissues of differing densities behave at differing tube voltages. DECT may have utility in evaluating response of HCC to LRTs with higher lesion-to-liver contrast-to-noise ratios on an iodine map, which can be helpful for detecting residual tumor.[18]

MR Imaging

MR imaging provides high-quality soft-tissue contrast and spatial resolution, allowing for multiplanar 3-dimensional reconstructions and maximum intensity projections. The use of functional parameters in MR imaging, such as flow, temperature, tissue oxygenation, dynamic perfusion, and diffusion, further assist in guiding therapy and assessing treatment response.[14]

MR imaging plays a particularly important role in patients with HCC. Contrast-enhanced dynamic T1-weighted imaging with diffusion-weighted imaging can be helpful in assessing treatment-related changes in HCC.[19] MR imaging may be superior to CT in evaluating patients treated with conventional TACE (cTACE) because the beam-hardening effects of the high-density ethiodized oil used in cTACE may obscure small enhancing tumors on CT. However, ethiodized oil does not adversely affect MR signal-intensity characteristics, so residual enhancement can be detected, especially when image subtraction is used.[9,20] Image subtraction can also be helpful in other situations. For example, lesions treated with RFA typically undergo coagulative hemorrhagic necrosis that can appear hyperintense on unenhanced T1-weighted imaging, making contrast-enhanced

evaluation challenging.[21] Using image subtraction techniques, MR imaging has been shown to be beneficial in depicting residual enhancement, with excellent correlation with histopathologic degree of tumor necrosis.[22]

Positron Emission Tomography

FDG-PET has become an indispensable tool for evaluating many types of cancer. PET has been incorporated into the response assessment criteria for Hodgkin and non-Hodgkin lymphoma,[23] and it has proven utility in detecting early response and predicting long-term response to imatinib in gastrointestinal stromal tumors (GISTs).[24] For cancers commonly treated with LRTs, such as metastatic colorectal cancer, FDG-PET may be more reliable than CT in the detection of liver metastasis or recurrence in the liver.[25] Gulec and colleagues[26] found that FDG-PET response in patients with colorectal cancer liver metastases treated with radioembolization was strongly associated with survival. On the other hand, FDG-PET has limited sensitivity in the detection of HCC, and its role in assessing response to therapy in this disease has not been validated.[14] At present, lack of widespread availability and lack of sufficient standardization prevent FDG-PET from being widely incorporated into many response criteria. However, it can be used as an adjunct to other imaging modalities following LRTs.

Contrast-Enhanced Ultrasonography

CEUS has been studied to assess response to LRTs including RFA,[13] TACE,[12] and combined techniques.[27] On postablation CEUS, nodules showing no contrast enhancement in the arterial phase correlate with complete necrosis on CT and nodules with persistent arterial vascularization are considered residual tumor.[27] Potential benefits of CEUS include the following: (1) it is easy to use and (2) the high-density ethiodized oil used in cTACE does not limit CEUS interpretation, as can be the case with CT.[12] However, to date, microbubble contrast agents are not approved by the US Food and Drug Administration (FDA) for the evaluation of liver lesions, and this technique is rarely performed in the United States.

DIAGNOSTIC CRITERIA

Early attempts to define objective response of a tumor to an anticancer therapy date back to the 1960s.[28] Shortly thereafter, following a rapid increase in cancer-related research, it became apparent that a common language would be necessary to report results of cancer treatments in a consistent manner. In 1979, the first definitions of objective tumor response were widely disseminated and adopted after the publication of the 1979 *World Health Organization (WHO) Handbook for Reporting Results of Cancer Treatment*.[29]

World Health Organization Guidelines

According to the *WHO Handbook*, tumor size is determined by multiplying the longest diameter of a target lesion in the axial plane by its greatest perpendicular diameter (bidimensional cross-product) (**Fig. 1**). In the presence of multiple lesions, the sums of the cross-products are compared before and after treatment. Although tumors were assumed to be spherical, lack of sophisticated imaging technology in the late 1970s lead to the adoption of bidimensional measurements for the criteria.

Objective response is divided into 4 categories determined by 2 observations not less than 4 weeks apart:

1. Complete response (CR): Disappearance of all known disease
2. Partial response (PR): Greater than or equal to 50% decrease in size of measured lesions (**Fig. 2**)
3. No change or stable disease (SD): Disease between PR and progressive disease (PD) (ie, <50% reduction to <25% increase in size of measured lesions)
4. PD: Greater than or equal to 25% increase in size of measured lesions

The WHO criteria were widely accepted and used for more than 2 decades in response evaluation for solid tumors. However, over time several deficiencies were identified, including lack of guidelines on (1) thresholds for lesion size, (2) minimum number of lesions to be measured, and (3) type of imaging modality to be used. Moreover, calculations using bidimensional

cross-products were cumbersome, and minor errors had a significant impact on the estimation of tumor burden.[30] Several modifications, for example, Southwest Oncology Group (SWOG) criteria, were proposed,[31] which only resulted in further confusion.

There became an identified need to formulate a new criterion that would overcome the shortcomings of the WHO guidelines.

Response Evaluation Criteria in Solid Tumors Guidelines

Based on evaluation of more than 4000 patients from multiple collaborative studies, the RECIST guidelines were published in 2000 by a Task Force that comprised the European Organization for Research and Treatment of Cancer (EORTC), the National Cancer Institute of the United States, and the National Cancer Institute of Canada Clinical Trials Group.[5]

The RECIST guidelines updated the WHO definitions with the objective of again unifying criteria of response assessment. Significant changes in response categorization were avoided to enable meaningful comparisons with the WHO guidelines. Unlike WHO, RECIST defines the minimum size of measurable lesions, number of lesions to follow, and imaging technique to be used and uses simpler, unidimensional rather than bidimensional measurements for the evaluation of tumor burden.[5] The RECIST guidelines require lesions to be categorized as measurable or nonmeasurable based on a single measurement of the longest tumor diameter in the axial plane (**Fig. 3**). Lesions that measure more than 10 mm on CT are considered measurable. Measurable lesions are further classified as target or nontarget lesions based on size and suitability for reproducible measurements. The original RECIST guidelines allow up to 5 target lesions per organ and 10 lesions in total. Nontarget lesions are also important, as their unequivocal progression implies PD.

Response is categorized by the percentage change in the sum of the diameters of target lesions as follows:

1. CR: Disappearance of all target lesions
2. PR: Greater than 30% decrease in the sum of diameters of target lesions (**Fig. 4**)
3. SD: Changes between PR and PD
4. PD: Greater than 20% increase in the sum of diameters of target lesions, or the appearance of new lesions, or unequivocal progression of nontarget lesions

The cutoff for PD is larger in the RECIST guidelines than in the WHO criteria; the WHO criteria

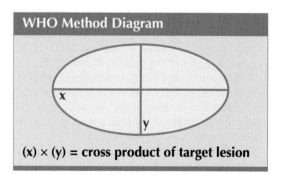

WHO Method Diagram

(x) × (y) = **cross product of target lesion**

Fig. 1. Bidimensional cross-product of target lesion using WHO guidelines.

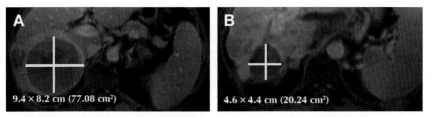

Fig. 2. WHO partial response. Greater than 50% reduction in tumor cross-product pretreatment (*A*) and post-treatment (*B*).

define PD as 25% or more increase in the sum of the cross-product of lesion diameters, equivalent to a 40% increase in tumor volume. In the RECIST guidelines, PD is defined as greater than 20% increase in diameters, corresponding to a 73% increase in tumor volume. **Table 1** highlights the major differences between WHO and RECIST.

RECIST was widely adopted by the oncology community, especially for clinical trials, and has been accepted by regulatory authorities such as the FDA as an appropriate guideline for tumor assessments.[30]

However, as with the WHO criteria, several issues were identified with the original RECIST guidelines, including the (1) total number of lesions to be assessed (ie, if <10 lesions could be assessed), (2) assessment of lymph nodes, (3) use of newer imaging technologies (MR imaging and FDG-PET), and (4) use of RECIST in trials of LRTs and noncytotoxic drugs that did not necessarily result in tumor size reduction.[30] In addition, unidimensional measurements were used based on the assumption that lesions are spherical, which is not always true. New technologies that enabled 3-dimensional volumetric measurements could be more accurate, especially with infiltrating, confluent, or ill-defined lesions. A prospective database of solid tumor measurement data obtained from various trials that consisted of more than 6500 patients was obtained by the RECIST working group. Using this database, several modifications were made to the original RECIST guidelines, RECIST 1.1.[32]

Response Evaluation Criteria in Solid Tumors 1.1 Guidelines

In RECIST 1.1, the maximum number of target lesions was reduced to 2 lesions per organ and 5 lesions in total, thus simplifying response assessment. RECIST 1.1 maintains the 4 major response categories from RECIST 1.0. The definition of PD was modified. In addition to a 20% increase in the sum of diameters of target lesions, an absolute increase of at least 5 mm is required in small lesions. With lymph nodes included as target lesions, even if CR is achieved, the sum may not become zero because normal lymph nodes are defined as those with a diameter of less than 10 mm. RECIST 1.1 therefore recommends that the target pathologic lymph nodes be recorded in a separate section, and to qualify for CR, each lymph node must have a short axis of less than 10 mm. This criterion eliminates a major drawback of RECIST 1.0, in which visible, nonpathologic lymph nodes could not be categorized as CR. For all other response categories, the short-axis measurement of lymph nodes is included in the sum of target lesions. RECIST 1.0 did not have a consensus on how to measure when a lesion splits or when multiple lesions coalesce. In RECIST 1.1, when the lesion splits, the longest diameters of the fragmented portions should be used to calculate the target lesion sum. If lesions truly coalesce and are not separable from one another, the vector of the longest diameter should be used as the longest diameter of the coalesced lesion. RECIST 1.1 also recommends that unequivocal progression of nontarget lesions be representative of overall disease status rather than measurements of a single lesion. **Table 2** highlights the major differences between RECIST 1.0 and RECIST 1.1.

The WHO and RECIST guidelines, both based on changes in tumor size, remain the most widely used guidelines for assessing imaging response to therapy in clinical trials.[30] However, assessments

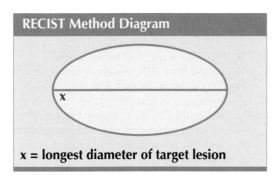

Fig. 3. Unidimensional measurement of target lesion using RECIST guidelines.

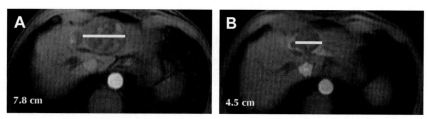

Fig. 4. RECIST partial response. Greater than 30% reduction in tumor diameter pretreatment (*A*) and posttreatment (*B*).

based solely on changes in tumor size can be misleading when applied to newer therapeutic interventions (eg, TACE for HCC) or anticancer drugs (eg, imatinib for GIST) because the purpose of many of these therapies is to cause tumor necrosis, regardless of lesion shrinkage.[14,24] The use of tumor measurements without considering necrosis is a major yet unanswered pitfall of WHO and RECIST. Furthermore, the introduction of novel therapies without direct cytotoxic effects has imposed an additional challenge in the assessment of treatment response using traditional size criteria (eg, bevacizumab for metastatic colorectal cancer, temsirolimus for renal cancer, and sorafenib for HCC).[33–35]

Several modifications are therefore necessary before any single criterion becomes the standard for the evaluation of tumor response. New tools and imaging techniques, such as functional MR imaging, PET, and CT perfusion, have to be aggressively studied before possible incorporation into guidelines such as RECIST 1.1.[30] Because a single response evaluation criterion is unlikely to be useful for all tumor types, developing individualized response criteria based on tumor types may be more practical; this has been particularly true for HCC, one of the most common types of cancer treated by interventional radiologists.

Assessing Imaging Response to Therapy in Hepatocellular Carcinoma

LRTs are playing an increasingly important role in the treatment of patients with HCC.[1] However, recent studies have shown a poor correlation between the clinical benefit provided by LRTs and conventional methods of response assessment. Extensive tumor necrosis (ie, one of the goals of LRTs) may not be paralleled by a reduction in diameter of the treated lesion.[6] In response to these limitations, a panel of experts on HCC convened by the EASL amended the response criteria for HCC to take into account tumor necrosis induced by treatment.[6]

Table 1
Comparison between WHO and RECIST guidelines

	WHO Guidelines	RECIST Guidelines
Imaging modality	Not specified	CT and MR imaging recommended
Definition of measurable lesion	Measurable in 2 dimensions No minimum size	Measurable in 1 dimension; ≥10 mm on spiral CT
Method of measurement	Bidimensional cross-product (see Fig. 1)	Unidimensional (see **Fig. 3**)
Number of lesions to be measured	Not specified	Up to 5 target lesions per organ and 10 in total
Response definitions	CR Disappearance of all known disease PR ≥50% decrease in sum of cross-products SD Changes between PR and PD PD ≥25% increase in sum of cross-products	Disappearance of all target lesions >30% decrease in sum of diameters Changes between PR and PD >20% increase in sum of diameters; new lesions; unequivocal progression of nontarget lesions

Table 2
Comparison between RECIST 1.0 and RECIST 1.1 guidelines

	RECIST 1.0 Guidelines	RECIST 1.1 Guidelines
Number of lesions to be measured	Up to 5 target lesions per organ and 10 in total	Up to 2 target lesions per organ and 5 in total
Lymph nodes	Not specified	Target lesion >15 mm (short axis); <10 mm nonpathologic
Target lesion response	CR Lymph nodes not specified	Lymph nodes must be <10 mm (short axis)
	PD >20% increase in sum of diameters; new lesions	>20% increase in sum of diameters; new lesions; absolute increase >5 mm
Nontarget lesion response	Unequivocal progression = PD	Unequivocal progression representative of overall disease status rather than measurements of single lesion
Progression-free survival	General comments	More specific comments on use in phase 2 and 3 trials

European Association for the Study of the Liver Guidelines

The EASL (necrosis) guidelines were published in 2001 and are based on the percentage change in the amount of enhancing tumoral tissue posttreatment. The guidelines consider estimation of the reduction in viable tumor volume (recognized by nonenhanced areas on cross-sectional imaging) the optimal method to assess local response to treatment (**Fig. 5**). Viable tumor is defined as the uptake of contrast agent in the arterial phase of CT or MR imaging.

Objective response is based on the WHO definitions:

1. CR: Disappearance of intratumoral arterial enhancement (**Fig. 6**)
2. PR: Greater than or equal to 50% reduction in intratumoral arterial enhancement (see **Fig. 6**)
3. SD: Changes between PR and PD

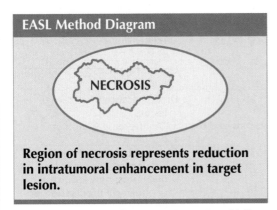

EASL Method Diagram

NECROSIS

Region of necrosis represents reduction in intratumoral enhancement in target lesion.

Fig. 5. Measurement of necrosis using EASL guidelines.

4. PD: Greater than or equal to 25% increase in intratumoral arterial enhancement

The concept of viable tumor proposed by the EASL guidelines was subsequently endorsed by the American Association for the Study of Liver Diseases (AASLD). The AASLD practice guideline on the management of HCC published in 2005 stated that the evaluation of treatment response should take into account the induction of intratumoral necrotic areas in estimating the decrease in tumor load and not just a reduction in overall tumor size.[36]

Because of the growing complexity of assessment of benefits in HCC, a group of experts convened by the AASLD developed a set of guidelines aimed to translate the concept of tumor viability and necrosis posed by the EASL guidelines in a more updated RECIST framework: the modified RECIST assessment (mRECIST) for HCC.[2]

Modified Response Evaluation Criteria in Solid Tumors Guidelines

The mRECIST assessment for HCC addresses many of the shortcomings of the EASL guidelines by defining methods for (1) image acquisitions, (2) target lesion selection, and (3) target lesion response, by adapting many of the strengths of the RECIST guidelines.

mRECIST uses the single largest diameter of the viable tumor (defined as the component enhancing during the arterial phase) and is more practical for clinical use.[2] To be selected as a target lesion using mRECIST, an HCC lesion should meet all the following criteria: (1) the lesion can be classified as a RECIST measurable lesion, (2) the lesion is suitable for repeat measurement, and (3) the lesion

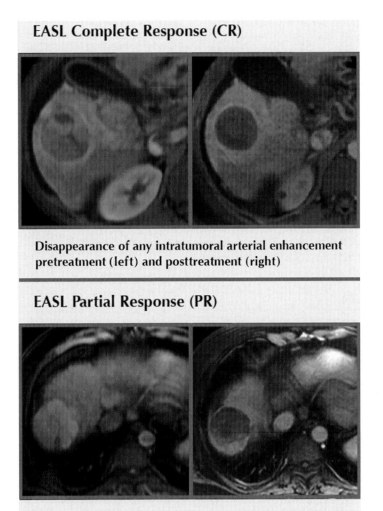

EASL Complete Response (CR)

Disappearance of any intratumoral arterial enhancement
pretreatment (left) and posttreatment (right)

EASL Partial Response (PR)

>50% reduction in intratumoral arterial enhancement
pretreatment (left) and posttreatment (right)

Fig. 6. EASL complete and partial response.

shows intratumoral arterial enhancement on contrast-enhanced CT or MR imaging.

Assessment of target lesion response is defined as the following:

1. CR: Disappearance of any intratumoral arterial enhancement in all target lesions
2. PR: Greater than 30% decrease in the sum of diameters of viable (enhancement in arterial phase) target lesions, taking as reference the baseline sum of diameters of target lesions
3. SD: Changes between PR and PD
4. PD: Greater than 20% increase in the sum of diameters of viable target lesions, taking as reference the baseline sum of diameters of target lesions

Several studies have shown mRECIST to be superior to RECIST in predicting HCC response to LRTs.[37,38] Measurement of the 2 largest target lesions has been shown to be adequate for the assessment of HCC response to TACE when using mRECIST.[39,40] In 2 studies of patients with HCC treated with TACE, mRECIST criteria independently predicted overall survival.[38,39] Response assessments based on EASL and mRECIST criteria approximately 1 month after drug-eluting bead TACE have been shown to predict survival, with better performance by the mRECIST guidelines.[37] In addition, a recent study showed that EASL and mRECIST responses are independent prognostic factors for survival after TACE, whereas there was no significant association between survival and RECIST 1.1 response.[41]

The EASL and EORTC have endorsed the use of the mRECIST guidelines for the assessment of

HCC response based on dynamic CT or MR imaging performed 1 month after LRTs.[42] However, the mRECIST criteria have several limitations: (1) they have not been validated for assessing HCC after other LRTs, including RFA and radioembolization; (2) it remains difficult to measure lesions with intervening viable and necrotic components; and (3) many patients with multiple HCCs are treated in stages, so tumors are treated at different time points, which decreases the value of these criteria when assessing LRTs.[14]

The lack of consensus and introduction of new imaging techniques has led to further modifications and combinations of the previously described criteria, including the primary index lesion and EASL × WHO Scoring System guidelines.[43,44] The major limitation of all of these guidelines is limited data to date.

Primary Index Lesion

Given that the single common factor for most patients undergoing LRTs is that they have at least 1 dominant first-treated lesion, the concept of measuring response in the primary index lesion was introduced as an alternative biomarker for response in HCC.[43] Response is measured using WHO, RECIST, and/or EASL in the primary index lesion, defined as the lesion targeted during the first treatment session. In contrast to WHO, RECIST, and EASL guidelines alone, this method relies on response in 1 lesion only in the setting of multifocal disease. In addition, it incorporates anatomic and necrosis criteria, such as mRECIST. Preliminary data show that response in the primary index lesion alone resulted in statistically significant correlations with disease progression and survival. In addition, among this group of patients, agreement for classification of therapeutic response was high between size criteria (WHO and RECIST guidelines) but low between each of these and EASL.[43]

European Association for the Study of the Liver × World Health Organization Scoring System

Recognizing the significant differences and potential advantages of both anatomic and necrosis criteria for response, a recent analysis combining both criteria was performed with pathologic correlation.[44] Numerical values were assigned to the defined response classes. The data show that the product of EASL and WHO response (ie, the EASL × WHO Scoring System) demonstrated better receiver-operator characteristics than the individual guidelines for assessment of tumor response.

Future Directions

Modern imaging acquisition techniques permit volumetric (ie, 3-dimensional [3D]) quantification of tumor burden. Both anatomic and necrosis (3D EASL) methods have been described.[7,45] An important theoretic advantage of volumetric measurements is that they permit measurement of overall tumor burden in an organ, thereby eliminating the arbitrary guideline of measuring 2 or 5 lesions per organ. However, 3D measurements require proprietary software, can be time consuming, and may not add significant value compared with 2-dimensional (2D) methods.

Functional imaging has the potential to revolutionize oncological imaging. The most common functional imaging tool today is FDG-PET. Although FDG-PET has been incorporated in the tumor response criteria for lymphoma,[23] its use in assessing other solid tumors is limited by availability, cost, and poor spatial resolution. False-positive (eg, inflammatory and infectious pathologies) and false-negative (eg, small lesions, non-FDG avid tumors) results also limit the overall accuracy of this modality.

Diffusion-weighted MR imaging is a functional MR imaging approach that can detect alterations in motion of water molecules resulting from compromised cell membrane integrity or edema. This apparent diffusion of water molecules is quantified by the measurement of apparent diffusion coefficient values. Diffusion-weighted MR imaging has been described as an alternative parameter to assess HCC tumor response following TACE and radioembolization.[9,19] HCC tumor response assessed with diffusion-weighted imaging may precede anatomic size changes and may assist in early determination of the response or failure of LRTs for HCC.[19]

Potential metabolic imaging abilities of MR imaging are also being explored. In addition to blood oxygen level–dependent imaging, an indirect measure of angiogenesis, and dynamic contrast-enhanced MR imaging, a direct measure of tumor angiogenesis, macromolecular MR imaging contrast agents have been found to be promising for the detection of tumor angiogenesis and its response to antiangiogenic therapy in experimental animal studies.[46] Other molecular imaging methods aimed at detecting and quantifying tumor angiogenesis include stem cell imaging (labeling endothelial progenitor stem cells and tracking their behavior in vivo) and use of contrast agents targeting the endothelial cell surface markers to be used with MR imaging, PET, single-photon emission CT, or optical imaging.[47]

Although experience with these novel techniques is limited, they show promise as ancillary tools in assessing radiologic response to therapy.

PEARLS AND PITFALLS

With advances in cancer therapy, there is an increasing demand for accurate criteria to assess the beneficial effects of these novel treatments. Knowledge of the advantages and limitations of various tumor response evaluation criteria is crucial to provide the best possible care.

World Health Organization Guidelines

Method summary

- Multiply the longest diameter of target lesions by the greatest perpendicular diameter (bidimensional).
- Measure the percentage change in the sum of the products of the perpendicular diameters of the target lesions.

Advantages

- Standardized assessment of tumor response to therapy and reporting of results
- Anatomic
- Widely used and validated

Limitations

- Differences in interpretation of WHO guidelines resulted in a situation in which response criteria were no longer comparable among research institutions.
- It does not take into account changes in tumor viability.
- Not all disease is measurable (eg, lymphangitic carcinomatosis).

Response Evaluation Criteria in Solid Tumors 1.0 and 1.1 Guidelines

Method summary

- Target lesions 10 mm or more on CT
- Measure the longest diameter of target lesions (unidimensional)
- Maximum of 5 lesions per organ and 10 lesions in total (RECIST)
- Maximum of 2 lesions per organ and 5 lesions in total (RECIST 1.1)
- Measure percentage change in the sum of diameters of target lesions

Advantages

- Unidimensional (in contrast to WHO guidelines)
- Reproducible

- Anatomic
- Widely used and validated

Limitations

- There is low reliability in evaluating response in certain tumors (eg, malignant pleural mesothelioma).
- The optimal number of lesions that should be measured remains uncertain.
- It does not take into account changes in tumor viability.
- Not all disease is measurable (eg, blastic bone lesions).

European Association for the Study of the Liver Guidelines

Method summary

- Measure the percentage change in tumor necrosis (recognized by nonenhanced areas) in target lesions.

Advantages

- It takes into account changes in tumor viability.
- It may serve as an earlier surrogate for therapeutic benefit when compared with anatomic criteria (ie, EASL response has been shown to be achieved earlier than WHO response).

Limitations

- The guidelines do not describe methods to measure tumor necrosis.
- Enhancement is assumed to represent viable tumor.
- Results are not necessarily reproducible.

Modified Response Evaluation Criteria in Solid Tumors Guidelines for Hepatocellular Carcinoma

Method summary

- Measure the percentage change in tumor necrosis (recognized by nonenhanced areas) in target lesions.

Advantages

- The guidelines take into account changes in tumor viability.
- The guidelines describe methods to measure tumor necrosis.
- The guidelines may serve as an earlier surrogate for therapeutic benefit when compared with anatomic criteria.

Limitations

- Enhancement is assumed to represent viable tumor.
- There are limited data to date.

Volumetric Techniques

Method summary

- Measure the percentage change in overall (volumetric) or viable (3D EASL) tumor volume of target lesions.

Advantages

- The techniques may permit measurement of overall tumor burden.
- The techniques may overcome difficulties measuring confluent or irregular lesions in 2D techniques.

Limitations

- Volumetric techniques may not add significant value compared with 2D techniques.
- They require volumetric software.
- They are time consuming.
- Definitions of response are not as clearly defined as 2D techniques.

WHAT THE REFERRING PHYSICIAN NEEDS TO KNOW

Since imaging response following LRTs has been shown to predict patient survival times, one of the goals of LRTs should be to achieve a radiologic response. Assessing imaging response to LRTs, however, can be challenging and is evolving.

The WHO and RECIST guidelines, both based on changes in tumor size, remain the most widely used guidelines for assessing imaging response to most cancer therapies, including LRTs.

In HCC, studies have shown a poor correlation between the benefit provided by LRTs and conventional methods of response assessment. Extensive tumor necrosis (ie, one of the goals of LRTs) may not be paralleled by a reduction in tumor size. In response to these limitations, the EASL and mRECIST guidelines for HCC were introduced to take into account the amount of intratumoral necrosis following treatment.

Tumor size and necrosis guidelines are the gold standard for assessing imaging response to LRTs. Newer imaging modalities (eg, functional MR imaging, FDG-PET) and biomarkers of response (eg, serum tumor markers) show promise as ancillary tools in assessing response to therapy.

SUMMARY

LRTs have proved valuable in the treatment of patients with cancer, most commonly in the liver. Accurate assessment of response to these therapies is crucial because objective response can be a surrogate of improved survival. Imaging plays an essential role in the objective evaluation of tumor response to most cancer therapies, including LRTs. Assessing imaging response to LRTs, however, can be challenging and is evolving. This article reviews the different criteria used to assess radiologic response to LRTs, with special attention to imaging assessment after treatment of HCC.

REFERENCES

1. Llovet JM. Treatment of hepatocellular carcinoma. Curr Treat Options Gastroenterol 2004;7(6):431–41.
2. Lencioni R, Llovet JM. Modified RECIST (mRECIST) assessment for hepatocellular carcinoma. Semin Liver Dis 2010;30(1):52–60.
3. Memon K, Kulik L, Lewandowski RJ, et al. Radiographic response to locoregional therapy in hepatocellular carcinoma predicts patient survival times. Gastroenterology 2011;141(2):526–35, 535.e1–2.
4. Miller AB, Hoogstraten B, Staquet M, et al. Reporting results of cancer treatment. Cancer 1981;47(1):207–14.
5. Therasse P, Arbuck SG, Eisenhauer EA, et al. New guidelines to evaluate the response to treatment in solid tumors. European Organization for Research and Treatment of Cancer, National Cancer Institute of the United States, National Cancer Institute of Canada. J Natl Cancer Inst 2000;92(3):205–16.
6. Bruix J, Sherman M, Llovet JM, et al. Clinical management of hepatocellular carcinoma. Conclusions of the Barcelona-2000 EASL conference. European Association for the Study of the Liver. J Hepatol 2001;35(3):421–30.
7. Prasad SR, Jhaveri KS, Saini S, et al. CT tumor measurement for therapeutic response assessment: comparison of unidimensional, bidimensional, and volumetric techniques initial observations. Radiology 2002;225(2):416–9.
8. Miller FH, Keppke AL, Reddy D, et al. Response of liver metastases after treatment with yttrium-90 microspheres: role of size, necrosis, and PET. AJR Am J Roentgenol 2007;188(3):776–83.
9. Kamel IR, Bluemke DA, Eng J, et al. The role of functional MR imaging in the assessment of tumor response after chemoembolization in patients with hepatocellular carcinoma. J Vasc Interv Radiol 2006;17(3):505–12.
10. Kamel IR, Reyes DK, Liapi E, et al. Functional MR imaging assessment of tumor response after 90Y microsphere treatment in patients with unresectable

hepatocellular carcinoma. J Vasc Interv Radiol 2007; 18(1 Pt 1):49–56.

11. Khan MA, Combs CS, Brunt EM, et al. Positron emission tomography scanning in the evaluation of hepatocellular carcinoma. J Hepatol 2000;32(5):792–7.

12. Kim HJ, Kim TK, Kim PN, et al. Assessment of the therapeutic response of hepatocellular carcinoma treated with transcatheter arterial chemoembolization: comparison of contrast-enhanced sonography and 3-phase computed tomography. J Ultrasound Med 2006;25(4):477–86.

13. Chen MH, Wu W, Yang W, et al. The use of contrast-enhanced ultrasonography in the selection of patients with hepatocellular carcinoma for radio frequency ablation therapy. J Ultrasound Med 2007; 26(8):1055–63.

14. Yaghmai V, Besa C, Kim E, et al. Imaging assessment of hepatocellular carcinoma response to locoregional and systemic therapy. AJR Am J Roentgenol 2013;201(1):80–96.

15. Iannaccone R, Laghi A, Catalano C, et al. Hepatocellular carcinoma: role of unenhanced and delayed phase multi-detector row helical CT in patients with cirrhosis. Radiology 2005;234(2):460–7.

16. Wald C, Russo MW, Heimbach JK, et al. New OPTN/UNOS policy for liver transplant allocation: standardization of liver imaging, diagnosis, classification, and reporting of hepatocellular carcinoma. Radiology 2013;266(2):376–82.

17. Silva AC, Morse BG, Hara AK, et al. Dual-energy (spectral) CT: applications in abdominal imaging. Radiographics 2011;31(4):1031–46 [discussion: 1047–50].

18. Lee SH, Lee JM, Kim KW, et al. Dual-energy computed tomography to assess tumor response to hepatic radiofrequency ablation: potential diagnostic value of virtual noncontrast images and iodine maps. Invest Radiol 2011;46(2):77–84.

19. Rhee TK, Naik NK, Deng J, et al. Tumor response after yttrium-90 radioembolization for hepatocellular carcinoma: comparison of diffusion-weighted functional MR imaging with anatomic MR imaging. J Vasc Interv Radiol 2008;19(8):1180–6.

20. Kloeckner R, Otto G, Biesterfeld S, et al. MDCT versus MRI assessment of tumor response after transarterial chemoembolization for the treatment of hepatocellular carcinoma. Cardiovasc Intervent Radiol 2010;33(3):532–40.

21. Kierans AS, Elazzazi M, Braga L, et al. Thermoablative treatments for malignant liver lesions: 10-year experience of MRI appearances of treatment response. AJR Am J Roentgenol 2010; 194(2):523–9.

22. Kim S, Mannelli L, Hajdu CH, et al. Hepatocellular carcinoma: assessment of response to transarterial chemoembolization with image subtraction. J Magn Reson Imaging 2010;31(2):348–55.

23. Cheson BD, Fisher RI, Barrington SF, et al. Recommendations for initial evaluation, staging, and response assessment of Hodgkin and non-Hodgkin lymphoma: the Lugano classification. J Clin Oncol 2014;32(27):3059–68.

24. Choi H. Response evaluation of gastrointestinal stromal tumors. Oncologist 2008;13(Suppl 2):4–7.

25. Agarwal A, Marcus C, Xiao J, et al. FDG PET/CT in the management of colorectal and anal cancers. AJR Am J Roentgenol 2014;203(5):1109–19.

26. Gulec SA, Suthar RR, Barot TC, et al. The prognostic value of functional tumor volume and total lesion glycolysis in patients with colorectal cancer liver metastases undergoing 90Y selective internal radiation therapy plus chemotherapy. Eur J Nucl Med Mol Imaging 2011;38(7):1289–95.

27. Pompili M, Riccardi L, Covino M, et al. Contrast-enhanced gray-scale harmonic ultrasound in the efficacy assessment of ablation treatments for hepatocellular carcinoma. Liver Int 2005;25(5):954–61.

28. Gehan EA, Schneiderman MA. Historical and methodological developments in clinical trials at the National Cancer Institute. Stat Med 1990;9(8):871–80 [discussion: 903–6].

29. World Health Organization. WHO handbook for reporting results of cancer treatment. Geneva Albany (NY): World Health Organization; sold by WHO Publications Centre USA; 1979. p. 45. WHO offset publication no 48.

30. Shanbhogue AK, Karnad AB, Prasad SR. Tumor response evaluation in oncology: current update. J Comput Assist Tomogr 2010;34(4):479–84.

31. Green S, Weiss GR. Southwest Oncology Group standard response criteria, endpoint definitions and toxicity criteria. Invest New Drugs 1992;10(4): 239–53.

32. Eisenhauer EA, Therasse P, Bogaerts J, et al. New response evaluation criteria in solid tumours: revised RECIST guideline (version 1.1). Eur J Cancer 2009; 45(2):228–47.

33. Hurwitz H, Fehrenbacher L, Novotny W, et al. Bevacizumab plus irinotecan, fluorouracil, and leucovorin for metastatic colorectal cancer. N Engl J Med 2004; 350(23):2335–42.

34. Hudes G, Carducci M, Tomczak P, et al. Temsirolimus, interferon alfa, or both for advanced renal-cell carcinoma. N Engl J Med 2007;356(22):2271–81.

35. Llovet JM, Ricci S, Mazzaferro V, et al. Sorafenib in advanced hepatocellular carcinoma. N Engl J Med 2008;359(4):378–90.

36. Bruix J, Sherman M, American Association for the Study of Liver Diseases. Practice Guidelines Committee. Management of hepatocellular carcinoma. Hepatology 2005;42(5):1208–36.

37. Prajapati HJ, Spivey JR, Hanish SI, et al. mRECIST and EASL responses at early time point by contrast-enhanced dynamic MRI predict survival in

patients with unresectable hepatocellular carcinoma (HCC) treated by doxorubicin drug-eluting beads transarterial chemoembolization (DEB TACE). Ann Oncol 2013;24(4):965–73.

38. Shim JH, Lee HC, Kim SO, et al. Which response criteria best help predict survival of patients with hepatocellular carcinoma following chemoembolization? A validation study of old and new models. Radiology 2012;262(2):708–18.

39. Kim BK, Kim KA, Park JY, et al. Prospective comparison of prognostic values of modified response evaluation criteria in solid tumours with European Association for the Study of the Liver criteria in hepatocellular carcinoma following chemoembolisation. Eur J Cancer 2013;49(4):826–34.

40. Shim JH, Lee HC, Won HJ, et al. Maximum number of target lesions required to measure responses to transarterial chemoembolization using the enhancement criteria in patients with intrahepatic hepatocellular carcinoma. J Hepatol 2012;56(2):406–11.

41. Gillmore R, Stuart S, Kirkwood A, et al. EASL and mRECIST responses are independent prognostic factors for survival in hepatocellular cancer patients treated with transarterial embolization. J Hepatol 2011;55(6):1309–16.

42. European Association for the Study of the Liver, European Organisation for Research and Treatment of Cancer. EASL-EORTC clinical practice guidelines: management of hepatocellular carcinoma. J Hepatol 2012;56(4):908–43.

43. Riaz A, Miller FH, Kulik LM, et al. Imaging response in the primary index lesion and clinical outcomes following transarterial locoregional therapy for hepatocellular carcinoma. JAMA 2010;303(11):1062–9.

44. Riaz A, Memon K, Miller FH, et al. Role of the EASL, RECIST, and WHO response guidelines alone or in combination for hepatocellular carcinoma: radiologic-pathologic correlation. J Hepatol 2011;54(4):695–704.

45. Duke E, Deng J, Ibrahim SM, et al. Agreement between competing imaging measures of response of hepatocellular carcinoma to yttrium-90 radioembolization. J Vasc Interv Radiol 2010;21(4):515–21.

46. Barrett T, Kobayashi H, Brechbiel M, et al. Macromolecular MRI contrast agents for imaging tumor angiogenesis. Eur J Radiol 2006;60(3):353–66.

47. Barrett T, Brechbiel M, Bernardo M, et al. MRI of tumor angiogenesis. J Magn Reson Imaging 2007;26(2):235–49.

Index

Note: Page numbers of article titles are in **boldface** type.

Radiol Clin N Am 53 (2015) 1089–1092
http://dx.doi.org/10.1016/S0033-8389(15)00127-X
0033-8389/15/$ – see front matter © 2015 Elsevier Inc. All rights reserved.

Moving?

Make sure your subscription moves with you!

To notify us of your new address, find your **Clinics Account Number** (located on your mailing label above your name), and contact customer service at:

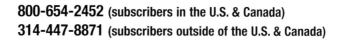

Email: journalscustomerservice-usa@elsevier.com

800-654-2452 (subscribers in the U.S. & Canada)
314-447-8871 (subscribers outside of the U.S. & Canada)

Fax number: 314-447-8029

Elsevier Health Sciences Division
Subscription Customer Service
3251 Riverport Lane
Maryland Heights, MO 63043

*To ensure uninterrupted delivery of your subscription, please notify us at least 4 weeks in advance of move.

ELSEVIER